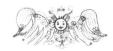

The
HOLISTIC
Caregiver

A guidebook for at-home care in late stage of Alzheimer's and dementia

Sabrina Mesko

BESTSELLING AUTHOR of *HEALING MUDRAS*

ARNICA PRESS

By Sabrina Mesko

HEALING MUDRAS
Yoga for Your Hands
Random House - Original edition

POWER MUDRAS
Yoga Hand Postures for Women
Random House - Original edition

MUDRA - Gestures of POWER
DVD - Sounds True

CHAKRA MUDRAS DVD set
HAND YOGA for Vitality, Creativity and Success
HAND YOGA for Concentration, Love and Longevity

HEALING MUDRAS
Yoga for Your Hands - New Edition

HEALING MUDRAS - New Edition in full color:
Healing Mudras I. ~ For Your Body
Healing Mudras II. ~ For Your Mind
Healing Mudras III. ~ For Your Soul

POWER MUDRAS
Yoga Hand Postures for Women - New Edition

MUDRA THERAPY
Hand Yoga for Pain Management and Conquering Illness

YOGA MIND
45 Meditations for Inner Peace, Prosperity and Protection

MUDRAS for ASTROLOGICAL SIGNS
Volumes I. ~ XII.

MUDRAS for ARIES, TAURUS, GEMINI, CANCER, LEO, VIRGO, LIBRA, SCORPIO, SAGITTARIUS, CAPRICORN, AQUARIUS, PISCES
12 Book Series

LOVE MUDRAS
Hand Yoga for Two

MUDRAS and CRYSTALS
The Alchemy of Energy protection

YOUR SPIRITUAL PURPOSE
Intentions and Choices

The
HOLISTIC
Caregiver

A guidebook for at-home care
in late stage of Alzheimer's and dementia

Sabrina Mesko

BESTSELLING AUTHOR of *HEALING MUDRAS*

ARNICA PRESS

The material contained in this book has been written for informational
purposes and is not intended as a substitute for medical advice,
nor is it intended to diagnose, treat, cure, or prevent disease.
If you have a medical issue or illness, consult a qualified physician.

ARNICA PRESS
www.ArnicaPress.com

Copyright © 2021 Sabrina Mesko

Photography by Sabrina Mesko

Photos on page 124,149, 214, 247 by Shutterstock

Symbol by Kiar Mesko

Printed in the United States of America

Manufactured in the United States of America

ISBN: 978-1-955354-05-9

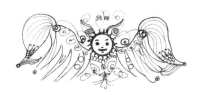

To the Caregivers of this world…

My Mother and I dedicate this book to all of Earth's angels,
who sacrifice so much, while bravely caring for a Loved One…

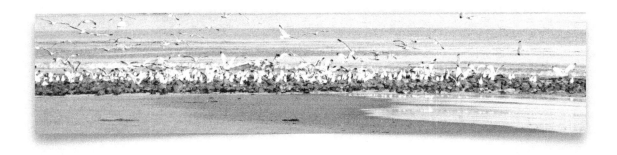

TABLE of CONTENTS

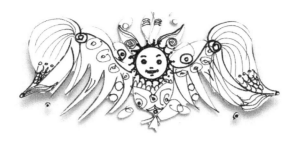

I n the times of ancient Egypt,
the Symbol of an angel winged Heart Scarab,
was placed on the heart of the departed,
for their protection in the world beyond.

In those cultures it was a deep honor and a blessing,
to care for an elder who was nearing the heavenly gates.

You are now called to journey on this well-traveled path,
where other noble and kindred spirits before you,
carried out this honorable assignment.

You and I are inspired by a great sense of duty
to respect every and each moment of one's life.
This was embedded in our Souls, in ancient times of long ago.

When we care for our loved ones with deep respect,
we cherish their beautiful presence, wisdom and love,
and celebrate the magnificence of their Soul.

We all travel towards the faraway horizon
and each one of us shall one day turn to dust.

But your acts of selfless kindness, compassion and love,
shall remain forever embedded in the fabric of your Soul.

May your Light shine brightly as you help others in need,
for in Spirit, we are all One…

INTRODUCTION

Dear Caregiver,

If the whirlwind of life has thrown you into the unexpected duty of a primary caregiver, this book is for you. It is here to help you bravely move forward and ease your daily and sometimes hourly challenges. It offers every practical solution to the difficulties you're facing and lays out a complete holistic maintenance program for your loved one and yourself. Because without your stamina, resilient health, and unwavering inner harmony, there is nothing. Without you, the ship will sink. So you need support in every which way - physical, mental, emotional and spiritual. And you need tons of love, because you give so much love to the one you care for.

Here you will find answers to your most pressing questions for practical, immediate solutions when everything seems overwhelming. It doesn't have to be. You just need to pace yourself. And you need someone to stand by you, give you some options and cheer you on. I will do that, this is why I am here.

There are numerous books about caregiving for people with Alzheimer's. Many of them describe their own path of caring for a loved one and I applaud their genuine efforts to share their insights.

This book is different. It lays out a very thorough holistic caregiving method to help sustain yourself and your loved one through the lengthy caregiving journey. As a Holistic Healing modalities professional, I created this unique program, when caring for my dear Mother. This book addresses every singular aspect that plays a decisive role in how you will manage care, ease discomfort, survive caregiving and later return to a thriving life.

It takes into account the physical, mental, emotional and spiritual elements that play a decisive role in this complex dynamic. It strives to infuse you with spiritual strength to persevere when you are weary, tired, sad, feel somewhat lost and are just about ready to give up. This book will hold your hand and help you remain the captain of your ship, no matter how turbulent the storm.

But it will also do much more than that. It will considerably improve the life of the dear one you are caring for. It will guide you how to ease, avert and somewhat reverse their journey into the delicate, vulnerable and increasingly fragile state. It will offer you numerous options how to resolve an issue that may seem unsolvable, but can often be resolved within minutes. You will find immediate answers and solutions which will help eliminate much suffering for everyone involved. This is my intention.

If you are not the family primary caregiver, but are simply perusing this book for more information for your caregiver friend or a relative, you are very welcome to stay and learn as much as you can. This book is in no way here to make anyone feel ridden with guilt, that they could have, should have, or must care for someone better than they did or are attempting to. You can only care for someone else as much as you are capable of, physically, mentally, emotionally, financially and spiritually. You can only try to do the best you can, and the rest is not up to you. The rest is up to God.

Knowing how you can help your loved one is the key and now you have more options, choices, suggestions and great solutions. This is what you need, right at this very moment. I know, because I have been there. But at the time, I could not find a single book that would explain how to manage the most obvious of tasks, like cleaning an elder adult with incontinence. Nobody wants to talk or write about that. Here you will find step by step guidance, support and crucial insights to manage such care.

You will learn techniques for communicating with your loved one when they cannot speak and express the source of their discomfort. You will find out how to observe and look for clear signs that will help you understand if you loved one is feeling peaceful or is in distress. You will read how to see beyond the obvious and engage logical steps, so you can approach your loved one with clear intention and help them participate in their care. This is ever so important.

Caregiving is not a battle, it is about proper sensory communication. Are you really paying attention and considering what your loved one is conveying? Or are you just trying to get through a task while disregarding their effort to participate? Even if a person's mind does not function at their optimal capacity, they respond to basic sensory stimuli and express comfort or pain. You need to learn to understand this in a very perceptive way.

Not everything in this life is as it seems. In fact, things that matter most may be the unseen, unspoken, intangible ones. Love, care, compassion, selflessness, service, kindness, gentleness, sacrifice, resilience and patience, patience…and more patience. That is what is required.

But everything always returns back to love. Love is chased by its polar opposite, which is fear. When you are a caregiver, love sustains you and fear chases you. This is the inner battle that goes on, daily. The fear of the inevitable dreaded end, the fear of how you will survive this challenge and the persistent fear that there will be nothing left of you when all this is over. The ultimate fear of all fears is fear of death. This is what you are facing, every day. It is an unpleasant, unwelcome and most visceral fear.

And then there is love. The love you hold in your heart that guides you and sustains you through the caregiving stumbles, setbacks, weary days and desperate nights…The love in your heart and soul. This is who you are, you are the giver of love.

I am here to assure you dear caregiver, that if you give it your very best, at the end of this difficult caregiving journey, you will be filled with indescribable love and deep inner calm. And that is an immeasurable treasure.

There will be no regrets, no guilt, no resentment…you will be in a state of deep spiritual awareness. Fear won't be able to touch you, for you have looked it right in the eye and learned that the only thing to fear, is fear itself. Once you stare death in the eye, it loses the dreaded hold over you. A deeper understanding of our mysterious existence is perceived in an unspoken way. You know that life is precisely that…a secret enigma. Caregiving will give you that gift of deeper knowledge and spiritual perception. It will reshape your heart, mind and spirit-life in profound ways and you will never be quite the same. You will know that each day and minute matters and will live your life fully, wisely and in constant awareness.

I consider this book a collaboration. It was written as a result of a years-long unplanned journey, that my Mother and I endured. I cared for her through a lengthy odyssey of her difficult early-onset Alzheimer's, until the very final breath of her life. Day after day we walked on this path and fought the battle together, stoically navigating through this indescribably challenging process.

While she is no longer in human form, she is with me as I write this book for you, dear reader. We are here to help ease your way. Together, my Mother and I learned how to travel through this deeply strenuous passage and gathered valuably precious information that can help you weather the storm. Now, our gift to you is finally in your hands.

The positive difference this book will make in your life is the only consolation we have. If we can ease the way for you, we have won. Our laborious odyssey was not in vain. May you benefit and learn from us, so that your path is lighter, safer and easier with this most precious knowledge. We are holding the Light for you, so that your step forward is secure and your path is brightly lit.

We dedicate this book to every cherished caregiver, for your brilliant Soul will forever light up the vast sky.

Blessings and peace,

Sabrina

WHAT IS HOLISTIC CAREGIVING?

**IN HOLISTIC CAREGIVING,
WE CARE FOR THE HUMAN BODY AS A WHOLE, INTEGRATED UNIT
AND STRIVE TO MAINTAIN IT IN OPTIMAL BALANCE AND HARMONY.
IT WILL HELP ALLEVIATE SUFFERING AND PREVENT NEW AILMENTS.
THIS PRINCIPLE APPLIES TO YOUR LOVED ONE AND THE CAREGIVER.**

Holistic Caregiving is an integrative total care system. Your body functions as a whole unit and your physical, mental, emotional and spiritual states closely influence each other.

Dementia does not only affect the abilities of the mind, but the entire being, including the physical and emotional state. In advanced, late stage of illness, the entire body is affected. The loved one is immobile and incapable of taking care of themselves. Therefore the entire being needs to be properly supported and sustained. Keep in mind, every part of human body is cellularly interconnected. If a specific area of one's constitution is predisposed to weakness and suffers from an ailment, their overall state will be affected. As a result, the entire being requires multi-layered, all-encompassing care.

In order to help maintain an overall level of comfort, proper attention needs to be applied to three main areas; physical body, mental functioning and emotional states. By addressing only one aspect and ignoring others, the care is incomplete. *Holistic Caregiving* takes into account your loved one's entire picture and all elements that contribute to their final condition.

As a result, the *Holistic Caregiving* approach requires your dedicated and systematic care that includes using natural remedies for alleviating any ongoing discomforts. At the same time, specific preventative measures are put in place to help avert future decline. This will facilitate your loved one's optimal functioning under the given circumstances. It will also help prevent an onset of additional ailments and further deterioration. Overmedicating is a common challenge and since seniors metabolize drugs differently, the combined effects of too many medications can be especially harmful. Natural remedies and care are the key.

Do not assume that someone in the advanced stage of Alzheimer's does not require holistic care, since there is no hope of recovery. It is a common misconception, that if you care for someone very well, they will live longer and therefore suffer longer.

I have heard this uninformed remark countless times. I cannot express enough how mistaken that concept is. When someone suffers from an advanced illness with no chance of recovery or regaining their healthy operating ability, they still need the best holistic care. It will help prevent further overall physical decline that would cause them great suffering. It will also vastly improve the quality of life they have, regardless of how limited it seems. Your loved one can live through their days in comfort and peace, or in pain and suffering. *Holistic Caregiving* will assure them peacefulness, ease, alleviation of discomfort and dignity.

For example, if a person is bed bound, they can quickly develop bed sores which are raw open wounds that can get infected and cause great pain. That person will not die faster, but will unnecessarily physically suffer. If you can prevent bed sores, you will completely eliminate pain and suffering, assuring them a physically comfortable sate. The person will not necessarily live longer, but they will certainly live better. Especially in the final part of one's earthly sojourn, a good quality of life, void of unnecessary suffering is of great importance. It is in fact, a luxury.

THE BENEFITS

Holistic Caregiving system is an optimal approach to long term caregiving. In addition to greatly improving the loved one's overall condition, the method in this book is an essential guide for preserving the overall health of the family caregiver. You will find detailed and easy to follow answers for everyday caregiving challenges and step-by-step guidance for solutions and effective natural remedies.

Holistic Caregiving can also be used and applied by professional caregivers in facilities. It is an excellent method to help increase the quality level of care in nursing homes, as well as protect professional caregivers from long term burn out.

The healthy lifestyle principles, organic diet, natural supplements and remedies will support both the caregiver and the loved one. As a caregiver, you need to endure this demanding journey without damaging consequences to your health. By learning to offer high quality care to your loved one, you can preserve your own valuable health as well.

In addition, *Holistic caregiving* introduces detailed sensory observation tools to help you understand your loved one. Learn how to establish a resilient mindset and find answers to difficult spiritual questions that arise through this experience. The book you're holding in your hands is the definitive guide to help you improve the quality of life for your loved one, as well as yourself.

ABOUT UNCONDITIONAL LOVE

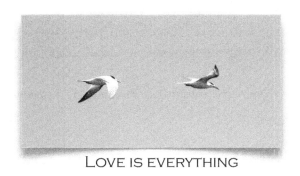

LOVE IS EVERYTHING

In this book, we will call the person we care for, Your Loved One. Why? Because what you do for them requires an incredible amount of love. They are in fact your very-much-loved person.

When someone tells you they care about you, what they are really saying is that they love you. They love you enough to not want you to suffer, be in need or in pain. So what they feel for you is love…caring love.

IF YOU ARE SOMEONE'S CAREGIVER, YOU ARE REALLY THEIR LOVE - GIVER.

And that is a privileged position to have, for you are offering them a most precious and invaluable gift. And even though it may seem difficult to understand, you are the fortunate one. You have an opportunity for selfless service to another human being. This is a mighty virtuous task.

We all need and deserve love. We long for it our entire life and search for it in all different places... with partners in love relationships, with our parents, children and friends. Some of us search for it in careers, work or strive to acquire wealth and power, all in hope that this will bring us the most precious and desired currency - love.

But love as the greatest power of the Universe has very specific rules and the many fine nuances of its expression are beyond complex. Giving love selflessly and receiving love openly is what helps us comprehend this mighty power. When you care for someone, you are embodying precisely these principles, you are the selfless giver and the loved one is the open care receiver. This is your dynamic.

If you care for your parent, you were probably the receiver as a child and they were the selfless giver. If you care for your partner, you were always bonded by love. Nevertheless, you are experiencing the full circle of what love truly is. It is a flowing, moving energy between two people. The balance is delicate and perhaps in some way, you are both learning, experiencing and living the highest, purest and fullest principles of love.

This book is written with massive amounts of love and is a product of deep, dutiful and loyal love. Therefore it is really about love.

Life treats everyone differently and each one of us has a very unique story and an invisible path we follow. There are many predestined moments that meet us at various intersections. And as always, we are presented with choices. Even if it appears like we have none, there is always a choice.

Do not underestimate the power of your decision, for the consequences may be vastly different and quite profound. Each and every moment of our lives can be decisive, nothing is unimportant and everything matters.

Nobody has a permanently happy and lucky life, for we all experience suffering. Some more, some less. And while your personal suffering seems unbearable at times, there is always a soul in this world that is suffering indescribably more than you are, at this very precise moment. Remember that and know that amidst all your heavy burdens, there are still traces of luck and love in your life. This awareness will help you soldier on thru the gravest moments you may be facing.

PRACTICE GRATITUDE FOR BLESSINGS IN DISGUISE AND YOU WILL OVERCOME ANYTHING.

In my life I've experienced incredibly fortuitous moments and opportunities, as well as immense challenges and extreme difficulties. Nothing came easy and everything required hard work and persistent effort.

I consider myself extremely fortunate and for that, I am eternally and deeply grateful. But I am not sure you'd want to walk in my shoes, for sometimes my step was heavy and the road incredibly steep. We each have our life assignments and as they say, God only gives you what you can carry, nothing more and nothing less. But sometimes, the load seems unbearably heavy and your knees are about to give in. But you always pull through, you overcome and stand solid in your core at the end of the storm.

One of those immeasurably challenging life circumstances I faced, was when I was taking loving care of my beloved Mother. Throughout my life, she was my great protector, my biggest ally and closest friend. Watching her suffer through this debilitating illness filled me with anger and rage of helplessness, determination to save her, persistence to find a cure, exhaustion with battles, and bitter despair in realization, that nothing was going to pull her away from the inevitable abyss she was facing. In the end, I surrendered to doing all that could be done for her loving care, comfort and protection. The journey seemed endless, merciless and it took away just about everything I had. Except my love for her. Nothing was going to destroy that, ever.

It has been over ten years now since she transitioned into another world of existence and honestly, it has taken me this long to feel ready and share this book with the world. My grief was so deep that I needed time. I needed a decade to work through my sorrow and mold it into a shape that doesn't threaten my happiness.

Now, I feel it is incredibly important and valuable to share with you all the knowledge I gained.

IF I CAN EASE YOUR PATH IN ANY WAY, ALL MY EFFORTS WILL BE WORTH IT.

And I will seek refuge in knowing that something good and helpful came out of my Mother's journey. Something to help ease your way, while you and your loved one travel through this experience.

All the suffering my Mother endured, is perhaps a tiny dewdrop smaller if we can help someone else who is going thru this process now. So it is really my Mother and I together that speak to you on these pages, through sharing everything we learned and experienced together. She cannot speak, but I can do it for us both...and we hope it will ease your way, save you much time, energy, effort, and give you clear tools for navigating thru these stormy waters.

I feel it is tremendously important for me to clarify and affirm, that the information you will find on these pages is truly for everyone and anyone who has a loved one in a challenging situation fighting with Alzheimer's or dementia-like illnesses. It does not matter if your loved is at home or in a facility, you can benefit from this valuable information and take what you need. I am not in any way suggesting that this is the only way, I am only sharing with you some tremendously valuable information and giving you clear tools how to accomplish what you need.

Guilt is a constant companion for many who have a loved one in this predicament, feeling like they are not doing enough or not doing it right, or whatever else one thinks of.

GUILT IS AN UNNECESSARY BURDEN THAT CARRIES NO BENEFIT.

Everything seems wrong and the pain may expand into all areas of your life and affect all relationships that you have. That's right, every single part of your life is affected by this dynamic and you should just expect, know and accept that.

Why? Because knowledge is power and you need to pick your battles. Anger is not going to help you, information will. Depression is not going to save you, but a clear plan of action will ease your way, help you pace yourself and make best choices for yourself and your family.

What you will find here is a hands-on method and practical tools about the most essential holistic, all natural, shall we say, "organic" aspects of caregiving. This is not a book about caregiving legalities, it is not about choices of facilities, or medications, or some distant concept and philosophy that makes no sense when you are dealing with real life. There are countless books on that.

This book is about you needing a quick answer when "shiitake hits the fan," if you know what I mean...when you are alone in the middle of the night, with a seemingly unmanageable mess on your hands and are desperately clueless about what to do. Nobody will help you then, but your clear inventive spirit, your creative intuition and your hopefully fast common sense.

Some people hate to take responsibility for anything, they want quick solutions and a miraculous pill to make it all better or go away. If you are going thru a divorce and are stressed, do you think it is necessary to go to someone, only to hear the big proclamation that you are stressed? Did you not already know that yourself?

If you are a caregiver to a loved one, do you think you'll be stressed? I guarantee you that you will. Is your health going to suffer? Yes, absolutely. Your partnerships, your career, your entire life in a comfort zone will shift.

EVERYTHING WILL CHANGE AND BE DIFFERENT.
BUT YOU WILL MAKE IT.

You will get better thru this and at the end of this journey, you will feel at peace that you have done everything you personally could, and will have no regrets about it. That is the ideal outcome, more you cannot expect or want.

So while I feel privileged to be able to share with you my experience and gained knowledge, I do it with an immeasurable amount of love and compassion in my heart for all you have been thru, all you are enduring now, and all that lies ahead.

Let my strength, inner peace and love be your inspiration, for you must know that you shall get thru this journey like a stoic traveler, bruised and worn out, but incredibly wise, rich within your heart and exalted in your spirit.

CARING FOR YOUR LOVED ONE IS THE GREATEST GIFT YOU CAN BESTOW UPON THEM.

Sacrificing your precious moments of life while you remain a protector and caregiver, is something you consciously decided a long time ago. Now you are here to fulfill your unspoken, unwritten agreements of your soul. I do believe that being a caregiver to someone you love is on your soul's path, a true higher calling. It is the ultimate test and an essential aspect to experience on the evolutionary journey of your soul. It is a spiritual contract and you will fulfill your promise.

And while human emotions will overwhelm you, remain strong and never waver in your intention to love the one that needs you most. And remember, the seemingly endless time it takes for this journey, is meaningless in the grand picture of important things in life.

And perhaps it is helpful to consider, that when you suffer most, surely the knowledge gained can ease the pain for someone behind you. And then, when the moment comes, you can be the one to offer a helping hand to another, by sharing your hard earned wisdom, that you can only gain when traveling this road yourself.

No one can understand how it is when a loved one is disappearing in Alzheimer's or dementia, no one can imagine in a most intricate way all the dynamics that occur…no one EXCEPT someone who has personally been there, lived thru it and survived. Yes, you may find very helpful people who will stand by you, even knowledgeable professionals, but living thru this with your own family member is entirely different.

Many people can help tremendously, but to understand you completely in every nuance that your heart experiences, every shade of sorrow, every thought of despair? No, this no one can understand, unless they too have traveled this thorny and deserted path that seems endless and so barren of any hope.

I have been there and while I am the eternal optimist, I must confess this test is beyond severe. It is actually so relentless and harsh, that the human spirit is pushed to it's absolute limit.

**ALLOW ME THE PRIVILEGE TO INSPIRE YOU WITH HOPE
AND INDISPUTABLE ASSURANCE,
THAT YOU WILL ENDURE AND RECOVER.
YES, YOU WILL SMILE AGAIN.**

You must believe and know, that after all is said and done, you will find a way to pick yourself up and go on with your life. Yes, you will be forever changed, but nevertheless still here, still alive and perhaps able to help others behind you. Then the pain is hopefully less crippling, the anger less fierce and from this darkest night a different, kinder emotion will emerge. Compassion and profound understanding for all kindred spirits experiencing a similarly cruel and merciless journey.

I also want to remind you, that there is no winner in this dynamic. Everyone battles their own inner war, and while this illness takes over your family, some may act unkind, run away, hide or lash out in fear...we do not judge anyone, because they were too weak to fight this fight with their bare hands. Everyone can only do what they best can. And if that means nothing, so be it.

I do not judge anyone, I only want to help those of you who are here and ready to benefit from all I've learned, so that your path is eased. And if it's only one singular tiniest piece of helpful advice that you'll find on these pages, I am content, as is my Mother. This book is from us both.

When we spend our last years together at the end of her precious life, I shared with her my intention to write all this valuable information into a book and she was most pleased about it. In her moments of complete awareness, she listened with enthusiasm and encouraged me to do so. She was a journalist, a master of words, and always fiercely courageous to get out the truth.

That promise I made to her stayed with me, and I feel obliged to keep my word. And now I feel ready, for enough time has passed. I can breathe again and evoke the fondest memories of my Mother when she was still vibrant and healthy, a most beautiful and loving Mother, truly the best one in the world. I miss her so, no words will ever be able to describe. But she is with me always and forever. May our love live on eternally in all the good this book will offer to you.

So my dear caregiver, no matter what, always know that all your beautiful, kind and loving actions won't go unnoticed. Everything, every word, every thought and every loving intention are your greatest treasures and in spirit you are brighter than the most brilliant star.

**YOU ARE A TRUE GIVER OF LOVE,
YOU ARE AN ANGEL DIVINE.**

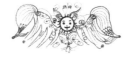

CHAPTER ONE

The Illness

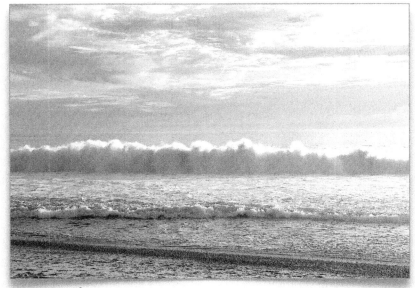

LIFE IS FULL OF UNEXPECTED WAVES,
SOME ARE GLORIOUS AND OTHERS LESS SO...

There is no perfect time to get sick. There is no time when you will be ready for this kind of illness. In my Mother's case, years went by before we realized that she had a serious health challenge.

She was always a healthy, strong, incredibly intelligent and capable woman, a renowned journalist, and leading simultaneous translator for the highest offices in the land. Her speed and linguistic abilities were simply staggering. She worked internationally, and was one of the very few women in such a position of high responsibility.

When the illness took hold, her strength and stamina slowly diminished, but she fought hard to overcome it and managed for a long while. However, in the end, the illness overpowered her. Our world came crashing down and small but old cracks in foundation created insurmountable gaps.

CHANGES

I will share with you the usually slow and deceiving progress of this hidden illness and how you can recognize it. This will help you reassess and understand, how long your loved one battled the disease and estimate the onset.

Why is his important? It will help you take into consideration any other events that may have contributed to this condition. The manifestation of an illness varies differently in each individual, depending on their natural weaknesses and strengths. Information is key to understanding and delaying this illness.

And while our focus in this book is on Holistic Caregiving in advanced, late and final stages of Alzheimer's dementia, it is important to review the illness's early phases and dynamics, so you may better understand the progress of this challenging ailment.

The first sign that something is amiss occurs with a change in one's general mental and emotional disposition. Since life is full of changes, we may have tendency to dismiss this shift. We may brush it off with an assumption, that everyone gets a bit forgetful and overly anxious in later years. But clearly this shift is not just a normal part of the aging process. The slightly annoying, confusing and upsetting changes can happen very slowly. Your loved one may become unreasonably moody, depressive, angry, confused, forgetful, unkempt and irritable. These changes can creep into their life over a long period of time, sometimes taking a few years.

You get used to these reoccurring developments and continue to mistake them for a part of the aging process. But what you are witnessing is the increasingly domineering nature of the illness itself.

The changes continue to steadily escalate, but you might have too many of your own life challenges and responsibilities to notice them for what they are. You may not be paying close attention and do not recognize that something is very amiss. Of course the sooner you realize what is happening, the better.

Why? Because you may still be able to do something about the illness. In addition to a few modern medicine - allopathic medications, there are numerous natural and alternative modalities and lifestyle changes you can implement in an effort to boost your loved one's overall state of health. You can help them keep healthy and functioning at their best capacity for as long as possible, thus effectively delaying the progress of the illness.

> **IT IS A COMMON OCCURRENCE, THAT BY THE TIME ALZHEIMER'S DEMENTIA IS RECOGNIZED, A MORE ADVANCED STAGE OF ILLNESS MAY ALREADY HAVE DEVELOPED.**

From then on, the downward spiral may progress rapidly, sometimes almost over night. This usually indicates that the early onset symptoms were smaller and ongoing through a long time span and were therefore easily overseen and went unnoticed. More than likely, this is the case.

You loved one's true personality is slowly disappearing in the process. Since each one of us in a very unique individual and we all have our own character and personality traits, the ongoing changes will most likely differ from person to person. But there is one similarity - the overall character traits or odd quirky tendencies become more exaggerated.

If a person was usually of a more quiet and shy nature, they will likely retreat even more, becoming oddly absent minded and disconnected. They may stop doing their daily chores, become despondent and depressed, attempting to hide their confusion and inner fear. They may become like your shadow, very co-dependent on you, refusing to make the most basic decisions for themselves, following you wherever you go and lingering around in desperate attempt of clinging to safety and the familiar. You become their safety blanket.

On the other hand, if the person was always in control and lived a life of high responsibility in career or work, their changes will veer in a very different direction. It is almost as if they subconsciously know that they are losing control of their life. They feel a deep-set inexplicable sense of weakness, an overwhelming state of stress, escalating and pushing them further into anger, as a result of daily obvious and embarrassing mishaps. Such a person will grow defensive, agitated, angry and will often lash out.

Something is wrong and they know it, but cannot face it. Everyone around them will not read this situation as they should. They will simply assume that the person is tired, stressed and growing crankier with age. They will dismiss the true underlying reason for increasing outbursts. Of course these are the two polar opposite examples, but there are endless versions in between.

The reality is, that this illness sneaks upon you like a dangerous and clever nocturnal enemy in hiding. Slowly and persistently it creeps into your life, first in small innocent and even funny spurts and then more aggressively and in full view. It becomes undeniable that something is very much amiss, but by the time you are ready to face that reality, it may be already very late in the game. The illness is already embedded in your loved one with full force. Negative and deteriorating mental and emotional changes that continually increase and intensify, should be paid attention to. They are sounds of alarm that something serious is going on which won't simply go away on its own. Usually, when changes increase and worsen, denial sets in.

DENIAL

The easiest reaction to your loved one's ailing health is denial. At some point, just about everyone is guilty of this. Why? Because the idea that your loved one is losing grasp is too frightening, too inconvenient, too disheartening and it is simply easier to stay in denial. It seems like maybe that way, we can all pretend the problem will go away and your loved one will get better, on their own. Or at least we hope they will not get much worse. On the other hand, recognizing and admitting that something is seriously wrong would require considerable attention and time and we are all in shortage of it.

There is also the decisive aspect of the loved one not being amendable or easy to deal with while facing any kind of confrontation about their increasing mental, physical and emotional challenges.

They may grow more stubborn than ever, fiercely denying anything is wrong. They may fight against any kind of practical or even medical intervention. This makes the entire circumstance quite challenging to deal with. Usually family members are inexperienced and ill-equipped to handle the situation and often take the loved one's denials and emotional outbursts personally.

As a family member you need to know that you are not alone in this rejection of reality. Your loved one probably furiously dismisses your ongoing concern with a wave of hand or even foolish jokes. This may go on for quite a while, perhaps even a few years. And since this illness often makes an extensive and prolonged entry, the changes become something we get used to. We regard them as our loved one's character traits, when in fact the illness is establishing a clear presence.

So when your loved one inevitably does or says something unpleasant or has an unreasonable and sudden outburst of anger, you may take it personally. This presents a great danger for conflict and possible estrangement. We are slowly losing them, they are becoming a different person, less present, reliable, cheerful or kind. They are in pain, they carry a secret inner turmoil and desperately need help. Very often the loved one lashes out at the person closest to them. Why? Because they are in fact the closest.

> **FOR MOST OF US IT IS TOO PAINFUL, FRIGHTENING AND DIFFICULT TO ADMIT, THAT A LOVED IS SUFFERING FROM DEMENTIA.**

Even when a family member realizes the magnitude of the illness, there may still remain other family members that are in denial. This dynamic can become quite counter productive, destructive and a source of great conflict. The family member in denial may try to fight, blame others and make a sad situation increasingly more difficult. As painful as this may be, facing the facts is the best option. It is like you are sitting on a sinking ship pretending all is well. It won't work. Unless someone takes charge, everyone will sink.

Refusing to accept the facts reflects the many things we don't want to face in ourselves. Maybe growing old is a factor, maybe the frightening realization that the family member who was always our protector and reliable provider may be disappearing or gone. Children that are entitled or spoiled are most often the ones in denial.

Why? Because their comfortable carefree lifestyle may be rapidly coming to an end. Therefore the initial state of denial that remains unresolved, may be an indication that future denials and conflicts are in sight.

MOOD SWINGS

Quite often the mental confusion and emotional imbalance your loved one is experiencing will cause them a lot of inner turmoil. They will feel out of sorts, their increasing episodes of forgetfulness and confusion will scare them and a sense of deep fear and sadness will set in. Any long discussions, followed by unreasonable explanations and senseless answers to your questions, will only increase their agitated and fearful state.

In desperate effort to regain their full command, the outbursts may increase and become more dramatic and difficult. This can be somewhat managed, but inevitably a sense of growing alarm will settle in the family dynamics.

ALL PREVIOUSLY UNRESOLVED OR LINGERING CONFLICTS WILL RISE TO THE SURFACE WITH LIGHTING SPEED.

Some family members will be more involved, others less and the basic communication with the loved one will become increasingly more complicated and frustrating. They may settle for one thing and then unexpectedly change their mind in the last moment, or entirely forget what the agreement was.

Increased confusion may set in when changing locations, going on vacation, having to meet others and missing appointments. Unexpected schedule plans or unplanned events will unsettle them. They may get lost in a parking lot or store and forget the basic daily errands. There will be keys lost, repeated phone calls with always the same questions and obvious staggering moments of forgetfulness. Buttoning shirts in wrong order, or wearing different color socks may at first seem comical, but with time really tragic. The sugar cravings will hit sky high. Taking care of household chores will become overwhelming. Their ability for basic hygiene will diminish. What stands on the horizon is a clear and decisive oncoming high-speed crash.

THE CRASH - BREAKING POINT

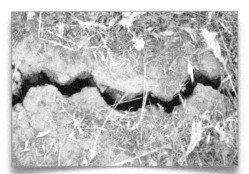

A SMALL FRACTURE MAY CAUSE A MIGHTY GAP

What comes next is a huge shift, a sort of a breaking point, major setback or a new symptom that is so dramatic it is impossible to pretend that everything is fine. This inevitable fracture will break the thin ice you have all been skating on. It may be caused by a seemingly innocent occasion on any regular day, when something goes very much amiss. It could be a million things; an unattended stove and near fire, a barely missed car accident, getting lost, falling down, or a sudden unreasonable emotional outburst or confrontation in a public place. It becomes clear that your loved one is unwell.

This dramatic shift will clearly mark the beginning of a new family dynamic. Your loved one has entered a fragile state of being. It is now clear that they cannot and should not be left alone. They need ongoing help, attention and experienced supervision.

Suddenly everyone's life in the family unit is changed forever. The domino effect that happens next is anyone's guess. Obviously a large or small family, a tightly knit or a complex and conflicted family will respond to this challenge differently. If you are suddenly the one in charge, this will undoubtedly be a difficult test. You will have to adjust to the new dynamic, get medical attention, try to balance the other family members that are experiencing a shock and remedy any ongoing or future family conflicts.

One hopes that everyone in the family unit will harmoniously get along or at the least remain supportive of each other in this new and difficult situation. But when illness, fear, and sudden upheaval disturb the family unit, this is not easy to sustain. Everyone has a different defense mechanism and way of dealing with challenges. Fear, sadness, anger, anxiety, blame, guilt and other unpleasant personality traits will emerge with immediate fury.

If the burden of resolving difficult issues and taking charge falls on your shoulders, you will have to brave the first of many storms that await. Who is ever prepared for this moment? It is something we never expect or even want to face.

THE WAKE UP CALL

W̶hat happened in my family was that one day, my Mother simply sat in a chair and did not really get up anymore. She stopped her regular daily activities or making any kind of decisions. She went into a completely passive mode. Even thou she was always the decider in the family, she suddenly didn't take the drivers seat. And just like that, over night, everyone in the family was forced into an unfamiliar position. Our lives suddenly came to a screeching halt and crashed into a thousand pieces.

This moment is a dramatic and big wake-up call. There is no denial that your loved one is ill, it is quite obvious that their memory faculty is impacted, they daily activities may suffer and life in general will change dramatically. Suddenly your independent loved one is incapable of being on their own. They may insist furiously that they are fine, but you all know that is not so. They need help and supervision. You will need to deal with this and find proper solutions. Someone will need to be present at all times, watch over them and pay attention to every detail to loved one's ongoing needs. This may take a while to set up, because it is very difficult to change one's life overnight and adjust to take care of an adult that has unexpectedly lost their independence. It is a struggle, there may be friction, anger, fear and resistance from your loved one. But the writing is on the wall: change has occurred and the family dynamics are forever altered.

A SHIFT IN POWER

One of the most significant challenges is the shift in charge, control and leadership of the family unit. Suddenly your loved one's lifelong position in family hierarchy and dynamics is altered. If that placement was prominent as in a parental or partner figure, every member will have to readjust. Nobody likes this process, for it involves an entirely unfamiliar territory. Fear, discomfort and an almost certain resurgence of any unresolved lifelong conflicts will ensue. Everything will blow right into the open.

This restructure will evoke elements of battle over control and power. An almost tribal role shifting will force every member to reassess and reestablish their new position. It is time to face reality, that the family unit is no longer lead or co-navigated by your loved one.

THERE WILL BE GREAT RELUCTANCE AND PERHAPS FRICTION IN REGARDS TO A NEW, UNKNOWN, UNTESTED AND UNFAMILIAR FAMILY HIERARCHY.

The functions carried out by your loved one who is now no longer capable of fulfilling them, will have to be divided, reassigned and this may cause much discomfort and unease.

The main emotion that usually prevails in such turbulent times is fear. Hopefully the love in the family will outweigh the fear and you will be able to find a new balance with shared responsibilities. The family breakdown and restructure will be additionally challenged, if the loved one refuses to acknowledge and accept their new weakened and fragile state. This will make the transition more difficult from every perspective; physical execution of duties and tasks, mental clarity about how to best proceed and certainly emotional pain while facing the new difficult reality.

There are certainly countless variables, but the general circumstances will always entail a major shift in family dynamics, sadly the presence of conflict and a profound emotional upset at the acknowledgment of this new painful reality. It is as if everyone that is insecure in their own right, will fall into fight or flight mode for their own survival. There will be much desire for control, and considerably less interest about responsibly fulfilling the new caregiving duties.

If you find yourself in the position of primary family caregiver, you have surely experienced at least a certain level of these shifts and changes before you arrived at the current situation in your life. By reflecting on the past dynamics and various phases of the way events unfolded, you will hopefully recognize with greater clarity, that whatever difficulties you experienced, they were all connected to the gradual onset, progressions and eventual reveal of Alzheimer's and dementia.

Let us understand, that every family is different and human nature is predictable when facing an existential upset. Disharmony is often more common than a perfectly united family with everyone getting along. Life is messy, families are difficult and personalities will clash.

They are all a variation of an expression of pain, emotional turmoil, fear, sadness, anger, and refusal to accept that we are all fragile and our life in this world is only a temporary journey with an inevitable departure.

> **FACING THE GREATEST FEARS WILL HELP YOU DIMINISH THEIR IMPACT AND RESTORE YOURSELF, SO YOU MAY PERSEVERE AND VICTORIOUSLY MANAGE WHATEVER LIFE SENDS YOUR WAY.**

Denial of the new circumstance will prove the most difficult challenge to overcome. Acceptance, clarity and immediate actions are required. Every passing day that your loved one lives without proper care, presents direct danger to their well being and safety. Time for delay and avoidance has run out. Your loved one requires ongoing care.

THE FAMILY BREAKDOWN

Let us hope your closest family members are capable of finding within their hearts the ability to put any unresolved personal issues aside. Ideally, they will generously participate and help establish a state of harmony within the family, so you can find solutions to new caregiving challenges together. If you help each other and hold together in this time of need, everything will be considerably easier. Sharing duties, putting old personal grudges aside, learning to curb selfishness and practicing loving and kind disposition towards loved one and each other - those are the qualities you need to call upon, promote and cultivate in order get through this ordeal as healthy and whole as possible. Consideration for others, deep self-reflection and compassion are necessary. Consciously eliminate pointless bickering, unnecessary hostility, rivalry, jealousy, envy and quarrel, for they will not only bring you down, but forever irreparably damage the remaining family unit.

> **IF YOU CAN HELP EACH OTHER, YOU WILL GROW CLOSER AND FIND SOLACE IN FACING THIS ORDEAL TOGETHER. IF YOU SUCCUMB TO CONFLICT, THE JOURNEY WILL WEIGH HEAVY ON YOUR MINDS AND HEARTS.**

Look within your soul and do everything you can to keep harmony. If that is not possible, then take whatever necessary steps and precautions you need, in order to assure a peaceful existence for yourself and your loved one. Secure an environment where their vulnerable state does not in any way put them in danger or cause them more suffering. Protect your loved one and yourself and establish a nurturing place of peace and harmony so that you accomplish two objectives; provide your loved one with best care possible and preserve your state of physical, mental and emotional health. The caregiving journey is extremely demanding and you do not need to waste your precious energy on unnecessary conflict. At this point in your life, peace is invaluable and an absolute necessity.

FAMILY RELATIONSHIPS

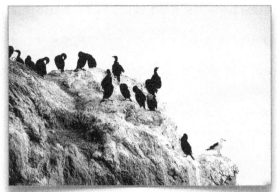

FAMILIES ARE COMPLICATED

Families are complex and colorful. Each family member has their own set of character tendencies, weaknesses and strengths. Keeping harmony requires effort, dedication and an endless supply of tolerance and love. Depending on how the family structure is set, parental figures in leadership positions face a tough juggling act. The children will hopefully behave according to the set rules, however, let us not dismiss the fact, that children can often override even the most dedicated efforts to guide them in a different direction.

If the family unit is exceptionally fortunate, they handle the crisis of this illness in an optimal way. Everyone helps and supports one another, and each family member contributes the best they can. They are unified in love for their loved one and the family, and manage this difficult chapter victoriously. They truly rely on each other, creating a powerful team that can endure any obstacle that comes their way. They support each other physically, mentally, emotionally, spiritually and financially. This illness may bring them even closer and they will cherish each precious moment they have as a united, strong, resilient and beautifully loving family. Yes, this kind of supportive family sounds simply lovely.

Unfortunately most of the time, this is not the case at all. The norm is the direct opposite. When one of the parents begins to suffer from this difficult illness, the entire family structure is toppled. Old order is broken and leadership can change overnight. Like a kingdom without a leader, this often results in a ferocious battle amongst the rest of the family. Grief, anger, fear as well as self-preservation, greed and control of power, become a source of deep family conflicts. Relatives from near and far may wish to get involved, offer their opinion or take sides. This is not helpful, but only adds to the conflict.

The most difficult battles often ensue between siblings who disagree on how to manage the family crisis. This conflict is very complex, as many elements play a decisive role. If one family member is more aggressive and feels entitled to a power grab, they will want to take control, while others less eager to fight, will take a carefully premeditated backseat.

It is unfortunately a very common occurrence that can turn incredibly ugly, sad and bitter. No matter what the ongoing family dynamics are, when the parent suffers from this illness, the priority must be to offer them the best care, delay the progress of illness and keep them in as good overall health as possible. At the same time, their assets need protection, and are to be used only for their care. If a parent has sufficient funds to assure good care for their needs, professional caregivers and all the services and supplies required, the funds must all be allocated for that. This will require careful management and ongoing oversight.

Unfortunately, this is where the conflict explodes, as adult children most often dispute about assets that are in fact not even rightfully theirs. All family members need to be very clear about the reality of the situation. Because this illness requires ongoing long-term, very involved and expensive care, it is highly probable that a large portion of loved one's assets, if not all, will be wiped out. Certainly if the family has unlimited funds, it will affect them less, but if opposite is the case, the family assets might quickly evaporate. This is a fact.

ANY EAGER PURSUITS OF PENDING INHERITANCE SHOULD BE ABANDONED. INSTEAD, CAREFUL ESTATE PLANNING MUST TAKE PLACE TO ASSURE LOVED ONE'S LONG-TERM COMFORT AND CARE.

In addition, if the other parent is still living, it is of crucial importance that their own financial security is not endangered or depleted. This is of course much easier said than done. While one parent suffers from this illness, the other parent is suffering under extremely difficult circumstance and needs to be protected in every possible way.

Protecting elderly loved ones from being taken advantage of, is an extremely challenging endeavor. Court battles ensue, adding more pressure to already difficult situation and further depleting funds for all involved. Siblings can become ferocious enemies and unforgiving opponents. Sadly, this is the most common occurrence, which is extremely damaging for all involved. The truth is that while the children argue about assets, the loved one often suffers neglect and is forgotten amidst this saga. Some people get enraged, unreasonable and embark on a destructive rampage, while others hide in the background, avoiding to pledge allegiance and conveniently wait for the outcome.

The biggest mistake is a lengthy battle with attorneys and courts, because the funds will get depleted, while the progress will be extremely slow. This could bring you financial ruin, bitter enemies in your own family and absolutely no resolve. It will result in total loss for everyone involved. Do everything possible to resolve any conflicts amicably, without long court proceedings and prioritize the comfort and safety of your loved one. Their assets must be allocated strictly for their own benefit, best care and comfort and assuring safety and comfort of the remaining parent. It is a huge assignment.

Try to work out the differences within the family dynamics and help each other out, so you can overcome this caregiving journey and the inevitable loss of loved one, with mutual support. If harmony is not possible, seek legal help with one primary goal in mind: to assure comfort and safety for your loved one, while they suffer through this long and difficult illness. Do everything you can to protect the remaining parent, who is entering a most difficult chapter of their entire life. This is not the time for selfish, immature arguing.

ESTABLISH PEACE AT ANY PRICE.
IF THAT IS NOT POSSIBLE, DISTANCE MAY BE YOUR BEST OPTION.

IN ORDER TO SUSTAIN THIS CAREGIVING JOURNEY,
YOU AND YOUR LOVED ONE NEED ABSOLUTE PEACE
AND SAFETY IN YOUR IMMEDIATE ENVIRONMENT.

ASSESSING THE LEVEL OF REQUIRED CARE

This illness is a slow progressing affliction, that eventually affects all areas of your loved one's life. Everyday Activities of Daily Living also called ADL, can be assessed by a professional to help establish the level of help and care your loved one requires. To give you a general sense of how ADL is measured, various factors are taken into consideration.

The Instrumental ADL (IADL) assessment measures individual's ability to manage their finances, use transportation, maintain their home and household with housekeeping, use the telephone, do the laundry, go shopping, care for pets, prepare their meals and remember to take their medication.

Another assessment measure is called Independence ADL and takes into consideration your loved one's ability to perform general tasks of self-care such as bathing, dressing, toileting, transferring from bed to chair and feeding. The most crucial ability - to retain self-control of one's continence, is also assessed. This gives the assessor a good idea what level of care your loved one requires.

> **IF AND WHEN YOUR LOVED ONE'S ABILITIES
> FOR INDEPENDENT SELF - CARE DIMINISH,
> THEY WILL REQUIRE AN ONGOING ADVANCED LEVEL OF CARE.**

When the illness becomes obvious and impossible to ignore, you will consult with your family doctor or specialist to properly test and diagnose your loved one. At this point, many other important matters will need to be addressed. Depending on the situation and dynamics in the immediate family, you will face the inevitable task of making various arrangements and ongoing crucial decisions.

Eventually, the primary caregiver who is best capable of caring for your loved one, has to be selected. The primary caregiver makes crucial decisions, however, if the family is harmonious, they can all work together and continually find an agreement on how to best proceed, always in the best interest of the loved one. Officially there is one Primary caregiver. Hopefully the large list of responsibilities can be fairly shared and divided among all family members. However, usually this is where much friction occurs and disharmony often comes in the way.

LEGAL MATTERS

Estate planning is crucially important. The main items are your Will, a Trust - if you so choose, Advanced Healthcare Directive, Durable Power of Attorney, and Beneficiary and Guardianship Designations. An advance healthcare directive, also known as living will, is a legal document in which your loved one specifies what actions should be taken for their health, if they are no longer able to make decisions for themselves, because of illness or incapacity.

> **IN AN IDEAL WORLD, YOUR LOVED ONE WOULD HAVE PREPARED ALL THE ESTATE PLANNING DOCUMENTS YEARS AGO.**

Unfortunately that is often not the case, which creates incredibly complicated, drawn out and expensive situations and becomes a source of great conflict.

When your loved one is diagnosed with Alzheimer's dementia, many important aspects of their life undergo an immediate and drastic change. You may be dealing with legal problems connected to your loved one's ability to make their own medical, financial, lifestyle, residence and basic caregiving decisions. In early stages of Alzheimer's dementia they will want to continue making decisions, but may be clearly incapable and could be vulnerable and even endangered. This denial may further delay a clear plan to save their assets and assure their protection and safety. If these issues are not resolved, which is most often the case, the loved one becomes increasingly more unreasonable when it comes to making important decisions.

When your loved one reaches the middle-stage Alzheimer's dementia, the situation will reach a critical point. This is when professional assessment will conclude, if your loved one is able to make their own decisions and who is their conservator or guardian, when it is clear they require one. If there are complex family dynamics or conflicts, you will most likely face immediate disputes around the loved one's conservatorship, their assets and estate. Since caregiving is a costly and demanding life altering undertaking, these details need to be rapidly addressed and properly handled. Unfortunately most often this becomes a source of great family conflict and long ongoing and extremely expensive legal battles that further deplete everyone's financial resources. The bigger the estate is, the longer and more expensive the battle. Designating a responsible party and person that will take care of everything is an incredibly complex and challenging process.

You will need professional legal advice and representation to help you manage through the many details and required proper paperwork to help resolve and obtain legally court approved documentation for conservatorship, including advanced health care directives and estate management. I suggest you deal with these issues as early as possible.

Ideally, this complex legal guardrails should be addressed before your loved one gets ill. This is crucial paperwork of vital importance that you should probably organize for yourself as well, so you can prevent any possible difficulties in the future, should you require any kind of help or care in your later years.

CONSERVATORSHIP

An incapacitated person who is unable to manage self-care, requires a representative. This is usually a designated court appointed "conservator of the person." They are in charge of medical and personal decisions for the loved one. This is most often the position of the family member, who is the primary caregiver. If there are disagreements around loved one's estate, the court will often appoint a separate "conservator of the estate," who will take care of and be in charge of the financial matters.

DESIGNATING THE PRIMARY CAREGIVER

If you are your loved one's primary caregiver, it is advisable to seek advice from legal council, who will help you attaining the legal position of "conservator of the person," As such, you primary obligation and duty is to look out for your loved one's best interest and follow all the rules of the law. This will entail providing the best around the clock care, safety and comfort of living arrangements, managing their physical needs, securing help, caregiving supplies, providing emotional support and mental engagement. It will include taking them to any required doctor's appointments, keeping track of all prescribed medication intake, logging daily events, preserving every document, notating every change in their condition and general state of health.

You may have to navigate through complex legal issues in order to protect your loved one's assets and do everything you can to assure their safety and optimal care. If there is friction in the family regarding options and decisions for your loved one's care and management of their assets, you will again require professional legal counsel to best protect your loved one's interest and well being.

In addition to professional legal and medical advice, you may also require assistance from a Senior Care manager. Read more in *Chapter Three: Keeping Your Loved One at Home.*

At the onset of this difficult situation, relatives and even friends may offer help, but when the reality of the magnitude, length of care and needed sacrifice sets in, the previously offered help will often vanish. There may be battles and lengthy frustrating discussions or arguments between the immediate family members. Some may agree and others may not. If your family has conflict, rest assured that you are not alone.

In fact, sadly this is the usual challenging outcome. It is quite rare to have perfect harmony and no disputes when deciding who will step into primary caregiver position and sacrifice so much of their life to manage such demanding care. Even if duties are shared, there is only one primary caregiver.

The most obvious conflicts will ensue about loved one's assets and financial management. If your family maintains harmony, you are extremely fortunate. If the opposite is true, console yourself with the sobering fact, that often people reveal unpleasant character traits when one needs them the most. You are not alone in this predicament. One word of consolation is, that if you remain standing alone with this entire situation resting on your shoulders, and there is no one else to help you, at least you will be able to maintain much needed peace in your immediate environment. In the bigger picture this may be easier than continuously negotiating basic decisions and task sharing.

It is also a fact, that some people are simply incapable of giving up their freedom and making the kind of sacrifice required, to care for a loved one in advanced stage of Alzheimer's dementia. As long as they do not interfere and adversely affect your dedicated primary caregiving process, it is perhaps better they stay distant and not add to your stress.

In the role of primary caregiver, you need to get all the help you can, so you can manage this delicate, complex and physically, mentally, emotionally and certainly financially extremely demanding situation. The estate of your loved one needs to be protected and used for their well-being and care. All family members need to understand and accept this fact.

If they do not, follow the advice of your professional legal counsel and protect your loved one, as well as yourself.

Long term caregiving at home or in a facility, is a very costly predicament. If your loved one has the means to be taken care of, this is where their means must go. If the long term care depletes all the assets of the loved one's estate, that is the reality. All potential heirs must understand and accept this fact. Proper planning must be in place about how the care will continue, if the funds run out. This may also affect your decision to keep and care for your loved one at home. It will be significantly less expensive, you can remain frugal with the funds and assure they are always provided for.

This is now the new realty. Your priority from now on is your loved one. They are helpless, vulnerable, fragile and probably frightened. It is time to care for them and protect them to the best of your ability.

CHAPTER TWO

Your Loved One and Your Past

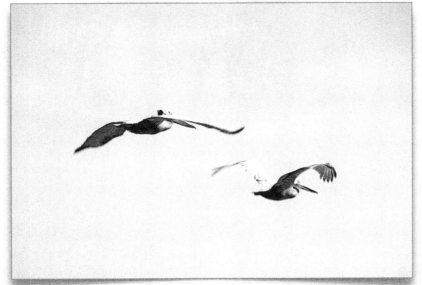

CHANCES ARE, THIS IS NOT YOUR FIRST LIFETIME TOGETHER,
YOUR BOND IS ANCIENT...

CAREGIVING FOR YOUR PARENT

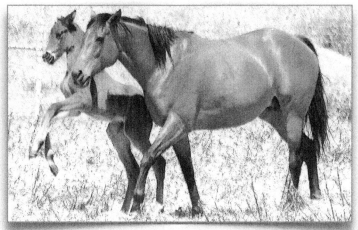

YOUR PARENT IS YOUR FIRST EXAMPLE
OF A RELATIONSHIP

I have always been extremely close to both of my parents. My Mother was my very best friend and I am endlessly grateful for ever opportunity she gave me through my childhood and early years. To me, she was simply the best Mother in the world. She did and would have done anything for me, so I never hesitated in doing the same for her. I consider myself very lucky to have had such a great Mother. And in return, she got lucky with me.

I know very well, that this is not always the case. Sometimes this illness creates and opportunity to heal any past conflicts between the parent and child, and other times the divide grows insurmountable and all ties get broken. No matter what your situation is, do the best you can. Know that your decision will affect you for the rest of your life.

What is required is absolute inner peace, resolution, acceptance and most of all forgiveness for any wrongdoings that may have happened. No parent is perfect. Neither is the child. You need to be an unconditionally loving , reliable and committed caregiver.

YOUR PAST FAMILY DYNAMICS

The bond between parent and child is sacred. No matter how you look at it, the two of you began your relationship the instant your own life began, and have undoubtedly impacted each other's lives tremendously. If you were adopted, you may have not known each other from the very first day of your life, but nonetheless, you were together from the start.

Our parents are our role models and whatever relationship dynamics transpire, we carry them deeply within our being. But all parent-child dynamics are incredibly different, some of them difficult and complex. Whatever happened between you and your parent before this illness is now in the past, for you are entering a new phase. From now on, your relationship takes on a very different shape. Roles are changed, often reversed and expanded. No matter how you look at it, now it is your parent that needs your protection, support, care and undivided attention. If you feel that your parent did not provide, offer and display all those qualities to you as a child, and this still upsets you to this day, you need to give it some serious thought, before making a decision about at-home care giving.

IF YOU PLAN TO BE THE PRIMARY CAREGIVER FOR YOUR PARENT, IT IS ABSOLUTELY ESSENTIAL THAT YOU RELEASE AND MAKE PEACE WITH ANY CONFLICTS YOU MAY HARBOR FROM THE PAST.

Now it becomes essential, that you re-evaluate yourself, and let your heart and mind thoroughly and honestly decide, if you can handle this challenge that destiny has handed you at this juncture in your life. You need to resolve and forgive anything that presents a problem for you, so that you may move on and truly embrace this new and demanding role in your life. Under no circumstances is it advisable to embark on this very demanding, sacrificing and challenging journey as a primary at-home caregiver, if you harbor any kind of past negative emotions towards your parent.

Thru daily new challenging caregiver situations, those old conflicts could easily resurface and become potentially, yet unintentionally very harmful to your parent. In all fairness, you cannot expect to be repeatedly awakened at 3 AM and have to clean your incontinent soiled parent calmly and lovingly while they scream in your ear, when you still harbor angry or resentful feelings towards them in any way. On one of those challenging nights you could snap, blow up at them, loose control and unwillingly harm them. When one is beyond physical exhaustion, all sorts of negative emotions can resurface.

Such is human nature. This assignment is difficult enough without additional challenging aspects and unresolved old grudges. If you would like to work thru a past minor conflict with your parent and have decided to make amends and care for them, then you have to really work on your forgiveness.

It is better to be honest and admit, that due to your past experiences and unresolved inner conflicts with your parent, you cannot take on this heavy responsibility. Perhaps you could remain helpful in a different role, by being supportive to your other sibling that ends up being the primary caregiver. Or, if the parent enters a facility, you could regularly visit them and demonstrate your care that way. You could still be helping in many ways, but not hands-on. It will be more beneficial to everyone, if you honestly face your feelings at this point, admit them and keep your distance.

HONESTLY ASSESS YOUR ABILITY TO FEEL COMPLETELY AT PEACE AND READY TO OFFER THE SELFLESS SERVICE YOUR PARENT WILL REQUIRE FOR THEIR DAILY CARE.

This is the decisive juncture where many people who have a strained relationship with their parent, subconsciously create some kind of a conflict within the family or with the sibling, who does end up caring for the parent. Instead of honestly admitting that they do not want to and are not capable of taking on the responsibility and burden of their parent's care, they create a discord. This helps them justify their avoidance, distance or complete abandonment of helping out. They may argue with the caregiver-sibling, accuse them of wanting to take charge or control, when in fact they are relieved that they found an excuse to abandon the entire challenging situation. Whatever the reason may be, the unresolved old conflict with the parent overrules their response and reaction. They simply can't step up or be honest.

There are of course countless other possibilities and reasoning why certain family members are incapable of becoming a helpful caregiver, or even part of a broader support system. Selfishness, entitlement, fear, ignorance, denial and greed all rear their ugly head and quite often the child is simply incapable of making any kind of sacrifice for their parent.

OF COURSE THERE ARE ENDLESS SITUATIONS WHERE THE CHILD TRULY DOES WANT TO CARE FOR THEIR PARENT AT HOME, BUT IS SIMPLY UNABLE TO DO SO.

There could be a very understandable reason, perhaps their own young family needs them, the partner is not supporting the idea, or their career is too demanding. Maybe they are the main provider, are under dire financial pressure and have an overloaded schedule as it is. Perhaps they are dealing with their own health challenges and can't take on additional stress. Maybe they live very far away. So you see, there is no blame game. It is just the reality of situation. But nobody wants to get stuck in this scenario completely on their own, in addition to a conflict with their siblings. You need to help each other in any and best possible way that you can.

IT IS NEVER A CONVENIENT TIME TO BECOME THE PRIMARY CAREGIVER.

Perhaps you are one of those people, who led a very distanced life and has a really non-existent relationship with your parent. Suddenly you are presented with the last opportunity to get closer, repair and mend your relationship and make peace. If your desire for that is very strong and heartfelt, this new dynamic presents a wonderful opportunity for you to do exactly that. It happens often that a child can finally heal the past and reach a peaceful and loving relationship with an ailing parent at this point in life, even though they were not particularly close before. Again, it has everything to do with your heartfelt intention and desire.

CAREGIVING IS AN EXCELLENT OPPORTUNITY FOR HEALING YOUR PARENT - CHILD RELATIONSHIP.

Keep in mind, mid-stage dementia patients may often for no apparent reason become verbally abusive, but the behavior in later stages is very different and much more peaceful. But if you - as a child caregiver to your parent - have perhaps lived thru difficult dynamics with them before, it is essential that you are strong enough not to take this bad behavior personally. Remain calm and know, that it stems from your parent's illness, previous pain and most likely deep fear. Remember that they cannot control their emotional outbursts, therefore remain detached and never take it personally.

If you cannot stay neutral, but feel hurt by your parent's outbursts, then caregiving may not be for you. However, in late stage dementia, these outbursts will most likely be very infrequent or completely absent. The worst phase of that side of the illness happens earlier on, and now they are probably quite tranquil and quiet. These outbursts can be caused by many factors including overmedication in facilities, since a high dose of an antidepressant can cause agitation and restlessness. As always, there will be challenges, but clearing past negativity and making way for peace, love and forgiveness can be incredibly rewarding.

On the other hand, if your relationship with your parent was and is loving, positive and very close, you will feel an overwhelming desire to care for them and do everything possible for their wellbeing and comfort. You may be naturally the kind of person that always takes care of everybody. As a result, it might be expected that this new responsibility falls on your shoulders, yet again. Be aware and prepared that this assignment is far more demanding than anything you have experienced before. You will be in the trenches and sometimes it will seem like there is no way out.

No matter what your unique situation is, once you have made the heartfelt decision to assure your parent's final years are spent under your care and in the comfort of your home, you have taken on an extremely demanding assignment. You will love, care, protect and watch over them and I applaud your courage and dedication and send you my deepest heartfelt prayers. You have embarked on possibly the most difficult journey of your life.

Is there an upside to it, you ask? Oh yes, there is, but not in a way one might expect. You will feel inner happiness in knowing that you are there for your parent or loved one in need.

> **A DEEP SENSE OF PEACE IN KNOWING THAT YOU ARE ASSURING YOUR LOVED ONE'S COMFORT, WILL BE BESTOWED UPON YOU.**
>
> **AS A RESULT, YOU WILL EXPERIENCE MOMENTS OF PROFOUND INNER JOY, THAT CANNOT BE DESCRIBED, PREPLANNED OR EXPECTED.**
>
> **YOU WILL LEARN TO UNDERSTAND ANOTHER KIND OF SELFLESS LOVE.**

When you least expect it, you might feel a beautiful and profound calmness that will undoubtedly confirm you are doing the right thing. Through the hardest moments, you will realize deep within, that even though this journey is lonely, you are truly never alone. The key to help you persevere is that your actions come from your heart and that you learn to make peace with the seemingly never-ending aspect of it. You cannot be in a rush.

There is no calculated schedule, no sure answers and no real break until the long journey is completed. More often than not, this will take many years. That is what this mission is about. Endless unconditional love, unshakably dedicated selfless service, massive inner strength and an unending supply of resilient, patient determination.

CAREGIVING FOR YOUR PARTNER

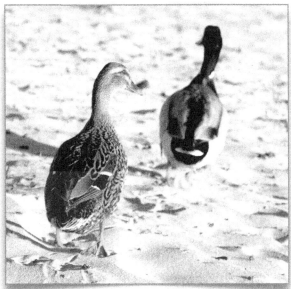

YOUR PARTNER IS THE MANIFESTATION OF YOUR HEART

I have watched my dear Father care for my Mother through the early onset and mid-stage of her illness. His unconditional love, dedication and sacrifice was truly remarkable. My Mother became entirely dependent on him and I saw her love for him reach new levels that no words can describe. It took a heavy toll on him. They bravely endured this final, extremely difficult and sad chapter of their love story, that was truly " in sickness and in health, until death do us part." But do not assume that every partner has the stamina and physical, emotional and mental ability to withstand such a journey on their own. If you have found yourself in this unenviable situation, you need all the help you can get.

At the crucial breaking point when my Mother's illness took the turn for the worse and she entered the late stage, I took over and relieved my Father of his heavy assignment. The roles changed once again. I became the primary caregiver and did not allow him to exhaust himself any further. I feared I would lose them both. So I took the reins into my own hands and drove the carriage through the final passage of the rugged and harsh territory ahead. The journey was too demanding for him, but I pulled all the inner strength I had and somehow managed. Of course everything else in my life came to a screeching halt. A total and complete standstill and undoing of everything my life had been about. A vanishing of all dreams of the future. Just one day, an hour, or a minute at a time. This is what primary caregiving at this point of illness requires. All or nothing. So hold on tight my dear, hold on tight.

YOUR LOVE RELATIONSHIP DYNAMICS

If you become a primary caregiver to your partner, everything from your past shifts into a brand new dynamic. Similarly as in parent - child caregiving dynamic, your roles are entirely different now. This shift may be tremendously difficult and not everyone can step into the role of a primary caregiver for their partner. If your loved one who is now ill was the main breadwinner, the domineering and driving force of the relationship and family, this shift may be tremendously challenging for you.

On the other hand, if the loved one was your dedicated and devoted partner who took more of a backseat role while taking care of all seemingly mundane tasks while you were the main provider, your situation will again become very contrasting and challenging in a different way. The roles will shift, transform and become something new, unfamiliar and most likely very uncomfortable.

Another important aspect that plays a decisive role is your deep emotional bond. The challenge of watching your partner until the end of life, now helplessly and slowly slipping away can be a great source of sadness and sorrow. Your emotions may shift from a sense of anger, fury, profound sadness, despair and abandonment as you watch them leave in a very slow, sad and intensely painful process. You are facing a deeply challenging emotional journey. To help you manage, do not be afraid to share your grief with friends and family and ask for help. You need to reach out, get informed and organize the care as best you can.

It is also important to mention that it is highly likely your relationship with your partner who is now in need of your care, may have been somewhat difficult and challenging for the past few years, before you recognized the presence of the illness.

MOST LIKELY, YOUR LOVED ONE HAS BEEN CHANGING FOR QUITE SOME TIME AND THEIR DISPLAY OR EXCHANGE OF AFFECTION TOWARDS YOU MAY HAVE BEEN LIMITED OR ABSENT.

Perhaps your partner's troubled emotional state was increasingly more difficult to tolerate and you assumed their moods had to with their aging personality shifts. It is possible you mistakenly assumed they were upset with you or their affection towards you diminished, when in fact they were trying their best to face the increased inability to handle simple daily tasks.

They were trying to hide their diminishing ability to remain in charge or in control of their emotions, behavior, mindset and physical mishaps. Perhaps they were angry at themselves and lashed out at you, since you are the closest person they have.

Now that you know the real source of this unpleasant and difficult behavior, it is time to put aside any harbored feelings of upset or hurt and step into the position of the stronger partner who understands and sees the larger picture. Your loved one is ill and they need to be provided with comfort, loving care and protection. This is now your priority. Healing the previous frustrating phase of your relationship is possible, once you understand the true source of ongoing conflicts or changing personality and behavior. It is essential that you do not hold any grudges, or resentment towards them. Step into a position of the wise and caring partner who is ready to deal with the challenging predicament your life has presented. This way you be able to navigate through the primary caregiver duties and demands.

Understand that your partner's previous difficult demeanor had nothing to do with you, but was a direct result of the beginning and advanced stages of the illness.

REACH INTO THE DEEPEST CORNERS OF YOUR HEART AND REMIND YOURSELF OF THE LOVE YOU CARRIED FOR EACH OTHER THROUGH THE MANY YEARS.

Remember how and what you loved about each other when you first met. Remind your loved one of those beautiful times and you may receive a beautiful surprise. They will follow your lead and gladly revisit your beautiful memories.

Even in later stages of dementia, long term memory often remains intact and this may be a most beautiful and enduring way for the two of you to communicate, reminisce and carry on through this journey. See the bigger picture and focus on the love and beauty you were fortunate to enjoy throughout the years. Later on, this will bring you a great sense of gratitude and inner peace.

ARE YOU READY, WILLING AND ABLE
TO BE THE PRIMARY CAREGIVER?

Becoming a caregiver for an Alzheimer's dementia person is usually not something you can plan ahead. It is one of your life's assignments that comes upon you without a warning. You may fear that someone close to you will get such a diagnosis and have to endure such fate, but you can't really ever emotionally prepare. So when the events unfold and bring you to his point, you respond to this difficult predicament the best you can, in that moment.

Countless circumstances play a role in your reaction and determine what you are capable of enduring at that particular time in your life. If you stand up and take on this challenge with determination and warrior-like spirit, it is essential to be as informed as you possibly can, so you can properly prepare and avoid magnifying the difficulties ahead.

A GOOD QUESTION TO ASK YOURSELF IS THIS:
AM I READY, WILLING AND ABLE
TO BECOME THE PRIMARY CAREGIVER?

This mission will require your physical, mental, emotional and financial preparedness. If you take on his assignment, you need to examine dynamics that will play a decisive role. How you will be able to manage, last, endure and sustain yourself through this journey?

YOUR PHYSICAL STRENGTH

STRENGTH

If you are physically strong and in good shape, you will be able to handle the physical demands and have the stamina and power required. However, do not underestimate how fast your great physical shape can change, when you are the primary caregiver.

You may quickly gain or lose weight, strain your back, begin feeling tired and suffer from chronic adrenal fatigue, arthritis, high blood pressure and hormonal imbalance. The lack of sleep will leave harsh consequences. However, disciplined self-care will help you prevent this from happening so you can manage to remain strong and in best shape possible.

> **IF YOU HAVE THE PHYSICAL STRENGTH TO HOLD YOUR LOVED ONE AND PERFORM BASIC CAREGIVING DUTIES ON YOUR OWN, YOU ARE AT A GREAT ADVANTAGE.**

WEAKNESS

If you are physically weak, frail, have your own health challenges, or are considerably smaller in size than your loved one that requires care, you will definitely need the help of another person, a professional hired caregiver. Let's be clear, I have met physically small, but mighty strong caregivers that were incredibly efficient in care of my Mother who was tall. Size does not matter, strength and professionalism does. In this case, you can still be the primary caregiver, but assistance will be needed on an ongoing basis. You will adjust the level of help depending on the needs of your loved one.

Perhaps you can begin with hired caregiver help a few days per week, however, in the late stage of illness when incontinence changes are required as frequently as every three hours, you will need a caregiver every day. You could manage smaller duties, most likely even basic night-time incontinence changes, but the most physically demanding tasks such as getting your loved one out of bed in the morning, showering and continuous incontinence care will require physically capable, prompt and efficient ongoing professional assistance.

You will be able to manage and keep your loved one in your home, but you won't be dealing with all the physical aspects of care yourself.

YOUR MENTAL STAMINA

STRENGTH

Let's no underestimate the importance of mental stamina and grit. You will require tremendous mental resilience to endure the demands of primary caregiving. This means an ability to make quick decisions, find a remedy as needed, assess various ongoing dynamics of care, perfect your observation skills, act calmly and responsibly in times of distress, and manage all intricate details and dynamics of care.

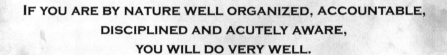

IF YOU ARE BY NATURE WELL ORGANIZED, ACCOUNTABLE, DISCIPLINED AND ACUTELY AWARE, YOU WILL DO VERY WELL.

WEAKNESS

On the other hand, if you have a scattered mind, are impatient, easily flustered, preoccupied with yourself, disorganized, overburdened with countless responsibilities, unable to stick with a set schedule, unreliable, incapable of displaying a strong sense of responsibility, you will not be able to be a stand-alone primary caregiver. You may want to, but it is simply not going to work and very quickly some circumstance will test your ability for self-control.

In such a case, you will require the help of a professional Senior Care case manager that will help you navigate through the many organizing decisions you will have to make. This does not mean you can't have your loved one at home, but you will require professionals in management as well as ongoing caregivers to take complete charge and handle every detail of your loved one's care.

So, your mental shortcoming will not prevent you from being the primary caregiver, but you will require professional help every step of the way.

YOUR EMOTIONAL BALANCE

STRENGTH

Some of us are emotional more resilient and others are more fragile. If you are emotionally balanced, stable and solid, you will be able to hold on through the various difficult and demanding phases that await. However, emotional strength alone is not sufficient for your assignment. What is required is a loving disposition towards the loved one. This experience will become a true test in your ability to love unconditionally, with compassion, and be willing and capable of a major sacrifice.

What does that mean? For the duration of your caregiving assignment, your own elementary emotional needs may not be easily fulfilled. The basic desire for a loving partner will be challenged. The desire to have privacy in your home will be compromised and your sense of freedom will be on an indefinite hiatus. To put it simply, your dreams will be on hold.

Of course you may hear well-intentioned suggestions from friends, how you need to pay attention to your own emotional needs, make an effort to go out and be social, go on a little vacation, but in reality this may not be possible. Maybe you can try, but to a very, very small degree. It may in fact cause you more stress than relief.

If you care for your parent, it will be very difficult to avoid direct repercussions on your own personal relationship dynamics. Primary caregiving requires a great emotional sacrifice. You have to be able to endure through this demanding period of your life, find ways to cope, so you can remain emotionally balanced. If you are caring for your partner, your emotional connection will undergo a significant change. As a result you may feel cheated, punished, or simply saddened about your obvious and tangible loss.

You will need to tap deep into your capacity for emotional resilience and find elements that still bring you some joy and help you sustain the love for your partner that is now so very different and utterly vulnerable.

IF YOU CAN FULFILL YOUR HEART'S DESIRES, YOU WILL MANAGE WELL. PERHAPS YOU ARE BLESSED WITH A GREAT AND LOYAL PARTNER. MAYBE YOU HAVE A WONDERFUL CHILD. PERHAPS AN ADORING PET. IF YOU REMAIN CREATIVE, AND NURTURE A SOURCE OF HAPPINESS AND JOY, YOU HEART WILL ALWAYS THRIVE.

WEAKNESS

If you are emotionally frail, exceedingly sensitive, easily brought to tears, feel personally overly responsible for everyone else's pain, are overwhelmed by guilt or sadness watching your loved one suffer from this illness and simply cannot face the inevitable end, then you probably won't be able to be a hands-on primary caregiver without professional help.

This is an intense assignment that requires serious emotional stamina and endurance. However, with professional assistance of a Senior Care manager and ongoing support of hired caregivers, you can still have your loved one at home.

There is another very important aspect to understand. As I explained previously, your past and current emotional relationship dynamics with the loved one are of utmost importance. If you hold any old grudges, cannot forgive something that happened in the past, you are not the ideal candidate for the position of a primary caregiver. In a moment of frustration, impatience and fatigue you could easily break down and fall into an old negative emotional pattern. Pent-up and unresolved unpleasant feelings would remerge and take over. This would make the loved one extremely vulnerable to abuse. Under no circumstances must that be allowed to happen.

You must be honest with yourself and your ability to resist snapping into an angry, revengeful and aggressive disposition towards your loved one. If you still harbor any kind of anger, irritation and resentment towards your loved one, you cannot be the primary hands-on caregiver.

Under very specific circumstances, if their cohabiting in your home would not interfere with your life, for example if they lived on a separate floor, a guesthouse or closed off wing of the house, you could still have them in your home, but only with professional Senior Care manager in place as well as ongoing caregivers.

> **WHEN FACED WITH THE CAREGIVING DYNAMIC YOU WILL BE FORCED TO EXAMINE YOUR OWN WEAKNESS AND STRENGTH. AN OPPORTUNITY FOR GROWTH IS ALWAYS THERE, IF YOU ARE OPEN.**

FINANCIAL ABILITY

Last but not least, the financial situation plays a decisive role in what kind of care your loved one will receive. This is much more complex than assuming that a family with an endless supply of funds, will naturally offer the best care for their loved one. Unfortunately in many cases, the personal wealth factor does not automatically assure best care. More often than not, the family may have quite complex and deep-set financial conflicts of interest. In other words; someone could be quite wealthy, but their close relatives do not wish to spend the funds on care, and will therefore select a low quality nursing facility for them. Or they may have a large house, but will refuse to keep the loved one at home. Wealth does not guarantee a great caregiving set-up. One the other hand, a family may have very limited funds and yet they provide loving, comfortable and best possible care for loved one in their own home. These are the two extreme, but very common examples.

When a person is affected by this illness, they are not able to effectively make their own financial decisions. In worst case scenario in a family with complex interpersonal dynamics, control issues and old unresolved conflicts, simple greed may take over and prevent a good outcome. It is a very sad, but very common problem.

THERE ARE COUNTLESS COMPLICATED VARIATIONS IN FAMILY DYNAMICS. MONEY ALWAYS TRIGGERS UNRESOLVED EMOTIONAL ISSUES AND OLD CONFLICTS, THAT RESURFACE WITH A VENGEANCE.

No matter what the case is, if your loved one has some funds, they need to be properly used for their best care. The heirs usually struggle with this reality, and cannot overcome their own personal self-interest. Professional caregivers are an expensive proposition. Facilities vary in level of comfort, quality and related cost. People that have strong narcissistic and self-centered personalities, simply cannot accept that their possible inheritance will diminish when used for loved one's necessary care.

No matter how complex your individual circumstances and family dynamics are, if you are the primary caregiver, you will have to face and navigate through the financial situation which will affect the ability to hire caregivers, Senior Care managers and provide all the needed comforts of at-home care. You can find the pros and cons of keeping a loved one at home or in a facility in chapter: *Hiring Caregivers*. If you have very limited funds, you have to make a decision about the care considering all factors, including your own ability to financially weather the storm and provide for your own survival. These are very complicated issues and cannot be generalized.

If you have your loved one at home, you need to know the basic costs of monthly care. Explore various options; the caregiving cost with no outside help and the consequences on your own limited ability to earn a living. Explore the option of getting weekly caregiving help from other family members, even if just a few hours. However, that is rarely doable. Calculate the cost of hired help and what are the financial benefits when your freed-up schedule allows you to continuously make a living. These are you two very basic options.

It is also important to consider the time factor and duration of this illness. Each individual is different and numerous facts play a decisive role in overall health and longevity. However, the reality is that the early stage of this illness can take between two to four years, middle stage two to ten years, and the late, severe or advanced stage anywhere between one and three years. This is a long illness, therefore careful planning is an absolute necessity.

> **SEEK GUIDANCE FROM YOUR FINANCIAL CONSULTANT
> AS WELL AS HEALTH CARE SERVICES ADVISOR,
> TO EXPLORE WHAT GOVERNMENT ASSISTANCE PROGRAMS
> ARE OFFERED IN YOUR STATE,
> AND HOW YOUR LOVED ONE AND YOU CAN RECEIVE FINANCIAL HELP.**

If you keep them at home, inquire about various government programs that cover some costs for the caregiver, who may be a family member. Medicaid programs will usually cover some assisted living costs for eligible residents, nursing care and hospice care. There are new laws and regulations continuously changing. Some of them could greatly benefit you, so do keep informed and up to date.

FINAL THOUGHTS

After assessing all these different aspects of your physical, mental, emotional and financial situation, you will be able to proceed and make the best decision for your loved one's care. Always remember, that every and each situation is truly unique and you may be able to find a good solution to have your loved one at home, remain their primary caregiver and still manage a balanced life as best possible. There will be many ongoing adjustments as the care level will continuously change and shift. But if you stay informed, well organized and are ready willing and able to give it your all, you will succeed.

CHAPTER THREE

Keeping Your Loved One at Home

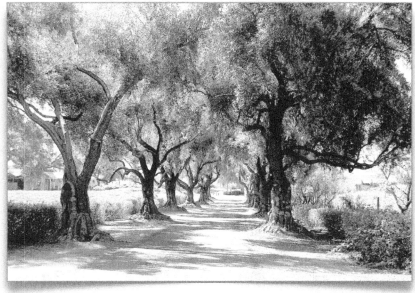

LIVING AT HOME IS A BLESSING...

After a long journey thru different countries, nursing homes and a hospital, the final chapter of my Mother's care presented a possibility to take her back to living at home. I was both thrilled and frightened of this prospect. It seemed that there was much organization, experience and time needed to prepare everything properly. But I went forward with it and got into the trenches.

Had I known then all that I know now, it would have been considerably easier. But I only had a slight idea about the scope of needed care, and there was no one to tell me what to expect. Despite hiring a professional caregiver to help us with Mother's back-to-home transition, I was left alone within 24 hours when the caregiver decided the job was more demanding than she wished. So I was left to my own devices.

I searched thru all the literature I could get, but did not find a simple description on how to care for a late stage Alzheimer's patient at home. A simple and extremely important daily task of changing a grown up's incontinence pad or diaper seemed a topic no-one bothered to describe. It may seem like a logical procedure, but it is not. Anyone who shrugs their shoulders and says that this should be "as easy as changing a baby's diaper," is beyond ignorant. Honestly, a remark like that may infuriate you. People always assume something is easy-peasy, until they face the challenge themselves. For two years that I cared for my Mother at home, I learned hands-on the most valuable solutions to everyday problems. My education and knowledge of Holistic Healing modalities, helped me create a unique program.

Many I discovered myself, but basically I look at this experience with deep gratitude towards my dear Mother. It was thru her illness, that she speechlessly taught me everything I know about this today. So the information you read here is the result of her direct contribution. I was just the instrument to do the work. My Mother and I unite on this pages sharing with you this information that hopefully assists, alleviates and guides you thru every day obstacles and challenges that this circumstance presents.

Due to difficult stage of my Mother's illness and other dynamics, my Mother endured a long journey experiencing international nursing facilities at their best and worst. Through this odyssey, I gained direct knowledge of complex nursing homes dynamics and countless caregivers of international scope. I leaned this invaluable information hands-on in real life, and not as an author writing a book based on interviews.

When after a long transatlantic flight I landed with both my parents in Los Angeles, my Mother was in very late stage of her illness. The journey was indescribably exhausting for me, but my Mother was comfortable, enjoyed herself with all the friendly flight service attendants and delicious food perks of first class. Flying first class was the only realistic option for our circumstance. Mom was thrilled to be traveling. At that time, my Father and I decided to keep her at home. A long and strenuous journey thru her care followed, but she stayed at home with us till the end of her life. I have peace in my heart, that she was loved, cared for and protected by both of us. And most importantly, she was well aware of it.

THE DECISION PROCESS

This is certainly a life altering decision. You have to take into consideration many factors. First and foremost is the state of your loved one's health. If they require professional medical attention at all times, you do not have much of a choice. If your professional life and means of livelihood is such, that doesn't allow the possibly of tending to them, there is nothing to decide. If your personal family situation with an uncompromising partner or troublesome children makes it unfathomable to care for your loved one, the decision has been made for you. If your health does not permit to take on any kind of strain or stress, it all adds up to the same result - your loved one cannot be cared for in your home.

There are certainly cases where all those obstacles are ignored and the family still decides to go for it. They rearrange their home, abandon or change their careers, ignore partner's pleas, de-prioritize their children and dive into the all-consuming caregiving river. But the unpredictable current is much more violent and disturbing than one expects.

> **THE SITUATION REQUIRES DEEP, ONGOING AND DRAMATIC SACRIFICES. TIME SCHEDULES SHIFT, PRIORITIES ARE OVERTURNED AND LIFE CHANGES DRASTICALLY.**

As always, your resilience thru it all depends on your personality, abilities, disposition and stamina. It reveals the level of your strength and tests your inner convictions, principles patience and resilience.

I believe that if one is determined, they can do anything. The question is, at what price? But we rarely think of that ahead of time. I also believe, that if one is a detached person who is mostly concerned about their own well-being and has a good dose of self-centeredness, they will never go thru this. They will not be able to decide to care for a parent or loved one at home or be supervising their care in a facility. And they probably won't be reading this book neither. If it doesn't concern them what to do with their loved one, how they may feel, how they are sleeping, do they have nightmares about being abandoned, are they alone and soiled, then they are simply unable to feel compassions and care.

But you, my reader, are as far from that as the North Pole is from the South Pole. You do care. You worry and you want the best for your loved one. The fact is that no matter where your loved one will be, whether a nursing home, an institution, a board and care facility… anywhere, you will always worry.

You will visit them, fight for their comfort, peace, respect, attentive care and safety. No matter what kind of facility your loved one is in, your supervision will always be needed.

If your relationship with your loved one is challenging and you cannot, and do not want them in your home, you can still care for them in a different way by making sure they are in a good facility, well taken care of and comfortable.

LET'S NOT BE QUICK TO JUDGE SOMEONE
WHO PLACES THEIR LOVED ONE INTO A FACILITY.

IT DOESN'T MEAN THEY DON'T LOVE THEM EQUALLY AS MUCH,
AS SOMEONE WHO HAS THEM AT HOME.

KEEP IN MIND, EVERYONE'S CIRCUMSTANCES ARE DIFFERENT,
AND WE EACH HAVE TO LIVE WITH THE CHOICES WE MAKE.

A very particular combination of circumstances will make it possible for you to have your loved one at home. There are certainly also heartbreaking cases when the loved one is living at home, but is not cared for properly and is suffering in neglect. So you see, what I am concerned about in this book is the best care for them, no matter where they are.

THE HOLISTIC CARE SUGGESTIONS YOU'LL FIND IN THIS BOOK,
CAN BE APPLIED TO YOUR LOVED ONE'S CARE ANYWHERE,
IN A FACILITY OR AT HOME.

BUT IN YOUR HOME, YOU'LL BE ABLE TO IMPLEMENT THEM SMOOTHLY.
AT HOME, YOU ARE IN CHARGE.

Let us review a few different options, in regard to where your loved one lives.

*S*ome people have good experiences and are satisfied with their loved one in a nursing home. I am not one of those people. I have always been supremely demanding when it came to providing care for a loved one. At mid-stage of her illness, my Mother was in a facility and I visited her every day. I stayed with her for at least four hours, made sure she was clean, fed, felt all right, took her medicine and never felt abandoned. Nevertheless, there were times I found her soiled, hungry, in discomfort and wondering about all alone, upset, lost and confused. This occurred despite the fact that the facility was of high quality and highest standard.

I agonized over it and felt heartbroken. I was polite with the staff as I called on them to immediately correct the mishaps, I spoke to the supervisors and directors in charge, showed up every day, and if there was anything wrong with my Mother, I let them know immediately. It bothered them greatly that I saw and noticed everything. Their pace and style were cramped by my constant supervision and presence. But I didn't care. I was making sure my Mother was all right. Nothing was going to stop me.

But by having to deal with me on an ongoing daily basis, the staff knew better and treated my Mother with extra care and respect. If not, I was going to find out, one way or the other. My Mother could not speak to them, but I could. I fended and fought for her.

When I left her at the end of the day, I continued to worry into the evening and called to ask if she was sleeping. I called again first thing in the morning asking how was her night, how she was doing and if she got her medicine. My Mother was in a very complicated stage of her illness and was not easy to deal with. I feared they would just increase the sedatives to have less stress with her. This is why I inquired about her ongoing response to medication. The problem was that very often, I was not told the truth. The morning caregiver would assure me that all was well, and then in the afternoon at my regular visit, a different caregiver would reveal that my Mother had a bad night, did not get her medication and ate nothing.

This only escalated my worry and the whole circle became continuously more stressful. The driving back and forth to the nursing home each day didn't help much neither, so all my days revolved around this all consuming worrisome situation. Certainly to be fair, there are positive sides to nursing facilities as well. If you are fortunate with the right combination of good staff, attentive doctors that are present and quick to respond to medicine adjustments, and of course a clean and comfortable environment, it may be a great solution.

NURSING HOMES PROS AND CONS

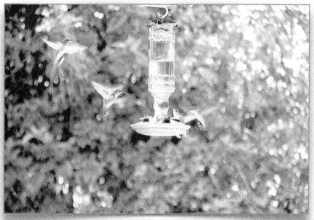

CAREGIVING REQUIRES COMPASSION,
KINDNESS AND LOVE ...

POSITIVE ASPECTS OF NURSING HOME

There are certainly many positive aspects to having your loved one in a nursing facility, especially at the mid-stage of the illness or if your lifestyle and family dynamics make it impossible to care for them at home.

BENEFITS

You know your loved one has constant professional care

Someone else is responsible for them

They are under medical supervision with qualified staff at all times

You can maintain a sense of normal personal life and schedule

You can keep your job and financial security

You can sleep at night

You can go on vacations

You don't have to deal with day and nigh-time incontinence clean up and diaper duty

You can see your loved one any time during the day

You can possibly bring them home for a day visit

You can maintain your health

You don't have to worry about any supplies

You are still enjoying your personal freedom

This may be your best option for mid-stage Alzheimer's dementia patient

NEGATIVE ASPECTS OF NURSING HOMES

DISADVANTAGES

Your loved one may not be properly cared for and tended to

You don't know 100% reliably how they are doing

It may take days before wrong dosage or medicine is adjusted, causing irreversible set-back

They may not be eating since nobody is spoon feeding them for more than 5-10 minutes

They may get into altercation with other residents, get injured, resulting in overmedication

They may have complete insomnia and will be overmedicated

They may be suffering in pain and you don't know

They may be soiled and nobody notices for a few hours

They may be calling for you and you can't hear them

They may have a lucid moment that your are missing

They may be in complete discomfort and unable to communicate

They may be lonely and feel abandoned

They may be suffering

If you worry about all these very real possibilities, the worry alone reduces your positive aspects considerably. And frankly, the worry is a constant.

> **A NURSING FACILITY MAY NOT BE THE BEST OPTION FOR A LATE - STAGE ALZHEIMER'S DEMENTIA PATIENT.**

The reality is that unfortunately all the negative possibilities above do apply. The fact that the facility is being paid a substantial monthly fee does not guarantee that your loved one is secure, fed, not in pain, not overmedicated, receiving proper care or even feeling comfortable and safe. To be fair, an Alzheimer's patient in mid stage of illness can be very difficult to manage. They usually reside in locked dementia units and often aimlessly wonder about the unit halls, sometimes falling and breaking bones, or hitting their head requiring stitches or even surgery. When in need of surgery the anesthesia alone can prove detrimental for their continuous cognitive decline and they rarely recover and return to their previous mental state.

Keep in mind, it is quite challenging to supervise each and every patient non-stop. Since the unit is locked, the residents cannot easily escape, but are nevertheless left to wonder about on their own. Possible altercations with other residents are not uncommon.

They need to be properly supervised, they present a flight risk and will most likely need medication to help them settle down. The dosage of the sedatives is very often too high, which can send them into a rapid downward spiral. They could be sleeping through days and nights, not eating and getting seriously dehydrated. This will further expedite their cognitive and overall decline. The facility is often slow to adjust the medication, because the doctors in residence may be present only on certain days the week, so your loved one may have to wait a few days to have a simple adjustment of the sedative dosage. Due to the nature of illness, the dosage may require a careful continuous adjustment until finding a perfect balance. This may be too time consuming for the staff, thus causing them to avoid adjustments altogether.

However, if your loved one is in advanced stage of illness, it will be challenging for them to receive sufficient care by the regular staff. Why? Because your loved one requires ongoing non-stop care and that is not possible with the regular schedule and staff set up.

> **IN A FACILITY, THERE IS SIMPLY NOT ENOUGH STAFF ON HAND TO CARE FOR EVERYONE INDIVIDUALLY, AT ALL TIMES.**

In advanced stage, Alzheimer's patients are usually moved to specific units that are not locked but open, since the flight risk is obviously eliminated in immobile and bed-bound patients.

In a facility, everything revolves around clearly set schedules. Understandably, this is the only way the care can be managed. Therefore your loved one is awakened at a particular hour, regardless of their personal preference. This could be as early as six or seven in the morning, which may automatically unsettle them and start their day in upheaval causing them great anxiety. The result? Increased medication.

Your loved one is bathed and incontinence-cleaned on a set schedule, regardless of their personal needs. They get fed only at meal times and not whenever they feel hungry. Personalized care is unfortunately not possible in the regular facility setting.

However, a late stage Alzheimer's patient requires personal one-on-one attention throughout the day. Therefore they need an additional personal caregiver, at additional cost to you, and supplied by the facility. This is the only way you can be assured that your loved one is truly kept clean, fed and properly tended to. Keep in mind, it may require up to two hours for your loved one to slowly and comfortably get thru a meal.

At that stage, the level of hygiene care required in order to avoid any bed sores, demands a one-on-one personal caregiver that changes them immediately, as needed. The regular staff at the facility cannot possibly offer that kind of attention, as there is always a shortage of personnel, no matter how nice the facility.

FOR PROPER CARE OF ADVANCED ALZHEIMER'S IN A FACILITY, YOU ARE FACING THE EXPENSE OF THE REGULAR NURSING HOME FEES, IN ADDITION TO THE COST OF A PERSONAL FULL - TIME CAREGIVER FOR EXCLUSIVE ONGOING CARE AND ATTENTION THAT YOUR LOVED ONE REQUIRES 24/7.

Thus the cost of proper care in a facility with the extra caregiver expense quickly gets into the stratosphere. If you do not provide the extra personal caregiver, your loved one may suffer from malnutrition, become a high bedsore risk and undergo consequential rapid and painful decline. A good nursing home facility will let you know in advance that your loved one needs the additional personal one-on-one caregiver, before they will even accept them into their care.

CIRCUMSTANCES FOR KEEPING YOUR LOVED ONE AT HOME

Obviously you need certain conditions to be able to keep your loved one at home. First and foremost, it is crucially important at what stage of illness they are, at this particular moment when you are facing this difficult decision.

As mentioned previously, in the mid - stage of the illness, it may be completely impossible to keep your loved one at home. These patients are often inclined to argumentative behavior, feel restless and wonder about, suffer from severe insomnia and "sun downing," which refers to disturbing anxiety and increased restlessness at sundown. If your loved one is seriously unmanageable, you may have no choice, but to put them into a facility that has a proper locked unit for dementia patients. At that stage of illness, they will most likely not yet require an additional personal caregiver in the facility.

If they are calm and manageable thru early and middle stages of illness, you may be able to avoid this altogether, and keep them at home all the time. But unfortunately that is a less common occurrence.

They usually just need a quiet place to sit, rest or lie in comfortable bed. Most likely they are well beyond the point of wondering off on their own, getting lost or feeling aggressive, so you may be able to have them at home after all. They are most often immobile, sitting on a recliner and bed-bound. Unless they require other demanding health care service that you cannot offer at home, you could now begin assessing the possibility of taking them back into your home environment. You need to carefully evaluate, if your situation satisfies the required conditions.

You will certainly need an extra room with a separate bath. You will need a caregiver who will have the time to supervise them at all times. If that is you, realistically determine what that means and what may be required. If you have the option of engaging a private caregiver for at least a few hours on certain days of the week, this will prove enormously helpful. In fact, it may be a deal-breaker. And last but not least, you need to asses the finances and determine what your realistic budget for caregiving is. On that note, at home caregiving is a definite advantage and less costly.

THE COSTS

No one really likes to think about these daunting facts until they have to face them head on. These days, massive fortunes are spent on elder care and if there is a way to crunch down the stratospheric expense this illness creates, the at-home care is actually a surprisingly good option.

This has certainly proven to be the case during the Covid pandemic. Many family members were rightfully concerned about their loved ones feeling isolated and suffering a rapid cognitive decline in a facility that had to implement visitation restrictions. Therefore many families made the brave and wise decision to take their loved ones back into their home. The majority of these adjustments will remain in place even after the restrictions are lifted. Family members have adjusted positively to this necessary new arrangement.

To their surprise, many of them realized that at-home care is financially considerably less expensive. In addition, the constant worry about your loved one is simply eliminated. You know how they are doing, because you have them in your home. If you want to ask them a question or make sure they are comfortable, you can just do so yourself. This significantly reduces the level of stress, which is critically important.

I encourage you to seriously explore all options and know, that even if you are spending large sums of money for a facility, it doesn't necessarily mean everything is provided and taken care of, for your loved one. It may not be the ideal setting for them and it may be an overly expensive setting for you.

Make no mistake, even having your loved one at home proves to be costly and extremely demanding. But at least the expense is manageable and that way, you can make sure and be certain that they have the best of everything. And that is because you are the one that is responsible and in charge. They key is knowing ahead of time all that is needed and required, to make that option as easy and successful as possible for everyone involved.

> **THE BASIC EXPENSE FOR KEEPING YOUR LOVED ONE AT HOME IS CERTAINLY CONSIDERABLY LOWER THAN A FACILITY. FURTHER COSTS DEPEND ON YOUR DECISION TO HIRE OUTSIDE HELP.**

Whatever you decision is, the most important focus should be that the resources spent provide the best health and personal care for your loved one.

The fees for nursing facilities vary, but keep in mind what I mentioned previously; at this stage of illness you will need to add the personal one-on-one caregiver. The final amount will be frightening. If the nursing facility ranges conservatively on the average between $6,000 to $8,000 in monthly fees, then you can easily add almost as much for a monthly personal daily caregiver. In that case you are practically doubling the rate and looking at approximately $12,000 in monthly expenses for this arrangement in a decent facility.

It is important to understand that this is a demanding long-term illness that could go on for a few years, even in this final phase. At this rate, financial situations can become overwhelmingly critical. Fortunes are lost, savings and retirement accounts depleted, homes are repossessed and people go bankrupt. That is the brutal reality. However, getting well informed and planning ahead, will help you prevent this from happening.

IF YOU KEEP YOUR LOVED ONE AT HOME, AND CARE FOR THEM ON YOUR OWN, YOUR ONGOING RUNNING EXPENSES WILL ENTAIL BASIC LIVING COSTS AND SUPPLIES.

If you hire a professional caregiver from a private caregiving agency, they usually offer different care and schedule structures. The cost will depend on your geographical location and local pricing. If you do the caregiving alone, this expense is eliminated. There are some private health insurance companies that may provide for select caregiving services, but most will not pay for non-medical care services at home. This varies from insurance companies and state to state regulations.

Please check the regulations and offers for your specific needs in your geographical area. Nevertheless, the expense will be relatively small compared to the astronomical cost of facility and additional private caregiver services.

To help you properly prepare your home environment for your loved one's needs and care, there will be a one time set-up expense so that you have all required equipment and supplies. Unless the loved one's insurance covers possible home visiting doctors, that is an additional cost. Personal insurance or Medicare mostly always pays for hospice services, but that is the very final stage of illness and may not occur for a few years.

ALL IN ALL, THE EXPENSE IS CONSIDERABLY SMALLER WHEN YOU KEEP YOUR LOVED ONE AT HOME.

However, do keep in mind, there are other factors that cannot ever be reimbursed that will prove "expensive" in different ways, like the sacrifice of your years of time, energy and effort. That can never be repaid. Personal and relationships sacrifices, the toll caregiving will take on your health and most likely your diminished financial freedom. Your ability to work and the damaging impact on your career are only some of the un-reimbursable "expenses" that you will face. Family time will be affected, and if you are a late bloomer, the chance of creating a family of your own, will most likely be delayed or possibly lost.

I assume you know that and have somewhat made peace with it. But it is something that other family members, such as your siblings or relatives must also be made aware of. I must remind you, in order to avoid disappointment, do not expect others to truly understand the magnitude of the sacrifice and service you are providing for your loved one. Only a likeminded caregiver, a person who has traveled a very similar journey will have the slightest idea what you are experiencing. They will know, you will know, and God will know. That is just how it is.

GERIATRIC CARE MANAGER

Another very helpful professional that can prove invaluable through this complex caregiving decision process, is a Geriatric Care Manager. This could be a social worker, a nurse, or counselor that can offer assistance when making important care choices. They can help you find doctors that offer home visits, and various other resources you'll need.

The Geriatric Care Manager can help you in all aspects of caregiving, if your loved one is at home, or if they reside in a facility or nursing home. The Care Manager comes to your home and helps assess the situation, makes a care plan, arranges for various services, and continuously monitors any new needs or developments. This services usually work on an hourly fee basis, so this will be an extra added expense. However, especially at the beginning, it may be well worth it. They could help you set-up the at-home caregiving structure. Later, you can have them visit only occasionally, if the need arises.

**A GOOD GERIATRIC CARE MANAGER
CAN BE VERY HELPFUL AND A GREAT RESOURCE.
THEY WILL FORTIFY YOUR PROFESSIONAL CARE SUPPORT SYSTEM.**

Before hiring, ask about their references, agencies or organizations they may be associated or affiliated with, professional credentials, licenses and certifications, and if they carry a personal liability insurance. Inquire in writing about precise cost and fees for their services.

Finally, you need to assure they are aligned with your personal views on eldercare. Ask them directly of their philosophy about at-home-care versus nursing-home care. If the Care Manager works for a nursing facility, they may encourage you to place your loved one there. Inquire about their knowledge of dementia and associated care needs, how long have they worked in this field, how familiar are they with local area resources, are they easily available for emergencies, and how they plan to communicate with you.

YOUR LOVED ONE'S WISHES

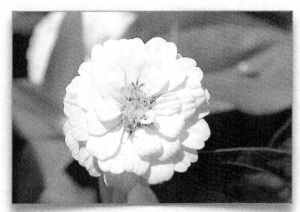

YOUR LOVED ONE WILL ALWAYS
PREFER TO LIVE AT HOME

In ideal circumstances, your loved one would be able to voice their wishes. Sadly this is often not possible. In most cases, your loved one would much prefer to stay at home in their familiar environment. As I mentioned, in early and mid-stage of this illness it is very difficult to care for your loved one at home. They require ongoing supervision, can be at risk of getting lost, falling or even mistakenly ingesting a dangerous substance.

The mid-stage of this illness is especially challenging, because they may often suffer from anger outbursts, aggressive frustrating bouts and in general refuse to hear your advice, suggestions, or dislike your watchful presence.

For your loved one, it is emotionally very stressful to move away from home, leaving behind all that is familiar and their homes full of memories. They will struggle with the fear of the unknown, foreign, surrounded by strangers and living with restricted freedom. If at that mid-stage of illness they require care in a facility, then you can be involved with regular visitations and pay close attention to their everyday needs. Later, when they enter a less challenging phase, you could move them back into your home, if at all possible.

BY KEEPING YOUR LOVED ONE IN A PEACEFUL LOVING HOME ENVIRONMENT, THEY WILL STILL BE ABLE TO INTERACT WITH FAMILY MEMBERS, EVEN IF ONLY IN A VERY LIMITED WAY.

Even if they cannot communicate beyond a few basic words, your loving care and presence will offer them comfort, safety and awareness that they are not abandoned, but very much loved. The approach of how to navigate through the various complex stages of illness and your loved one's needed level of care, will greatly fluctuate and change as you go along.

Many decisive circumstances must be taken into consideration; such as the dynamics of harmony or conflict in the immediate family, and how that could adversely affect or endanger the loved one. They certainly cannot reside at home, if the family is in severe conflict about care and your loved one is in any way endangered.

ALWAYS SELECT AN OPTION THAT WILL GUARANTEE YOUR LOVED ONE'S OPTIMAL SAFETY, COMFORT AND CARE.

FINAL DECISION

YOUR LOVED ONE IN A FACILITY

If you have decided to place your loved one into a facility, get familiar with all supervisors and have their contact information. Do your best to kindly inform the staff that you are going to be present as much as possible. If you live far away, call regularly, develop a good relationship with the tending doctors, the supervisors and head of caregivers or nurses in charge and always communicate respectfully, but firmly. Stay informed and be involved. Inquire about any medicine changes, dosages and reasons for prescribed medications. Do not become indifferent. Get regularly updated and request ongoing and current status report. It may be wise to hire the services of a Geriatric Care manager that can personally supervise your loved one's care on a regular schedule.

When you visit your loved one, be present for incontinence pad-diaper change and see for yourself if there are any bedsores. Pay attention to your loved one's overall physical condition and emotional state. Carefully and attentively observe every detail of care and note any problems or concerns that seem present.

IMMEDIATELY COMMUNICATE WITH THE SUPERVISORS ABOUT ANYTHING THAT TROUBLES OR CONCERNS YOU.

FIND THE RESPONSIBLE PARTY AND MAKE IT CLEAR YOU ARE AWARE AND INFORMED. BE PRESENT AND INTERACT WITH THEM REGULARLY.

If possible, be present at doctors' visits in the nursing home, communicate directly with them, develop a personal rapport so that you may call them if needed. If the supervisors become aware of your level concern and care for your loved one, they will definitely pay more attention to them.

You can also apply numerous holistic care and healthy diet suggestions from this book to your loved one in facility. Keep in mind, that regular disciplined holistic care will create positive long term effects. You cannot expect the same results from only occasional use of the suggestions or following these principles. If you have an addition personal caregiver for your loved one's care in the facility, instruct them to follow any holistic caregiving suggestions you'll find in this book. For example: preparing a serving of blended prunes or adding ground flaxseed to diet, may prove decisive in overcoming chronic constipation. Long term use of laxatives can lead to electrolyte imbalance, so whatever you can do to minimize overmedicated state is beneficial. Such seemingly small adjustments may make a decisive and positive difference.

YOUR LOVED ONE AT HOME

If you have made a decision to keep your loved one with you in your home, then prepare as best you can. Be aware, that there will always be adjustments and improvements. You will keep learning and discovering new solutions to challenges, but with dedication, patience and loving care, you will manage.

In either case, this time in your life will demand massive amounts of energy, compassion, stamina and strength. Take good care of yourself, so that you may endure this mission and come out intact and healthy. However, I forewarn you, internally, you will be changed forever. You will see life from a very different perspective.

Your ability to discern people will most likely greatly expand and your hard earned wisdom will be one of your greatest rewards. The most significant transformation will occur in your heart. In no way should my earnest words discourage you. They are meant to prepare you with valuable knowledge. I am your greatest cheerleader.

I BELIEVE THE MORE INFORMATION YOU HAVE, THE BETTER YOU WILL BE ABLE TO GUIDE AND NAVIGATE THRU THIS PERIOD OF YOUR LIFE.

AND THAT WILL PROVE GREATLY BENEFICIAL FOR YOUR LOVED ONE, YOUR FAMILY AND THE CAPTAIN OF THIS SHIP - YOU.

CHAPTER FOUR

Preparing Your Home

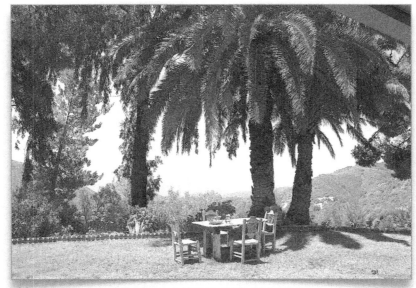

YOUR HOME CAN BE A HEALING AND PEACEFUL OASIS

*I*n my case, I was incredibly fortunate to be able to search for a house that could satisfy all of my Mother's specific care needs. It had to be large enough for my Dad and I as well, all on one level for easy access and with enough distance away from any neighbors.

We ended up living on a ranch in serene nature and some land. My Mother could make any noise she wanted, without disturbing the neighbors. Her room was in a separate wing with its own entrance. We custom built a lovely large care-specific bathroom for her and added a small kitchenette for caregivers. We installed a separate heating and air conditioning unit so we could adjust the temperature in Mother's room specifically to her needs. All of it was an immense undertaking, but her set-up was ideal.

Except for a few rare rainy days in winter, the weather in California was always perfect, so we kept her bedroom door to the rose garden open at all times. She spent her days and months comfortably sitting in her recliner, looking far into the distance, enjoying the fragrance of the rose garden, observing the hummingbirds and gazing at the lovely sunsets. Sometimes she seemed very absent minded, other times she would utter a few words expressing her marvel of nature. With Dad and I always at her side, she was completely content and at peace. This greatly consoled all three of us.

CREATING THE PERFECT SPACE

Once you've made the decision to care for your loved one in your home, there are many things that need to be done, adjusted and properly prepared. I suggest that you get the basics done immediately, and the rest of the details can be completed and added over time, even when your loved one is already settled with you.

Of course one does not always have a choice or all the needed resources to create the perfect environment. But keep in mind, as long as you have the proper space and conditions for easy hygiene care with all safety measures covered, you are in good shape. If you can offer them comfort, loving care and a peaceful, private space, you have provided the main and necessary basics. Everything else can be added in time and adjusted to personal preferences.

YOUR LOVED ONE NEEDS A SENSE OF CONSISTENCY AND SHOULD FEEL SECURE IN THEIR ENVIRONMENT.

BEDROOM SET - UP

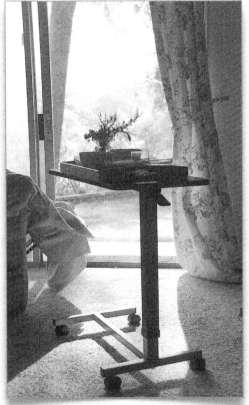

A TRANQUIL BEDROOM IS VITAL

Your loved one will definitely need their own bedroom. You cannot place them into a small, crammed room. There will be various supplies that require space, most likely a wheelchair, a shower chair on wheels and at times, two caregivers simultaneously. If you have one caregiver that comes to help you out, with yourself included, that makes two of you. And let's not forget your loved one makes three, and that's a crowd. There may be occasional visits from doctors, nurses, care managers, and maybe even friends or other relatives. Even if that is not the case, you will no doubt be spending time with your loved one in the room, so it is important to designate a comfortable space.

**THE ENVIRONMENT INFLUENCES OUR OVERALL STATE OF WELLBEING.
A BEAUTIFUL, FUNCTIONAL, CLEAN AND PLEASANT ROOM
WILL BECOME YOUR LOVED ONE'S SAFE HAVEN.**

First and foremost, their room needs to be peaceful, hopefully away from the main living areas of your home, or rooms with high traffic and daytime noise. You cannot expect your loved one to enjoy peaceful sleep, if there is the loud sound of TV or disturbing conversation into the wee hours, right next to their room. You need to think ahead of all possible situations that could disturb your loved one's peace. If it is possible, place them furthest from the main living areas, TV room or children's room.

Keep also in mind, that your loved one's behavior, their needs, and nighttime care will create a certain ongoing commotion. Various sounds from their room could be disturbing to anyone who's room is too close, especially children who might get upset.

The room should have easy wheelchair access and a direct access to a private bath. Your loved one must have their own bathroom. There are many safety precautions that need be in place for them, especially in the bathroom. You will also need necessary equipment or supplies on hand and ready at all times. It is essential that you keep everything in perfect order and remain very organized. It will be very difficult to manage care, if there are other family members using the same bathroom.

YOUR LOVED ONE'S BEDROOM MUST BE CONNECTED TO A PRIVATE BATH, FOR EASY ACCESS FROM BATH TO RECLINER OR BED.

That way they will never be caught in a draft after a bath, which could be potentially dangerous. All doorways need to be wide enough for an easy wheel-chair access. Same applies for any door that will used to get out of the house. Most doorways are wide enough, but if not, I suggest you adjust the doorways right away. If that seems too difficult for you, you can acquire a smaller size portable wheelchair, that is a bit narrower and usually easily fits also thru a narrow doorway. That is a most economical solution.

The room must have the layout to be easily aired out, which means a door-window cross draft possibility. That is essential when you need to air the room out, at least once a day. If you keep the room uncluttered, clean, pleasant and well organized, you will help eliminate a major challenge that is very often difficult to overcome in nursing facilities - a bad smell.

The key is to create a beautiful, pleasant, comfortable and spacious room. Ideally there should to be a nice large window or door with garden, patio or terrace access. If that is not possible, hopefully there is a nice and serene view.

Facing your neighbor's wall or a noisy street is definitely not ideal. Imagine yourself sitting in front of a window for hours. You would want to see something pleasant and relaxing. Give your loved one the best and most tranquil view possible. This will prove very helpful in fighting anxiety or restlessness. There will be times when your loved one might yelp, scream or make some kind of a disturbing noise. Directly facing a neighbor may prove to be very challenging as they could complain, call police and cause you extra stress. The very best layout for your loved one's room is a special wing with separate entrance for caregivers, and a fair distance from the immediate neighbors.

BEST COLORS FOR THE ROOM

The colors have a very powerful influence on one's feelings and overall state of well-being.

**LIGHT PASTEL COLORS ARE IDEAL,
SUCH AS SOFT AND PALE VIOLET, GENTLE, VERY LIGHT BLUE,
LIGHT PINK OR ROSE, AND VERY PALE, SOFT, LIGHT FOREST - GREEN.**

They will provide a soothing effect for the room. White color can be too sterile and bright and can agitate your loved one, who may be light-sensitive. I also suggest you absolutely stay away from anything too vivid or fiery such as red, orange, and yellow or any depressing darker brown or black colors.

Make sure the windows have nice coverings or curtains and the room can be kept dark when needed for sound sleep and to protect them from bright and hot sun. Before you move your loved one into their room, remember about their favorite colors and make an effort to paint or include that color with some accents to make it to their liking. You want them to feel at home and in a familiar, comfortable environment. If you have some of their own small, very personal articles, art or photographs, place them in their room. Later, you will be happy you did.

You would be amazed how many sleepless and restless evenings and nights will be eliminated with the proper colors and overall soothing and pleasant feeling of the room. Use the same judgment for all decorative elements and pay attention to that same principle. You want your loved one to enjoy a most pleasant environment at this stage of their precious life.

BASIC ROOM FURNISHINGS

BED

You need to acquire your loved one a nice and comfortable bed. In nursing facilities they usually offer small single-size beds. My experience has been, that it is considerably easier to do night changes in a larger bed, but most of all, your loved one will be more comfortable if they are in a queen size bed. You can also get a nursing care bed. Make sure the bed is accessible from all three sides. It is also very important that the feet of the bed do not face the door.

THE BEST SOLUTION IS AN ELECTRIC, FULLY ADJUSTABLE BED THAT HAS THE CAPACITY TO ADJUST THE HEIGHT OF HEAD OR LEGS WITH AN EASY PUSH OF A BUTTON.

It is very important to be able to adjust the bed if loved one needs an elevated head due to difficulty breathing, cough or anything else. This is especially important in the late and final stages of illness. I highly recommend you invest in a comfortable bed; after all, your loved one will be spending lots of time there and needs to be as relaxed as possible. A good bed will last you for years.

A high quality mattress is also essential and will help prevent the occurrence of bedsores. You can use a waterproof mattress or regular mattress, that will require a few layers of protective padding in addition to disposable pads you will be using on a daily basis. My Mother loved her ortho mattress electric bed. It was incredibly comfortable and soothing for the body, inducing deep state of relaxation, which was great help when falling asleep.

The more comfortable you make your loved one, the better it is for them and everyone else. Whatever bed you finally decide on, make sure to purchase the warranty for parts. Keep the warranty documentation close and handy in case you need to repair anything. You do not want to be stuck with an electric bed in the wrong position for any length of time. Usually the service man can come to you the same day and repair the problem.

As the illness progresses, the bed adjustments are going to become more important than ever. You loved one will be sensitive to the slightest change and you will be able to help them feel more comfortable.

YOUR LOVED ONE'S BED WILL REQUIRE SAFETY BEDRAILS.

RECLINING CHAIR

You need to purchase a great electrical reclining lounge chair, that can be easily controlled with a push of a button. It is important that your loved one can stretch their legs completely and have them elevated away from the ground. When you are getting them out of the reclining chair, elevate the chair and help prop your loved one to an almost standing position. That way, you will easily help them get up into a standing position and will also comfortably lower them into the seat, when you are placing them back into the sitting position. You will also be protecting your back and preventing your own injury, that can easily occur when you are lifting them up or transferring them from recliner to shower chair or bed. Over time, you will realize how very important a good reclining chair is. It is a necessity.

OVER BED TABLE - NIGHTSTAND

This is a small adjustable table on wheels that can be used as a nightstand, night **table**, **bedside table**, day-stand or **bedside** cabinet. It is very practical and can stand beside a **bed**, recliner or can be moved elsewhere in the **bedroom**.

ENTERTAINMENT CENTER

It will be of great value for your loved one to have the basic entertainment appliances such as a small TV, DVD and CD player. I am not encouraging you to have the TV on full blast all day with the disturbing news, but there will be times when a nice distraction for your loved one with an old movie will do wonders for calming them down, and even help reminisce about their youth. This will help them retain some level of long-term memory.

SOUNDS AND VISUALS FOR SERENITY

You can use very soft and soothing music to wake your loved one up to a pleasant cheerful mood in the morning, help them relax during the day and calm them down when they are falling asleep at night. The same tune will naturally put them to sleep. Peaceful, serene, light or soft music can be a great healing element. For that purpose, you will need a selection of soothing sounds of nature, easy classical music and maybe a small selection of your loved one's favorite songs and singers. Nothing too energetic, only soft, pleasant sounds.

I also suggest you subscribe to a classic movie channel for easy viewing of your loved one's favorite old time movies. If they get restless in the late afternoon, you can have them view their favorite film. You can also select programs with nature, ocean, birds, flowers or forest. Make sure all programs are free of violence or any disturbing elements. Keep everything light, cheerful, happy and peaceful. This way, even if your loved one can't enjoy certain things in real life, you can keep them entertained and they will surely cherish it.

ROOM TEMPERATURE, AIR QUALITY and MOISTURE LEVEL

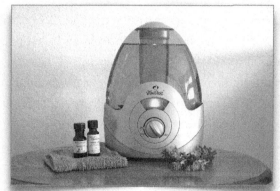

USE AIR HUMIDITY CONTROL DEVICES

Fresh air is essentially important for your loved one's new room. Obviously the fresher the air, the better everyone feels. A bad smell in the room is a clear indication that you are not sufficiently meticulous about hygiene. Your loved one is helpless and vulnerable, and you need to make the extra effort to provide them with top hygiene regimen.

The key is keeping your loved one as clean as possible at all times. The solution for good air is preventing any incontinence accidents, where permanent soiling can occur. If you are disciplined, organized and aware, you will be able to keep their room in pristine condition, without any unpleasant smells.

> **AIR THE ROOM OUT DAILY, WHILE MAKING SURE YOUR LOVED ONE IS NOT EXPOSED TO A DRAFT.**

I often hear people complaining that their elderly relative smells bad. All I can say is, there is absolutely no excuse for that. If you are the caregiver or have caregivers tending to your loved one, it is your sole responsibility to keep the loved one bathed, smelling fresh and feeling clean at all times.

One never complains that a baby smells bad. Why? Because usually we clean the baby immediately when their diaper is full. Same goes here. When someone is helpless and depending on you, then any indication of a bad smell is a direct result of your poor care. As I mentioned before, it is most useful if the room can be easily aired out. I suggest you do that after each morning routine, every time after a big change or clean up of incontinence, as well as in the evening after your loved one is in bed. Do not just spray the room with toxic air freshener and keep it closed off. Air it out every single day.

Weather and outside temperature must be considered, depending on your geographical location. The room has to be air conditioned and appropriately heated. If your home does not have air conditioning, you can acquire a portable one for your loved one's room. Remember, your loved one is extremely sensitive to temperature changes and when they cannot communicate their needs, it is again up to you, to notice any changes in the room temperature that may be uncomfortable. It is not easy to fall asleep in a room where you sat the entire day, has stale air or was never aired out. Especially when additional people or caregivers are present, the room needs to be regularly aired out.

The temperature must be carefully adjusted for the optimal comfort of your loved one. Keep in mind, that during caregiving duties you are physically active and will usually feel much warmer, than your loved one who may be receiving a bath. Therefore make sure it is never too chilly for them.

On the other hand, if the room feels warm to you, it might be much warmer for someone who is sitting on a recliner, immobile and covered with a blanket. Pay attention and adjust the temperature accordingly. Do not make the room temperature comfortable for you, but for your loved one. Observe and carefully assess their needs and comfort level.

Make adjustments to your loved one's personal preference. They have the final say, after all, it is their room. You have the freedom to leave the room, but they don't.

> **IF YOUR LOVED ONE IS RESTING AND IS COVERED WITH A BLANKET, THE IDEAL DAYTIME ROOM TEMPERATURE IS BETWEEN 70°F AND 73°F. WARMER CONDITIONS WILL CAUSE PERSPIRATION AND DISCOMFORT.**
>
> **BEST NIGHTTIME TEMPERATURE IS BETWEEN 69°F TO 70°F. THAT WILL ASSURE A GOOD BREATHING TEMPERATURE WHILE YOUR LOVED ONE IS COVERED WITH LIGHT BEDDING.**

Think logically: one cannot sleep comfortably in a room that's hot and stuffy. The better the air and the more appropriate the bedding, the better chances you as the caregiver will also have of a good night sleep, without night-time changing and disruptive wake-ups.

> **INAPPROPRIATE ROOM TEMPERATURE AND HUMIDITY LEVEL CAN HAVE SEVERE CONSEQUENCES FOR YOUR LOVED ONE. THE IDEAL HUMIDITY LEVEL SHOULD BE BETWEEN 30% AND 60%.**

If they are perspiring they could quickly develop skin problems and sores, since the skin is constantly moist and wet. They could also catch a cold, getting into a draft. Use logic and consider their optimal comfort. An uncomfortable temperature could also make them agitated and since they are unable to tell you, it can be very frustrating for all. Sometimes a room temperature adjustment will relieve all anxiety and restlessness.

ADJUST THE TEMPERATURE AND AIR HUMIDITY LEVEL, ACCORDING TO YOUR LOCATION'S CLIMATE AND SEASONS.

During winter months when you are using heat, or in exceptionally dry climate, I highly recommend a small room humidifier. Enough moisture in the air will provide comfort and help prevent dry cough and dry skin. If summers are exceptionally humid, air conditioner is essential, however, you can also use a dehumidifier.

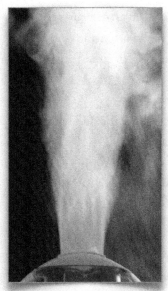

REGULATE AIR HUMIDITY LEVELS

Take into consideration also the previous habits and preferences of your loved one. If they loved sleeping in a cool room, by all means adjust the temperature to a bit cooler for nighttime, but of course provide proper covers for them. If they keep uncovering themselves, you will need to keep the room warmer. If they preferred their bedroom toasty and warm in the past, make sure that now they are not too hot, perspiring or getting agitated.

Remember also the fact, that in the past, your loved one could easily cover or uncover themselves whenever they wanted. Now, they are at the mercy of your intuitive observation skills in guessing their optimal comfort level and needs. Even if you have figured out their preference and behavior patterns in regards to room temperature, do still keep a close eye on them, because with this illness, their situation could change daily. That means that one night they could be cold and the next they could be hot and perspiring for no apparent reason. Always remain on guard and attentive.

CALMING AROMAS

Various aromatherapy oils can become real aids in uplifting or calming your loved one, in addition to being very helpful to you as well. You will need a natural and organic aromatherapy spray, made from pure organic botanical extracts. They will be helpful to quickly freshen up the room, after an incontinence change, in addition to always airing out the room. It is very helpful to use nice aromatic oils to help with a particularly difficult bad smell, which can sort of "stay in your nose." Have a small aromatherapy oil handy for such occasions, for your own needs. You can use it regularly to help improve the bad smell that seems stuck in your nose, and instantly change it to a more pleasant one.

Especially after an incontinence change the loved one can feel very unhappy, agitated and irritable. Use a pleasant aroma to shift their senses into a happier state. To calm them down at night time, you can let them enjoy the scent of rose, lavender or orange oil.

If they have trouble breathing due to a stuffy nose or allergies, offer them the scent of eucalyptus oil. You can soak a few drops onto a small cotton ball or handkerchief, and let them hold it in their hand or place it somewhere on their bed covers.

> **IT IS A GOOD IDEA TO HAVE A VARIETY OF AROMATHERAPY OILS.**
> **THEY WILL HELP IMPROVE THE MOOD OF YOUR LOVED ONE,**
> **WHEN THEY ARE AGITATED OR RESTLESS, AND HELP**
> **TRANSCEND THEM INTO THE BEAUTIFUL WORLD OF FRAGRANCE.**

Use the power of healing aromas as an effective aid and sensory healing tool. You could also have a small aromatherapy diffuser in their room for continuous fresh smell. However, be very careful, and only use a diffuser in a well ventilated area, as sometimes people can get an irritating cough, if they are too sensitive for strong aroma essences. Always use pure essential oils in minimal quantities of a few small drops. Limit the use of camphor, clove, lavender, eucalyptus, thyme, tea tree, and wintergreen oils to a bare minimum, since they are strong and may cause irritation.

Best essential aromatherapy oils to use for calming agitated states of dementia are peppermint, rosemary, bergamont, lemon balm, Ylang Ylang, geranium, ginger and lavender. They will help balance strong emotions in addition to having effective anti-viral, anti-bacterial, decongestant, and expectorant qualities. See chapter: *Holistic Caregiving Remedies* for detailed info.

The HEALING POWER of FLOWERS and PLANTS

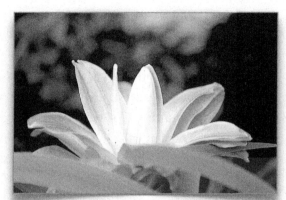

FLOWERS AND PLANTS RADIATE LIFE FORCE

Every few days I gave my Mother a small hand picked flower bouquet from our garden. Sometimes she held the roses in her hands, smelled them and a soft smile would appear on her beautiful face. She truly loved flowers. Of course we were lucky to be living in California, where roses thrive almost all year round, but you can get a small flower for your loved one anywhere in the world.

It is important to have some fresh and alive plant energy in your loved one's room. Pick a few low maintenance plants and place them in your loved one's view. Even one blossom will cheer them up. A pleasant smell can trigger a positive emotional response, which may help you gain a moment of communication with your loved one.

Bring the flowers closer to your loved one and gently explain which flower it is and how pretty it smells. Give them a moment and let them enjoy the scent for a bit. It may bring back a memory of their days in the garden, when they tended to their own blossoms years ago, or an old memory of flowers and nature.

You could remind them of a pleasant or happy event from their far past that is connected to a specific flower. It might help trigger a spark in their long term memory and help them speak a few words. But even is they offer you just a soft smile, your heart will be joyful. Cherish those moments. It will take your loved one back to a time when they enjoyed life and will remind you, that part of them is still here, somewhere deep inside.

SOOTHING LIGHT

It is essential to have excellent lighting in your loved one's room. You need a general good overhead light, that you can be used for necessary oversight of the entire room. However, you may use that light only when cleaning or if you need to see everything brightly in a moment of a night-time crisis.

You will need another standing adjustable light with a dimmer, for use during regular night changes. When you do a night change, you will never want to completely awaken your loved one, with a big bright and startling overhead light. The standing adjustable light should be positioned so it casts a bit of soft light on the lower part of the bed, and never any direct bright light on the face or upper area of your loved one.

YOUR LOVED ONE IS EXTREMELY SENSORY SENSITIVE.
KEEP THE LIGHTS SOFT AND COMFORTABLE.
A BRIGHT LIGHT COULD STARTLE AND AGITATE THEM.

In addition, a small adjustable night stand light could be very useful as well, so you can keep track of various night remedies, medicine and humidifier by the bed.

It is advisable that you also have a few soft, small nightlights. They are small electrical light fixtures, plugged into electrical socket and placed in dark areas for extra safety at night or in an emergency. These lights are important for you as well, and will help you when you check on your loved one at various times during the evening and throughout the night.

Your loved one will feel better having a nightlight, since total darkness could frighten and confuse them. Most importantly, keep in mind that your loved one is very light sensitive and a bright light will cause agitation. I highly discourage you from any kind of bright neon lights, especially above the bed. Just imagine how you would feel, if someone turned on such a disturbing light while you were sleeping or resting in your bed.

Pay attention to your loved one's reaction to a brighter or a darker room and light adjustment, and observe their preference. Properly adjust the lighting and always remember, keen observation and immediate adjustment is the key. With practice you will learn to do the night changes only with the soft nightlight, which will help your loved one to sleep thru and not even wake up. The better you become at this, the easier it will be.

BATHROOM

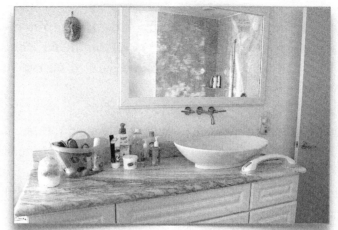

A SPACIOUS BATHROOM WILL SUPPORT YOUR CARE

Daily morning and bedtime routine are often the most challenging and energy consuming daily tasks for the caregiver, and certainly the loved one. That is why a proper bathroom is extremely important for at-home care. I had the fortune and the ability to transform a small room and create a completely new large bathroom addition, exclusively for my Mother's needs. Perhaps you can slightly adjust an existing bathroom to accommodate some of the needed bath requirements.

THE BATHROOM SHOULD BE SPACIOUS ENOUGH, TO COMFORTABLY ACCOMMODATE THREE PEOPLE: YOUR LOVED ONE, YOURSELF AND AN ADDITIONAL CAREGIVER OR HELPER.

THE BATHROOM WILL REQUIRE A WIDE ENTRY DOOR FOR EASY WHEEL CHAIR ACCESS.

More often than not, there will be only your loved one and yourself, or one assisting caregiver or helper, but under certain circumstances the care may require the help of two additional people. A spacious bathroom makes everything much easier, safer and more comfortable. If you cannot provide that ideal setting, make sure there is plenty of room to easily access the shower and toilet. You will need to be able to smoothly transfer your loved one from shower chair to the toilet and back to the wheelchair. A bathtub is not ideal for your situation, unless it is a walk-in tub, however, I do not recommend it for bathing. You need to be hands-on present and holding onto your loved one in the bathroom at all times. A window for easy airing of the bathroom would be preferred and ideal.

SHOWER

I recommend an open corner walk-in shower with no curb, flat floor and slightly inclined floor surface towards the middle of the centered shower drain, for proper drainage. Any good tile installing professional can do that for you. If you have a regular shower with a small elevated tile rim, you might consider taking the rim down, and adjusting the floor. Why? This way you can roll the shower chair straight into the shower. It will make care incredibly easier, especially with all the chair transfers that await.

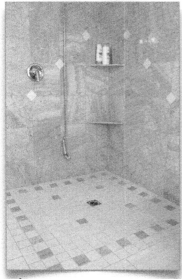

AN OPEN SHOWER WITH
SLANTED FLOOR

If this is not possible, a corner pre-fabricated shower may work, but you will need a shower chair in the shower. This will require a transfer of loved one from the portable rolling shower chair onto fixed shower chair in shower. This is doable.

In case you have a bathtub, you will require a shower chair in the tub and will need to transfer your loved one from the rolling shower chair or wheel chair onto the shower chair in the tub. This will be a most demanding transfer. I recommend you install a few shower grab bars for additional safety. If that is not possible, you may get a suction-cup grab bar that can be easily moved and repositioned to best suit your needs.

A handheld shower with a possibility of being mounted on the wall, will provide you with more control and ease of use. It is very difficult to safely shower your loved one, if they are in an enclosed single person shower; therefore an open shower is an absolute must. If you have a large, two person enclosed shower, you may be able to make it work, but you will need a handheld shower handle. Ideally, you have no shower doors or curtains. Prepare to get drenched and wear appropriate clothing that can be easily and quickly changed.

> **A SPACIOUS SINK WITH PLENTY OF COUNTERTOP SPACE AND STORAGE,
> WILL ACCOMMODATE ALL YOUR NEEDS.
> THE BIGGER THE SINK COUNTERTOP, THE BETTER.**

You will need easy access to the toilet from all sides and a possibility of mounted rails for safety. A higher toilet is preferred, so the loved one can be easily moved on and off the toilet. I advise you to get a soft cushion for the toilet seat. Elderly people loose muscle tone and can be extremely uncomfortable seating on a cold, hard toilet seat. You would be surprised how much screaming you can eliminate just with a comfortable toilet seat.

You should also place a few additional suction-cup grab bars and hand supports that can be removed or attached at various locations, such as your sink countertop, shower wall, or next to the toilet. Have a cabinet for a large selection of towels, the required incontinence necessities and all other bathroom supplies that are needed on a daily basis. Lighting in the bathroom should be good, but not extremely bright or disturbing.

SHOWER CHAIR

One of the most challenging care-giving tasks is giving your loved one the daily shower. Here again, I cannot stress enough the importance of proper equipment. The shower chair is a very essential item for a pleasant, comfortable and safe daily bath hygiene.

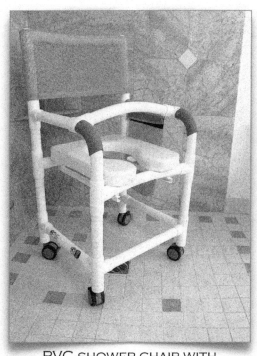

PVC SHOWER CHAIR WITH
ELONGATED OPEN SEAT
AND CLOSED SAFETY RAIL

It needs to be light but sturdy, so you can easily move it around. Avoid a chair with metal railing, as it is cold and uncomfortable to the touch. A strong plastic, waterproof, corrosion and slip resistant chair with good construction is the best option. The chair needs to be on wheels with the proper safety blockers, so that you can secure it and it won't move about, especially if your loved one is not sitting still, but fighting the shower episode. And that is usually the case.

Highly important is yet again the soft seat, so that your loved one does not suffer in pain while sitting on it. Hard plastic seats are not advisable. An open seat middle section provides the necessary easy shower handle access to the lower body, especially the groin area.

One cannot under any circumstances expect to have a fresh and clean loved one, if they are seating on a basic plastic shower bench or chair and can never really be reached for proper hygiene. Remember, an incontinent patient needs to be thoroughly washed daily!

The added possibility of a removable bucket underneath the chair, provides the extra feature for easy and accident-free transfer from bed to bath and back. During shower, you remove the bucket, as it is not needed. The feature of a handy open - close front safety rail is very important as well. It will prevent your loved one from falling out of the shower chair, which can easily happen when there is no handle present. In a split second they could come tumbling down, headfirst.

The safety rail also provides a nice handle for your loved one to hold on to. Otherwise they will be grabbing you, since they are desperate for a sense of security at all times. There is an additional low railing on the front a of the chair, where your loved one can place their feet and stay more comfortable. That way they do not have their feet on the cold bathroom floor.

The shower chair with sufficient height may also be rolled over the toilet, so that you can avoid difficult transfers from chair to toilet seat and back. Your loved one can simply remain in the shower chair, while you roll them over, when using the toilet. This multi function is very important and very helpful.

A side pocket can be useful for securing the handheld shower head, while soaping up. That way, once you have adjusted the proper water temperature, which is never easy, you will not have to continuously turn the shower on and off. Just find the ideal setting and leave the shower on until you are finished.

**A COMFORTABLE SHOWER CHAIR IS VERY ESSENTIAL.
THERE WILL BE TIMES WHERE YOU WILL HAVE TO GIVE A SHOWER
OR A LIGHT RINSE-OFF, A FEW TIMES A DAY.
YOU NEED ALL YOUR TOOLS TO BE SAFE,
PRACTICAL, EASY TO USE AND COMFORTABLE.**

The better prepared you are, the easier you will get thru these challenging times. A good shower chair will prove very valuable, since you will not be using it only in the shower. You will use it for transport in the morning from bed to the bathroom and back. Every detailed function of this chair will help you safely provide optimal hygiene care and will enable your loved one and yourself to get thru the shower and hygiene routines with ease and success.

When shopping for the best shower chair, look for these specifications:

- ❋ Built to fit standard toilet dimensions, for rolling over the toilet
- ❋ Reinforced design at all high stress points
- ❋ Fully water safe for showering and convenient cleaning
- ❋ Fast-drying removable mesh back sling
- ❋ Healthcare grade PVC
- ❋ Elongated open-front seat for comfort
- ❋ Anti-slip handgrips for added safety
- ❋ Push and pull handle built-in for easy transport
- ❋ Wheeled chair for portability
- ❋ Pocket pouch for placing shower handle during shower process
- ❋ Polymer plastics that inhibit bacteria growth

Invest into purchasing a good shower chair with all the described needed features, as it will help eliminate unnecessary discomfort while easing and shortening the daily bathing routine. Make the shower and daily body care a pleasant experience.

TOILET SEAT CUSHION

This is an added soft cushion that you can place on top of the toilet seat to assure greater comfort. It is usually secured with velcro strings. It will also help prevent your loved one from accidentally bruising or puncturing their delicate skin when using the toilet.

> **IF YOUR OPEN SEAT SHOWER CHAIR IS HIGH ENOUGH, IT CAN BE SIMPLY ROLLED OVER THE TOILET AND YOUR LOVED ONE DOES NOT NEED TO BE REMOVED FROM THE SHOWER CHAIR AT ALL.**
>
> **THIS MAKES THE PROCESS SAFER, MUCH MORE COMFORTABLE AND CONSIDERABLY EASIER FOR YOU.**

CHAPTER FIVE

Supplies and Safety

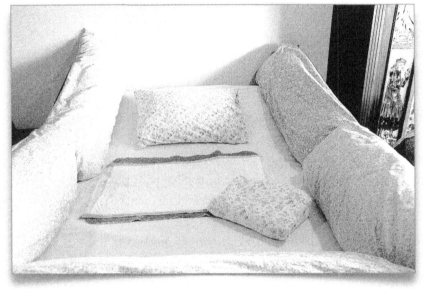

A QUEEN SIZE BED WITH BED RAILINGS,
LARGE PILLOWS TO PROTECT FROM THE EDGES,
WASHABLE INCONTINENCE BED PROTECTION PAD
AND DISPOSABLE BED PROTECTION PAD ON TOP

SUPPLIES

BEDDING

It is wise to have a good supply of extra bedding for emergency and unexpected changes.

Here is a list of minimal essential and must have's:
- 5 complete sets of sheets, pillow cases, preferably an organic cotton mix
- 1 flannel sheet and pillows cover set for colder nights
- 2 soft blankets
- 2 down comforters, in case one gets soiled or for colder nights
- 4 extra duvet - comforter covers
- 2 regular pillows
- 1 ortho pillow for head
- 4 smaller pillows for propping, various shapes
- 2 neck pressure relief pillows
- 4 very small pillows for hands
- 1 under knees half moon bolster, semi roll support pillow
- 6 extra long body pillows for safety precautions, placed at edge of bed railings
- 1 leg elevation pillow
- 1 high density memory foam leg rest for any ankle, leg, knee or hip pain
- 2 foot pillows - heel protectors, especially for final bed-bound phase

Place pillowcases on all specialty pillows for cleanliness and easy protection.

MEDICAL SHEEPSKIN

Medical sheepskin pelt is an excellent and natural way to help prevent bed sores and pressure sores by relieving the weight pressure on skin. The organic structure of wool fibers is soft and pliable, which helps the weight distribution and reduces the burden on pressure points. This is a vital point in preventing bedsores. Sheepskin also helps draw away the moisture, so the skin stays nice and dry. Sheepskin can be used on bed, chair or wheelchair. It is machine washable, so you can easily keep it clean.

INCONTINENCE SUPPLIES

If your loved one suffers from incontinence, change and wash your bedding multiple times a week and if needed, daily. Even if the bedding does not get soiled, I advise you to do that, as you will avoid bacteria and any lingering bad smells from permeating the room.

You will need at the minimum:

- ✻ A constant supply of disposable paper incontinence pads, to place atop the washable cloth bed-pads, they protect the bed and sitting surfaces from bodily fluids and are tossed after use
- ✻ 6 smaller leak preventable - waterproof washable bed pads (see photo below)
- ✻ 2 large size fitted sheets - leak preventable waterproof and washable

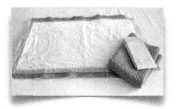

Read the Chapter *Incontinence Care* for details.

PROTECTING THE BED

In order to properly protect the bed, follow this order:

- ✻ Place the large, fitted, leak-preventable, waterproof, washable bed pad directly onto the mattress.
- ✻ Place the fitted cotton sheet on top of that.
- ✻ Place the smaller leak preventable washable pad in the center of the bed, where your loved one is lying - mid-torso.
- ✻ Place the self - adhesive paper disposable pad directly on top of that.

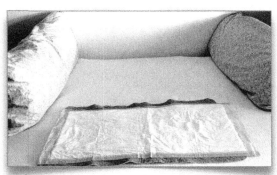

A GOOD SYSTEM TO HELP PROTECT THE BEDDING IS ESSENTIAL

Now the bed is properly prepared and protected. When changing the loved one, replace the paper disposable pad if needed. Freshly prepare the bed for each evening by changing the smaller pad on the fitted sheet and the paper disposable pad. In case your loved one is bed bound, change the sheets at least every other day. Change the smaller protection pad and disposable pad whenever there is a mishap or always at least once a day.

EATING SUPPLIES

When your loved one is eating, they will require a bib.

Have at least six washable bibs.

In order to prepare food, you will require a good quality blender.

BATHROOM SUPPLIES

In order to be organized and prepared for every possible situation or numerous bathroom visits a day, you need a good selection of various bathroom supplies. Proper organization will always be incredibly helpful.

Here is a minimal suggested list of towels you need:
* 4 extra large towels
* 10 regular towels
* 4 medium towels for the floor
* 20 washcloths for body
* 15 washcloths for face - use different color or pattern from body washcloths
* 4 non-slip bath mats - washable

BASIC TOILETRIES:
* Mild body soap - baby
* Mild hair shampoo and conditioner
* Gentle facial cream
* Deodorant, natural Crystal - Aluminum Free
* Natural lip balm
* Body lotion - hypo allergenic for dry skin
* Special rinse free soap
* Special bed - sore prevention healing cream
* Organic hand soap
* Hand disinfectant
* Organic hand cream
* Natural apple cider vinegar for foot bath
* Toothbrush and toothpaste if necessary
* Cotton Q-tips
* Nail clippers for toenails
* Nail scissors and nail files
* Soft hairbrush & comb
* Hair bands
* Hair dryer
* Kleenex
* Vaseline
* Organic aromatherapy spray

SAFETY

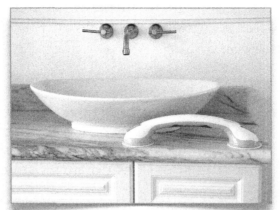

SUCTION SAFETY HANDLES ARE AN EASY
WAY TO OFFER ADDITIONAL SUPPORT

*K*eeping my Mom safe was always my primary concern. She used to be a very active individual and had a lot of physical strength. Almost as tall as myself, she was still about 5'7" at her age. She could topple over any tiny caregiver in a heartbeat. If she did not like something, she could make it fly across the room. Nobody could push her around, even while she was at her most vulnerable.

It was as is she was well aware of how her mind ailment betrayed her, despite her resilient natural inner strength and acute awareness. It upset her greatly. But if I spoke to her gently and clearly, while explaining to her how to help me transfer her from chair to bed, she would always do her best to help.

The bed was her safe haven. We completely surrounded her queen size bed with removable safety bars and added extra long body pillows on all sides. That way, even if she wanted to move about, she was protected by soft pillows. It provided great comfort and safety. She was at times very active or restless, but never ever fell out of bed or chair. And she looked super comfortable. That made me feel better as well.

Tucking her in each night and giving her a good night kiss made me happy. Despite the fact, that I was going to do a night change and see her again in a few short hours, we always did our good night routine. It was almost as if I became her Mother. That's what she used to do with me when I was little. She made me feel so safe and protected. Now it was my turn to return the love and offer her the same protection and gentle care. She seemed very content and peaceful.

Safety is without a doubt a major concern with your loved one. Again, may I remind you, that in this book we are only describing the late stage Alzheimer's dementia patient circumstances. For early stage dementia, the subject of safety would require a book of its own. However, for patient that is bed-bound and chair bound, there are other safety precautions that are equally important and necessary.

> **UNDER NO CIRCUMSTANCES**
> **SHOULD YOU LEAVE YOUR LOVED ONE ALONE**
> **WHILE UNPROTECTED, UNATTENDED,**
> **OR IN ANY WAY VULNERABLE TO A FALL OR INJURY.**
> **THE CONSEQUENCES COULD BE SEVERE.**

Guard them and protect them and prevent all falls and mishaps by remaining present, alert, attentive and observant. They can be left alone when they are safely tucked into their bed, with safety rails and pillows to assure comfort and security. They cannot be left unattended in a recliner for too long, unless they are taking a nap, which they may do quite often.

> **ALWAYS KEEP A WATCHFUL EYE ON YOUR LOVED ONE.**
> **BE PRESENT WHENEVER THEY ARE ALERT**
> **AND TAKE ADVANTAGE OF EVERY PRECIOUS MINUTE**
> **WHEN THEY ARE AWARE AND COMMUNICATIVE,**
> **EVEN IN THE SMALLEST OF WAYS.**
> **THOSE MOMENTS ARE A GIFT.**

The first challenge presents itself in the morning when you are getting your loved one out of bed. As I mention in the incontinence chapter, you need to be strong and versatile when lifting your loved one out of bed, especially first thing in the morning. Make sure you stretch and do a few gentle exercises, to properly prepare your body before lifting your loved one.

SAFE DISTANCE

If your loved one is very restless and kicks about, do not be surprised if they will reach for the free standing food-tray on wheels, that may be too close to them. You may find yourself cleaning food off the walls, carpet and various places where food does not belong. Be mindful of whatever objects are within their reach and make sure there are no safety concerns.

BED RAILINGS

When your loved one is placed in bed at nighttime, I strongly suggest you provide removable safety bed railings. You will place them on both sides of the bed as well as at the end of the bed near the loved one's feet. This railing is a special piece of light-weight equipment that is gently tucked under the mattress, between that mattress and bed-platform, or box spring. The railing helps prevent any falls, so you can rest assured that the loved one will not fall out of bed at night. If you have a nursing care bed, the railings may be included.

IMPORTANT: Bed railing should be always used with long body pillows to prevent any possible entrapment.

If you do not wish to use the bed railings, you must use roll guards or foam bumpers. Another option is to lower the bed and use concave mattresses. You must prevent the danger of loved one falling out fo bed or getting trapped in a bare railing. Huge soft long body pillows are an excellent option to assure safety from falling or entrapment.

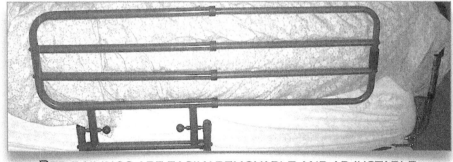

BED RAILINGS ARE EASILY REMOVABLE AND ADJUSTABLE

LONG BODY PILLOWS

Place long body pillows between your loved one and the bed railing, to assure maximum comfort and safety. Create a soft protective wall and prevent your loved one from getting caught in the bed-rail. You can also use them to help relieve pressure points, and help position loved on into a side sleeping position, which is the healthiest.

SMALL PROTECTIVE CUSHIONS

When your loved one is sitting in the recliner, they need to be properly protected with cushions, which will help prevent them from falling or sliding off. When the chair is reclined back so that her legs are stretched, it is pretty difficult to fall off. However, it depends on the mobility, behavior and stage of illness your loved one is in. In the late stage, they are mostly passive and will not have a desire to get up or out of the chair.

NON-SLIP BATH MATS

The bathroom should have a good supply of washable non-slip bathmats. In addition, you will need at least two rubber bathmats for the shower area.

BATHROOM GRAB BARS

They are very useful and can be placed vertically, horizontally or diagonally, depending on your needs. Provide a few round suction safety handles in the bathroom. They are really practical and better yet, they can be moved around as needed for your use. However, in late stage of illness your loved one will not be able to use them very much.

GRAB BARS FOR TOILETS

These are very helpful when transferring loved one from wheelchair or shower chair to the toilet seat and back, to the wheelchair or shower chair. They can be useful when sitting down, or rising from a seated position on the toilet. However, in late stage of illness your loved one will not be able to use them for getting up and down, but will lean on them for safety and to help prevent slipping off the toilet seat.

DUAL CONTROL LUMBAR SACRAL BODY SUPPORT BELT

You need to make sure that you protect your back and need the belt for added support and stability to your lower spine when lifting loved one or engaging in straining activities.

NON-SKID SHOWER SHOES

To eliminate worry about slipping and falling, wear most comfortable shoes that are slip-resistant.

ROOM MONITOR

There is a wide variety of wireless baby monitors or room monitoring devices that you can easily purchase. Some of the features include video, audio and intercom.

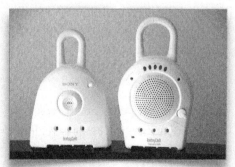

A ROOM MONITOR IS ESSENTIAL FOR NIGHTTIME SUPERVISION

There are also Wireless Caregiver Pager Call Button Nurse Alert Systems that facilitate your loved one pushing a button for your help, however, in late stage of dementia your loved one will not be able to use it. A simple baby room monitor is sufficient and will help you hear every sound they make during the day or night, so you can be immediately at their side, should they wake up and need you.

WHEELCHAIRS, WALKERS AND LIFTS

WALKER

This is another very useful tool that will prove very beneficial. It will help your loved one support themselves when walking or standing. In late stage of illness you may only be needing it to help your loved one support themselves when standing, while you are changing their incontinence pad. A walker is useful only in situation when your loved one is still able to stand up. In the final stage of the illness, when your loved one is very limited with body movement and ability to walk, I would not recommend it. There are a few different versions of a walker, a simple one with only four legs, a version with two wheels attached to the front legs, and a rollator model that has wheels attached to all four legs. I do not recommend this device in late stage of illness.

WHEELCHAIR

You will need a good quality wheelchair, even if your loved one spends most of the time in recliner or bed. Wheelchair can be used for any needed transport, when transferring, taking your loved one outdoors or even daily moving about the home and your loved one's room. I recommend a good quality, user friendly, lightweight and foldable wheelchair, that can be easily stored in the trunk of your car.

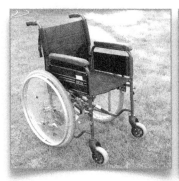 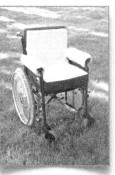 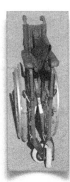

MAKE SURE YOUR WHEELCHAIR IS FOLDABLE, AND WILL FIT THROUGH ALL THE DOORWAYS OF YOUR HOME.

ADD SHEEPSKIN SEAT COVER FOR EXTRA COMFORT.

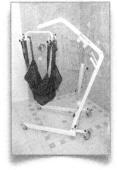

TOTAL BODY LIFT

If you have professional caregivers, they may find it easier to transfer your loved one from bed to chair with the help of a lift. Personally, I find it cumbersome and the edge of the sling that holds your loved one, can be too harsh for their sensitive and fragile skin. Total body lift is operated by either hydraulic-manual pumping or electric motor.

HOYER TOTAL BODY LIFT

CLOTHING

When my Mother became ill, I bought an all new wardrobe for her. None of her previous clothes were appropriate. She needed to be comfortable and wear only the healthiest most breathable fabric, such as cotton. Dresses and skirts or complicated blouses with a thousand buttons were out. Turtlenecks or fancy clothes were impractical, since she needed optimal comfort and ease of getting dressed.

Choosing her daily wardrobe was always my task, even when we had daytime caregivers. They repeatedly wanted to dress her according to their needs. If they felt hot, they chose short sleeves for her, regardless of the actual temperature. If they felt cold, they wanted to dress her in warm clothing. They did not take into consideration how she felt, but how they felt.

And she always felt differently than they did. Why? She was not very active and they were. They got hot, but she stayed cool and maybe even required a blanket. Or she got hot, but they stayed cool by having a cool drink.

As a caregiver of someone who cannot fend for themselves, you need to learn to expand your observation abilities. That is why I made the decision to supervise and choose Mom's outfit for the day. It was just too tiring to explain every day the same lesson.

Funny thing is, that people assume everybody dresses like they do. When they attempted to dress Mom into a sweatshirt without any undergarment, I was puzzled. The most ridiculous situation transpired when I found a caregiver actually wearing my Mom's summer shorts and her favorite sunhat, while my Mom sat in the hot sun without a hat!

As I felt my temperature rise, I approached the caregiver asking what was she thinking? Obviously she wasn't. When a few days later I found the same caregiver taking a lengthy nap on my Mom's comfy bed, while my Mom sat in the recliner unattended and alone, the caregiver was let go.

And then there is the almost unavoidable occasion when a caregiver tosses a delicate lambs wool blanket into the hot cycle of the washing machine. My Mom's favorite blanket emerged from the dryer the size of a postage stamp. Now my dog has it on his bed.

Healthy comfort is the rule. You may have to let go of the usual old clothing that your loved one was wearing. Making sure that they are comfortable is the ruling criteria and norm. Nice, fresh and clean smelling clothing makes everyone feel better. Pick pleasant colors, cheerful patterns and never use skirts or pants with tight belts, buttons or waistbands.

> **COTTON AND BREATHABLE, SOFT NATURAL AND ORGANIC FABRICS THAT GIVE A COZY AND COMFORTING FEELING WILL MAKE A BIG DIFFERENCE.**

If your loved one spends most of the day in the recliner, they will not need shoes, but just cotton socks that aren't too tight where they could impede the circulation. Socks should be changed daily. Everything your loved one wears should be washed after daily use unless it is a special unsoiled sweater or knitwear. When your loved one has incontinence, always wash their lounging sweatpants daily, even if they are unsoiled and seem clean. This way you will avoid any possibility of a bad smell. Incontinence must be managed with extra cleanliness.

DAYTIME WARDROBE

Long and short-sleeved cotton blend tee shirts with loose wide arms and broad open neckline will considerably ease the dressing challenge each day. All upper clothing such as tee shirts, sweaters and sweatshirts need to have a wide neck and sleeves. Make sure they are stretchy and a bit larger in size. Cardigan's also need to be stretchy and wide sleeved.

I suggest you have a comfortable supply of clothing for a one week uninterrupted changing routine. That means that if for some reason you cannot manage do to a set of laundry one day, you still have plenty to wear. Keep in mind that very often there is a soiling mishap and the loved one needs to be changed more times in one day. This is why you need that extra set. You need at least seven complete top to bottom outfits that will be washed once a week if you change your loved one's wardrobe each day only once.

The more you have, the less stress you will have with mishaps. Sweat suits and lounge wear that is soft, stretchy and loosely fitted will prove most comfortable and practical. If your loved one wishes to dress up and wear a skirt or a dress, use the same criteria. A cotton undergarment and variety of different tops matching with skirt or sweats can make it work.

NIGHTTIME WARDROBE

If your loved one is very restless during the night or is trying to remove or rearrange their incontinence pad, you need to get specialty clothing - a special nighttime full body pajamas. They close with a zipper that goes from the ankle of one leg all the way up and down the other leg to the other ankle. That way the loved one can be easily changed at night with simple unzipping. The zipper will prevent them from attempting to remove the pad, undress and have a mishap with the pad.

Once your loved one sleeps more peacefully or is bed-bound, I recommend a loose cotton nightgown or long nightshirt. Make sure the nightgown is not too long, but knee high. You need maximum comfort and practicality. When you do the changes at night, the short nightgown or nightshirt will be easy to handle or replace if needed. In the late stage of illness, the nightgown should have an open back for easy change. You can simply cut a regular nightgown in a straight line in the back, and create an open back nightgown, or purchase it online from an adaptive apparel store.

OUTDOOR WEAR

Depending on where you live, you will obviously adjust to various seasons. If it is possible, take your loved one outside, so they can enjoy some fresh air. In summer, you will need appropriate sunscreen, sun hat and light cotton blanket to cover them, if they take a nap in the shade. If you take them out in winter or live in colder climate, the stroll outside should be short, if at all advisable. Protect them against any wind or getting a chill. You will need a big coat that's easy to manage, warm shoes or furry boots, hat and gloves. Since they will be sitting in a wheelchair, they will feel colder than you, who are walking and pushing the wheelchair. No matter what climate you live in, provide plenty of fresh air and sufficient sunshine for them. Never leave them outside unattended, even while taking a nap.

LAUNDRY

There will be most likely one or two sets of laundry to do every day. One set of bedding and bath towels and the other set of soiled clothing. You will need a reliable washer and dryer. Always use mild detergent to avoid any allergies. Use the high temperature setting. Once a month, add white vinegar and baking soda to your wash in order to help preserve the freshness and keep everything smelling nice a clean. Have two laundry baskets for easy management of soiled and freshly cleaned sets.

IN CASE OF AN EXTENSIVE BOWEL INCONTINENCE MISHAP, TOSS AWAY ALL THE CLOTHING OR BEDDING THAT IS VERY BADLY SOILED.

CHAPTER SIX

Doctor Care and Home Visits

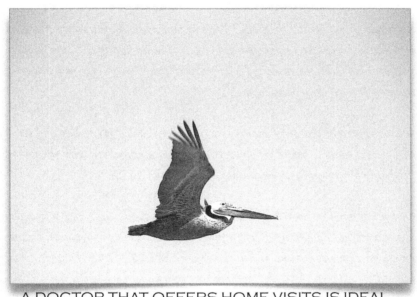

A DOCTOR THAT OFFERS HOME VISITS IS IDEAL

I had the fortune to find wonderful physicians for my Mother wherever we went. But it wasn't easy, I had to search high and low, as they say. Mom's doctors turned out to be my supporting rock, ever reliable and kind. They came to our home, so my Mother could stay comfortable in her own environment.

The family physician was a gentle and patient expert in her field of geriatric medicine, who devoted generous time and advice whenever I called on her. I feel truly fortunate to have had her stand by my Dad and I while my Mother's journey took her final turn.

The specialist, geriatric psychiatrist Dr. Daniel Plotkin that was supervising my Mother while she was living at home radiated a wonderful calm and kind heart. He studiously dedicated himself to exploring any and all possible approaches to make my Mother more comfortable. His vast knowledge and honest direct communication were of great value to me.

And what mattered to me was that both doctors also really cared about my Father and me. That was very comforting and I needed that. It helped me feel less alone and overwhelmed with the responsibility. They reminded me to think of my health, my endurance, my heart and my life.

Even though not much could be done for me at that time, just the thought that someone out there truly cared, noticed, was concerned and aware of my dedicated ever-consuming assignment, meant a lot to me. I truly felt they were my supporting team. When things were difficult, I knew I could call on them at any time and they would immediately return my call and visit in the shortest possible time.

My Mother liked them both and was relaxed and peaceful in their presence. She felt that they were an important part of the team that cared for her. I wish that everybody who cares for their loved one could have such supportive and caring physicians as I did. I urge you to go out there and search for them. It will make a great difference to your loved one and you.

FAMILY DOCTOR

If you care for your loved one in your home, it is an absolute necessity to find a family doctor that will make home visits. I know that is not always easy. Just like anything else in life, you need to make some effort and search for them. Finding a good and easily accessible doctor is essential. In this situation, where the main daily and nightly caregiving responsibility is on your shoulders, you need all the help you can get.

The more the illness progresses, any traveling and strenuous situations for your loved one where they would need to wait at the doctor's office, could prove extremely stressful for all. A seemingly innocent thing like being exposed to another patient who might have a cold or flu, could prove to be detrimental to your loved one.

INQUIRE WITH YOUR GERIATRIC CARE MANAGER, NURSING HOME, HOSPITALS AND FAMILY PHYSICIANS AND SEARCH UNTIL YOU FIND A DOCTOR THAT MAKES HOME VISITS AND SPECIALIZES IN GERIATRIC-ELDERLY PATIENTS.

There is another essential fact that will prove decisive in success of the tending physician. Unless you do your proper homework, you won't reap the optimal benefits of meeting and consulting with your expert physician in the comfort of your home.

YOU NEED TO KEEP A SUPREMELY WELL ORGANIZED LOG, WHERE EVERYTHING ABOUT YOUR LOVED ONE IS RECORDED. WHEN ANY NEW DEVELOPMENTS OCCUR THE DOCTOR WILL HAVE A TREMENDOUS ADVANTAGE OF REVIEWING ANY CHANGED CONDITIONS AND NEW SYMPTOMS. THIS WILL EXPEDITE PROPER AND EFFECTIVE DIAGNOSIS AND TREATMENT.

If you do your logging right, you will be able to figure out together with the doctor, wherein lies the possible problem that may have caused a change in the overall situation and well being of your loved one.

Keep in mind that a doctor is not God or a magician. They are a human being, just like you and I. But they are educated and equipped with vast knowledge and experience that can help prevent suffering and potentially save your loved one.

However, your observation, discipline, tenacity and dedicated care will be the essential element in maintaining your loved one in best possible condition.

Work with your doctor and together you will help your loved one feel comfortable. Open and honest communication will be of great importance. Educate yourself in any way you can about the various symptoms of this illness and the medications your loved one is taking. Read and research the possible side effects and log every observation. That will present immense help to your doctor, when making a proper and timely assessment. Ask any questions you may have, voice your doubts or fears and make an effort to understand and be involved. Inquire about any future therapy or medicine your loved one may require and could benefit from.

> **NEVER FOLLOW BLINDLY AND EXPECT ANOTHER PERSON TO BE ABLE TO READ YOUR MIND, GUESS WHAT YOU WANT AND NEED, OR WHAT YOU SIMPLY DON'T UNDERSTAND. COMMUNICATE, SPEAK UP, STAY INFORMED, BE AWARE AND RELIABLE.**

The goal here is the best situation for your loved one and nothing else. A good doctor will be happy about your informed involvement and will appreciate the help of your logging. But if you show no interest, are indifferent and carry an ignorant disposition towards your loved one's daily changes, in all honesty, you cannot expect a miracle.

One of your designated responsibilities is to be the eyes and ears for the doctor, when they are not around. Only then can you speak for your loved one. That way, you will avoid the most frustrating circumstance where your loved one may experience discomfort, but by the time the doctor arrives, suddenly all seems well. The doctor will have no information or reference point. Rest assured, that a few moments after the doctor's departure, the same discomfort could return, only for you to feel helpless when you can't help your loved one.

> **BY PROVIDING THE DOCTOR WITH YOUR SYMPTOMATIC TRACKING LOG, YOU WILL HAVE DONE AN ESSENTIAL PART IN ASSURING OPTIMAL CARE.**

A family doctor will address all of your loved one's physical issues, take blood for regular blood tests and supervise their general well being. They will prescribe general medication and unless any new situation requires more attention, they should usually visit your loved one at least once a month.

GERIATRIC PSYCHIATRIST & NEUROLOGIST

It is of great value and importance to be able to have a home visiting professional medical specialist of this kind. Alzheimer's dementia has many faces, stages and different battles. It is very beneficial to have a specialist, who can address the tremendously challenging task of adjusting the proper medication for your loved one's optimal comfort and well being.

This neurological illness is extremely challenging and affects every one in a different way. A usually wonderful, sweet person can turn into a volatile, aggressive and angry individual, who scratches, bites and yells obscenities. That is one of the ugliest faces of this illness. It is very difficult for family members to see and experience this and not be affected or take it personally.

IN THE LATER STAGES OF ILLNESS,
THE SPECIFICALLY CHALLENGING SYMPTOM
OF SEVERE AGGRAVATION OFTEN SUBSIDES,
AND A NEW CALMER PHASE SETTLES IN.

THE MAIN NEW DIFFICULTY FOR YOUR LOVED ONE
BECOMES NERVOUSNESS AND SENSORY HYPERSENSITIVITY.

You have to make an effort to understand, that it is the neurodegenerative illness and not the actual person you are dealing with at this point. The specialist will be able to asses what can be done to ease this awful state.

Proper medicine can be a real lifesaver. But yet again, I remind you that the log you keep about your loved one is of massive importance. It can very well be that your loved one is experiencing maddening nervousness or is yelling for no apparent reason, but yet when the doctor visits the person turns into the sweetest, calmest and easiest patient imaginable.

Little help will it be for you to resign and say: " Well, I guess they are feeling better now," only to experience the same agonizing spell a few hours after your doctor leaves. But when you provide the doctor with the detailed log notes of ongoing events, behavior patterns, challenging situations, nervous states, appetite and cravings, digestive issues, food intake, elimination and sleeping pattern, the doctor can with his knowledge and experience much easier and faster uncover the root of a reoccurring issue or problem.

In addition, you log will keep track of all reactions, response and effectiveness to the prescribed medication, which will help your physician asses if and what dosage of medicine works best, and at what particular time increments. By staying informed and educated, you will be able to work together with the medical specialist to manage the occasional temper, nervousness or any possible adverse reactions to the medicine. I cannot convey to you enough, how important your involvement in this process is.

If you are persistent and fortunate to find an excellent doctor like I did, count your lucky stars. With the help of your tediously kept log, they will be able to easily adjust and fine-tune the medication to such a degree, that it will make a tremendous difference in your loved one's life as well as yours.

ALWAYS STRIVE FOR MINIMAL MEDICATION OR POSSIBLY NONE.

**MASSIVE DOSES OF VARIOUS PRESCRIPTIONS
MAY CAUSE NUMEROUS ADVERSE EFFECTS
THAT NEED TO BE CONTINUOUSLY REMEDIED
AND CAN OVERWHELM THE DELICATE BALANCE IN THE BODY.**

AVOID OVERMEDICATING YOUR LOVED ONE AT ALL COST.

If the magic formula of keeping your loved one peacefully asleep through the night is discovered, it will save your life. And your life needs to be saved, because without you, who will take care of them?

By having wonderful and informative conversations with your doctor, you will be able to prevent or manage a probable middle-of-the-night anxiety attack your loved one may suffer from. You need to know what to do in every possible situation. Your doctor will help you prepare, so that you can act swiftly and immediately find a solution. Knowledge is the power that will help your get thru the most challenging of times.

EXCEPTIONS

If your loved one suffers from additional illnesses and symptoms, you will need to address them with proper specialists. If you need to bring your loved one occasionally to a very specific doctor who cannot make a home visit, make sure that it makes sense and is not an unnecessary stress on their overall state.

Do not exhaust your loved one with random tests when not necessary. Always consult your family doctor to help determine whether the suggested tests are truly necessary and in your loved one's best interest. Be selective and objective.

> **IT DOES NOT MEAN THAT IF
> YOU CONTINUOUSLY DRAG YOUR AILING LOVED ONE
> TO EVERY POSSIBLE MEDICAL TEST,
> YOU ARE A BETTER CAREGIVER.**

If the doctor truly believes the test or examination at the specialist or in the hospital is necessary and will make a decisive difference in your loved one's overall state, then by all means do it. But do not insist on it to make yourself feel better or to appease a nagging relative who thinks you could be doing more and better in your caregiving efforts. No matter what the side drama is, never forget who is the priority thru this journey. Always and only your loved one.

PREPARING FOR THE DOCTOR'S HOME VISIT

Your loved one should always be is a sufficiently well maintained state, so that no matter what day or hour the doctor shows up, everything is presentable and ready.

> **OPTIMAL CARE FOR YOUR LOVED ONE MEANS
> THAT THEY ARE ALWAYS CLEAN, COMFORTABLY DRESSED,
> AS CONTENT AS POSSIBLE UNDER THE CIRCUMSTANCES,
> PROPERLY FED AND HYDRATED,
> FEELING COZY AND PEACEFUL
> IN A WELL MAINTAINED ENVIRONMENT.
> THEIR ROOM NEEDS TO BE AIRED OUT, CLEAN AND FRESH AT ALL TIMES.**

Keep in mind that you will adapt yourself and your schedule according to your loved one's overall daily state. One of the important facts to remember is that the illness could sometimes create sudden unexpected changes, so it will become impossible to plan ahead with absolute certainty. If you always shower your loved one at 10 AM, there might come a time when that is not going to work for them anymore. They might be too sleepy and will be more comfortable with an afternoon shower time.

The luxury of having your loved one at home is that you are under no one else's schedule, but can adjust it at a moments notice, always according to your loved one's needs, wishes and preferences. That means that if your doctor is planning to visit in the morning and your loved one is too sleepy and bedridden, you will not be dragging them out of bed for a shower, just because of the doctors visit.

YOU HAVE TO RELAX YOUR SET SCHEDULE ACCORDING TO YOUR LOVED ONE'S NEEDS.

Your loved one certainly needs to be clean and dry, but not necessarily showered and all dressed up at that particular time. If you care for them well, they will be always presentable.

Once the illness reaches the last phase, your days will revolve around your loved one's momentary state. In short, keep in mind the optimal comfort of your loved one and do not compromise that for anything or anyone. A good doctor will understand that approach and encourage it as well.

HOW TO ADMINISTER MEDICATION

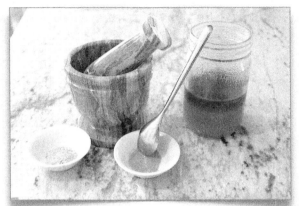

MAKE TAKING MEDICINE PLEASANT AND SWIFT

This can be a very challenging endeavor. It is very often the case, that when a loved one is in a nursing facility, the medicine intake is skipped. Why? Because dementia patients are rarely fond of taking medicine. So they rebel or put up a fight. They get aggressive with the caregivers, attempt to spit the medication out of their mouth and make some other effort to fight against it.

The nursing staff usually prepares the entire day's worth of medicine as scheduled for intake, for the whole list of patients. The specially marked pill containers help the staff keep track and regular schedule for timely medicine intake. When a patient spits a pill out, there is no other pill prepared for that day and that hour. So the medicine was officially given to them, yet, since they spat it out, they did not actually ingest it. That creates a major disruption in properly observing and delivering the prescribed dosage. It is difficult to assess the positive or negative impact of the medicine, when the intake has gaps and irregularities. One of the positive aspect of caring for a loved one at home is that you can personally make sure, that the medicine intake works and is successful.

I never trusted a caregiver with medicine intake for my Mother. Why? Because I knew very well her rebellious spirit and dislike of medications. So I personally made sure she took it regularly and was never overmedicated. The majority of elderly in facilities are without a doubt severely overmedicated or not taking the prescribed dosage. That can be entirely prevented when your loved one is at home and you are the responsible party. Work with your doctor to minimize the dosage, and then find the proper method to effectively deliver the medicine. You have the time, whereas the caregivers in facilities simply don't.

If you manage to eliminate the physical discomfort, due to any number of practical and easily eliminated causes, there is a good chance the strong anxiety medication or sedative, can be brought to a bare minimum. Remember, all medications do have side effects and very often these can be quite challenging. Apart from necessary medication for preexisting conditions such as blood pressure, heart, thyroid or any number of other ailments besides dementia, the anxiety medication can eventually be reduced and very possibly entirely eliminated.

A person suffering from dementia goes thru various stages and when they are in the mid-stage of illness, agitation is common, therefore you have no choice but to provide them with a calming medication, so that the anxiety subsides. But in later stage, while under your close and careful observation, the physician may feel comfortable to eliminate it entirely or suggest to use it only on as-needed basis.

Keep a log of everything that happens regarding your loved one's condition, especially any nervous outbursts, or a general sense of discomfort. Mark the date, time and duration of the agitated state and carefully examine what occurred or was different on that particular day and time, that might have added to their hypersensitivity. Was it a change in diet, a different caregiver, weather fluctuation, a temperature shift, different clothing that may feel uncomfortable? There is a long list of possible causes for discomfort and in order to truly understand what is the underlying reason, you need to have time and tremendous patience to research and find out the source of discomfort. See chapter *The Mind - Communication.*

Nobody enjoys taking medicine. Elderly can get especially set against it. Even if it is just a stubborn whim, they are not interested in taking medication. Instead of suffering through a long and nerve wrenching ordeal, you can completely eliminate this challenge and transform it into a seamlessly quick ritual.

Mortar and pestle are beautiful ancient tools used to crush, grind, and mix solid substances, usually herbs or medicine. They have been used in pharmacies for centuries. It is a most practical tool when you need to grind hard pills. Make sure the mortar cup is clean, dry and smooth. Place the pill inside and grind it into powder. Empty it carefully into a small pinch bowl or condiment cup, which is specifically designed to hold a single ingredient or condiment.

USE ONLY ONE THIRD OF A TEA SPOON - A SMALL SCOOP OF AN INGREDIENT SUCH AS HONEY, PEANUT BUTTER, JAM, SUGARLESS JELLO OR APPLE SAUCE. ADD IT TO THE CRUSHED PILL AND MIX IT INTO A SMOOTH PASTE. AS SIMPLE AS THAT!

If the pill is in capsule, open it up and blend it with chosen teaspoon of food. If you need to prepare a few different medicines, you should always crush each medicine separately and place onto a separate condiment cup. This way you can keep track of which medicine you successfully administered. Mixing each single medicine with your loved one's favorite food will accomplish two objectives: it will make a possibly bitter medicine taste better and its thick, sticky substance will help prevent it from being easily spat out. If your loved one suffers from diabetes use any good tasting and smooth sugar-free food.

Be honest and tell your loved one that this medication is needed, so that they will feel more comfortable. Sneaking and tricking a loved one into taking medicine will only make them more suspicious and angry. Treat them with respect and tell them you understand they may not like it, but it will taste fine and will help them feel better and less irritable. Tell them you understand that it is annoying and they dislike it, but you love them and want only the best for them. Always keep a precise log about all the medicine intake.

ADJUSTING MEDICATION

Your loved one's doctor may also provide you with an option of medication to be taken on as-needed basis, so you may use it only when and if continuous nervousness and escalated agitation or pain persists. Always communicate with your loved one and ask them how they feel. Even if their communication has diminished considerably, it is very probable that they can still answer with a Yes or No. Keep the communication going for as long as possible. I cannot express enough how crucial that is.

NEVER ALLOW A CAREGIVER TO DECIDE OR ADJUST YOUR LOVED ONE'S MEDICINE. YOU ARE SOLELY RESPONSIBLE FOR YOUR LOVED ONE. AN INCORRECT CHANGE COULD BE DETRIMENTAL TO THEIR HEALTH.

MEDICINE TAKEN ON AS - NEEDED BASIS SHOULD BE ADMINISTERED ONLY BY YOU WITH THE DOCTOR'S PERMISSION.

KEEPING A DAILY LOG

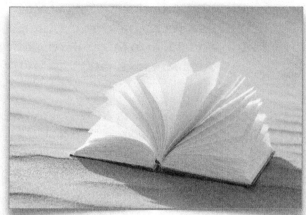

A WELL ORGANIZED CARE - TRACKING SYSTEM IS OF GREAT HELP

You may think that your daily caregiving routine and various tasks are always the same, not of great importance and that you will easily remember any changes. Let me assure you that it is impossible to keep track of everything in your head. A small seemingly meaningless detail such as a change in daily bowel movement, may be the cause of your loved one feeling unwell.

Your organized and clear daily notes are the key in assessing and maintaining your loved one's optimal well-being. You will need to implement an easy, very well catalogued tracking system. Logging various aspects of physical condition, mental disposition, daily developments and routines, plays a major role in understanding how your loved one feels, what agrees with them and what disturbs them.

You will be able to detect certain patterns and find some predictability in various fluctuations that occur. I know it may seem like additional work to keep a daily log considering your already overwhelming responsibilities, but I cannot stress enough how important this is. The notes will greatly help the doctor asses any possible problems that arise.

I STRONGLY SUGGEST YOU SET ASIDE FIVE MINUTES A DAY
TO MAKE THESE VERY VALUABLE NOTES
AND DOCUMENT ALL ONGOING AND ESSENTIAL INFORMATION.

YOUR LOGS WILL BE INVALUABLE.

MEDICATION LOG
DATE BEGINS: _____

DATE	TIME	MEDICATION	DOSAGE	NOTES

This very important log is for keeping precise track of daily medicine intake. If you need to administer the medication in the morning and at various times of the day, log the dosage each time right away and do not wait until the end of the day. This log is especially important for medication that is taken on an as-needed basis. In such case, write down the time, dosage and name of medication. Note if you noticed any improvement. Always immediately consult your physician when unusual reactions or changes occur.

CAREGIVING DAILY CHECKLIST
DATE BEGINS: _____

BASICS	MON.	TUE.	WED.	THU.	FRI.	SAT.	SUN.	
MEDICATION								
VITAMINS								
REMEDIES NEEDED								
MEALS								
SHOWER								
HAIR WASH - MIN. 1 X WEEK								
SKINCARE DAILY LOTION								
BED - PAD CHANGE								
NIGHT SLEEP PATTERN								
EXTRAS								
HAND & FOOT MASSAGE								
MOVEMENT MIN. 3 X WEEK								
MUSIC / MOVIE								
MOOD - TALK ACTIVITIES								
UPKEEP								
LAUNDRY DAILY								
ORDER SUPPLIES								
CLEAN ROOM 1 X WEEK								
NOTES								

This is a sample of empty daily checklist. This list will help you keep a great general oversight of all your daily duties. This is ideal for a basic oversight. For detailed tracking regarding other specifics, you can use specified logs.

CAREGIVING DAILY CHECKLIST
DATE BEGINS: FEB 9 - FEB 15

BASICS	MON.	TUE.	WED.	THU.	FRI.	SAT.	SUN.	
MEDICATION	✓	✓	✓	✓	✓	✓	✓	
VITAMINS	✓	✓	✓	✓	✓	✓	✓	
REMEDIES NEEDED	EXTRA PLUMS			EXTRA PLUMS	P. FLOWER DROPS FOR CALMING	EXTRA PLUMS		
MEALS	✓	✓	✓	✓	✓	✓	✓	
SHOWER	✓		✓		✓		✓	
HAIR WASH- MIN. 1 X WEEK						✓		
SKINCARE DAILY LOTION	✓	✓	✓	✓	✓	✓	✓	
BED - PAD CHANGE	✓	✓	✓	✓	✓	✓	✓	
NIGHT SLEEP PATTERN	3 -3.15AM AWAKE	FINE	RESTLESS	FINE	4:30 - 5AM AWAKE	AWAKE BUT CALM	FINE	
EXTRAS								
HAND & FOOT MASSAGE		✓		✓			✓	
MOVEMENT MIN. 3 X WEEK	✓		✓			✓		
MUSIC / MOVIE	MOVIE		MUSIC	MUSIC			MOVIE	
MOOD - TALK ACTIVITIES	TALK, WALK	QUIET & NAPPING	TALKING RESTING	NAPPING	AGITATED IN AM, PM BETTER	QUIET CALM	TALK, WALK	
UPKEEP								
LAUNDRY DAILY	✓	✓	✓	✓	✓	✓	✓	
ORDER SUPPLIES	✓							
CLEAN ROOM 1X WEEK					✓			
NOTES	GOOD DAY	QUIET DAY	ACTIVE DAY	QUIET DAY	HARD DAY	QUIET DAY	GOOD DAY	

This is an example of a filled-out daily checklist. You can adjust your notes as it best suits you, but keep them clear, simple and precise.

FOOD & LIQUIDS LOG - CUPS
DATE BEGINS: _____

		BREAKFAST	LUNCH	DINER	SNACKS
MON.	FOOD				
	DRINK				
TUE.	FOOD				
	DRINK				
WED.	FOOD				
	DRINK				
THUR.	FOOD				
	DRINK				
FRI.	FOOD				
	DRINK				
SAT.	FOOD				
	DRINK				
SUN.	FOOD				
	DRINK				

In this log you will keep a precise track of the amount of food and liquids that your loved one consumed in a day. I suggest that you count the amount in cups and half-cups. Make separate notations for food and drink. Inform your doctor if there is a drastic change in appetite, diminished liquid intake or severe thirst. Any changes in appetite could signal a dramatic change in your loved one's overall state of well being.

ELIMINATION MONITORING LOG
DATE BEGINS: _____

DATE	URINE X PER DAY	BM X PER DAY	DATE	URINE X PER DAY	BM X PER DAY

In this log you will keep a precise account of daily bowel movement - BM and urine. You will be marking BM by size in: small, medium, large and extra large. Mark urine by count. Take note of any changes in elimination such as diarrhea or constipation. Inform your doctor when severe constipation or diarrhea lasts more than three days. Both cases can cause dangerous consequences. Implement a healthy diet and use natural remedies to help balance elimination fluctuations. This will make a considerable difference.

NATURAL REMEDY LOG
DATE BEGINS: _____

DATE	TIME	PROBLEM	REMEDY	DOSAGE	RESULT

This log is important for notating any remedies that are taken on a regular or as-needed basis. For example: if there are issues with constipation, you can add to the diet prunes, flaxseed or Swiss Kriss herbal laxative. These seemingly small changes and additions can play a decisive role in helping resolve an ongoing issue or balancing a persistent health challenge. Keeping track of what was effective in a specific situation is most valuable. It will help you navigate through various challenging situations in the future.

DAILY VITAMINS LOG
DATE BEGINS: _____

DATE	TIME	VITAMIN	DOSAGE	NOTES

This log is for keeping track of any supplements and vitamins that your loved one is taking as part of their daily regimen. Make a list of supplements and keep track of what and how much was taken each day. Always consult your physician before changing, adding or eliminating any supplements or altering the dosage.

BLOOD PRESSURE LOG
DATE BEGINS: _____

DATE	TIME	BP		DATE	TIME	BP

Keeping track of blood pressure is especially important if your loved one suffers from high or low blood pressure. High blood pressure may also occur as a result of patient's nervousness or aggravation. If your loved one has been taking a high blood pressure medication for a long while and suddenly has low blood pressure, it may be time for reassessing the need for that medication. Inform your doctor immediately of any changes in blood pressure. Daily readings are recommended.

WEEKLY WEIGHT LOG
DATE BEGINS: _____

DATE	WEIGHT	DATE	WEIGHT

Keeping a log on body weight is pretty easy, since you only need to check it once every two weeks. If there are any noticeable weight changes, check it every week. I suggest you have a scale and with the help of caregiver or a friend, stand your loved one on the scale for just a moment. If a dramatic change in weight occurs, inform your physician right away.

EMERGENCY INSTRUCTIONS AND CONTACTS

For everyone's safety you should always have a list of main emergency numbers, clearly posted in a most visible place. This could be on the door, closet, cabinet, mirror or refrigerator. Anywhere where the list can be clearly seen will do.

The list should include the numbers for emergency, ambulance, firemen and security. The list must also include your loved one's doctors or a nurse, geriatric care manager if you have one, and hospice nurse if applicable.

Last but not least, the list must clearly display your very own number in case you are not present at the time of emergency, as well as a few numbers of a few trusted friends or neighbors that are familiar with the situation, know your loved one and hopefully live nearby.

Chances are you may never need to call any of these numbers for an emergency, but having the numbers clearly on display will ease everyone's anxiety and make them feel more prepared.

It is also important to always have the documentation of Advanced Health care Directive that your loved one designated before they got ill. Find more information on that topic in chapter titled: *The Illness*.

CHAPTER SEVEN

Hiring Caregivers

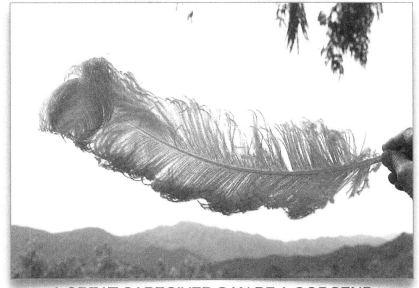

A GREAT CAREGIVER CAN BE A GODSEND

I have had my share of experiences with the caregivers. Thru the years I meet and worked with over sixty caregivers from all parts of the world. While my Mom lived with us at home, we went thru about forty of them. Why so many? That would require another book.

It was certainly not a usual caregiving experience at our house. Partially because of my background in holistic medicine and my intense involvement in my Mother's care, I was an ever watchful and demanding supervisor that didn't miss a beat. I gladly educated many of them in all sorts of techniques and approaches, but in the end, that did not offer me the relief I needed. The caregivers were getting paid to study and learn various caregiving holistic techniques from me. As long as it also benefited my Mom, that was sort of all right. But it was not ideal.

However, there are certain things that can't be taught, such as logic, fast decisive action and gentle, compassionate disposition towards the elderly. If I detected the caregiver had a natural gift and true heartfelt interest in their work, my energy investment when explaining intricate details and process made sense. But that was rare.

There were a few caregivers that were sweet people, but they were just not strong enough to handle the assignment for too long. This job can seriously burn you out, if you do not know how to protect yourself.

All this aside, I encourage you to search for that golden helper who will hopefully last you for a while and ease your journey. But remember, when your loved one is at home with you, the primary caregiver in charge that must always remain standing, no matter what upheaval is swirling around, that person is always going to be you. Prepare well and I will promise you, at the end of this journey, you will not regret it.

GETTING HELP

Even if you feel that you are a superhuman, you can benefit from having a good caregiver. Of course, like many things in life, it all depends on that challenging fact: how far does your budget reach? If there is a possibility that you can afford to hire outside help, even just once or twice a week, then by all means, get some relief. It will require a certain learning curve for you to find the best match. There are quite a few possible options, but chances are that you will need to change the caregiver every once in a while. Just as your loved one's illness will evolve, so will the level of care they require.

One fact will never change; by having your loved one live in your home, you are officially the primary caregiver. You are 100% responsible for their well-being. If you have a caregiver hired thru an agency, then that agency is liable for their caregiver's actions during the hours the caregiver is with your loved one.

> **WHEN YOU HAVE A FRIEND, RELATIVE OR PRIVATELY HIRED CAREGIVER WITH YOUR LOVED ONE, YOU ARE STILL THE LEGALLY RESPONSIBLE PARTY. THAT IS VERY IMPORTANT TO KNOW AND IS NOT TO BE TAKEN LIGHTLY.**

It means that you need to be very selective when entrusting anyone else to take care of your loved one, even if just for a few hours. You would not leave your helpless baby or a child with just anyone, would you? Well, this is equally demanding.

CAREGIVERS HIRED THROUGH AN AGENCY

There is a large selection of caregiver agencies that you can find thru Alzheimer's organization, doctor referral, nursing home, senior care manager, various newspapers, online or at medical supply store. You need to carefully review, inquire and find out anything and everything you can, about the services offered. Some agencies will make it all sound so wonderful: someone will show up ever day, cook, wash, feed, clean, go shopping, drive you anywhere and be there for you day and night. It seems like your life will become a careless dream. Of course that is not the case.

These are the facts you need to know before you decide to have your loved one in your home. If you are under the illusion that you will easily have fantastic, all-encompassing care for them, then you need to think again. At this point of your loved one's illness and the high level of care needed, you will have to tediously supervise any and all caregiving steps.

YES, A CAREGIVER CAN HELP YOU, BUT THE MAJOR RESPONSIBILITY IS ABSOLUTELY STILL ON YOU.

Agencies differ in quality level of caregivers they offer, and certainly in price. I suggest that you carefully interview a few agencies and assess their qualifications. Perhaps your loved one's primary physician may give you a good referral, but it doesn't hurt to interview a few agencies, just to make certain your expectations and your loved one's needs are met. Your communication with the agency supervisor is also very important. This will be the go-between person, interacting with you and the caregivers. They need to truly understand and be able to realistically accommodate your needs, while giving you a sense of reliability and professional assurance.

Once you have selected the agency, they will send you the caregiver they feel will best fit your overall needs. You can interview the caregiver and agree to a try-out period for a few days. This will require your full involvement while you go thru the process of familiarizing the caregiver with your loved one, their specific needs, habits, challenges and preferences. The caregiver also needs to become familiar with your home, your care supplies, your schedule and all the important details of your unique situation.

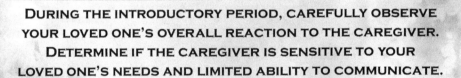

DURING THE INTRODUCTORY PERIOD, CAREFULLY OBSERVE YOUR LOVED ONE'S OVERALL REACTION TO THE CAREGIVER. DETERMINE IF THE CAREGIVER IS SENSITIVE TO YOUR LOVED ONE'S NEEDS AND LIMITED ABILITY TO COMMUNICATE.

Every detail of care needs to be assessed on your part. You need to determine how well the caregiver is dealing with all the duties and observe their behavior with your loved one.

If there is something in your caregiver's behavior or disposition towards your loved one that you do not like, immediately bring it to their attention and explain what they need to adjust. If they cannot or refuse to improve, correct and change their approach that same day, you should let them go. Inform the supervisor at the agency that you do not think this specific caregiver is a good fit for your home.

A good agency should send you a different caregiver, that is hopefully better suited for your loved one's needs. The next caregiver should come right away, on the following day. Otherwise you would be stranded alone with no caregiver and if you are not very experienced, it could be quite overwhelming.

Hopefully once a good match has been found, you may be able to keep that caregiver for a long time. When you get really good at assessing the caregivers, you will be able to know right away upon meeting them, if they are the right person for your loved one or not.

UPSIDE OF AGENCY CAREGIVER

A good agency is responsible for proper caregiver certification and education, all background checks, insurance, payroll taxes and so on. If a caregiver cancels and does not show up, the agency will usually immediately send you a replacement. Supposedly, you will never feel stranded and waiting, without help. If you want to change the set-up, add more caregivers or change to different hours, they will accommodate you. That is their job.

You will also receive the aid of a qualified senior care manager, who will help you assess the entire situation, follow your evolving challenges and assist with problem solving. You will feel that you have good backing, that will help you get thru this challenging time. Your support system will be in place, and this could be a considerable game changer.

DOWNSIDE OF AGENCY CAREGIVER

The agency will charge you 50% more of the hourly rate, than a private caregiver, who is not with an agency. The agency will pocket at least half the hourly fee. The contract you will sign with them will guarantee that you cannot ever "steal" a great caregiver, that you found thru them. I personally feel that is correct and proper, but you should be aware of this, so as not to go into any illusions of finding a great caregiver thru an agency and then stealing them away.

There is also another aspect to keep in mind: caregiving is a highly stressful job and caregivers suffer from burn out. If the level of your care is demanding, you may go thru all the caregivers in a smaller agency and in a few months or a year, they will not have anyone new to offer to you. At that point you could end up without a caregiver.

The other reality check is that the agency is obviously focusing on the most profit they can make from you. Therefore they may suggest your loved one's care level is too demanding for one caregiver. They will propose you hire two caregivers, when in fact one would suffice. By convincing you that care for your loved one is too challenging, or they are too tall, too heavy, or too difficult for one caregiver, and that they require two caregivers, the agency makes double the income.

Or perhaps they may suggest a longer working day, or an overnight caregiver. Keep in mind that they will usually encourage you hire them for more hours and additional caregivers. On some level this is understandable, since they are in business to make profit. But I find it exceptionally difficult to tolerate. If the agency starts sensing that your finances are drying out, they will quickly lose interest and be noticeably less concerned and caring about proper service for your loved one.

One more real sobering and harsh fact is, that when they see your loved one is approaching the very final stage, they know the client will be lost. At that time they really do not care much anymore. Of course you could be lucky and have an angelic agency that is an exception. But most of agencies are in it solely for the money, especially since there is much money to be made in their business.

My personal experience was such, that after a year with the agency and more than $100,000 spend for their caregivers, when my Mother began fading away, they just didn't care anymore. To them I was a tapped-out client. What happened next?

One day, without warning, their caregiver just simply did not show up, and I was left completely and utterly stranded with my dying Mother. The agency suddenly announced they had no appropriate caregiver for us, and deserted us in a heartbeat. It was a large national agency that prides itself in superior service.

Thankfully, I immediately called on hospice service, which helped, but they offered only a one hour daily visit. For the ongoing 24/7 caregiving, I was left completely alone. At that point, finding a new agency and training a new caregiver for the final, delicate stage of my Mother's care was not a good option. I chose to watch over my darling Mother myself, with daily short visits from a very kind hospice nurse.

My advice to you is to be aware that you are an interesting client to the agency, if it appears that you have the means, and a patient that will be around for a while. Life's reality truly is harsh, especially when it comes to strictly profit making from elder care.

CHANGING LEVEL OF CARE

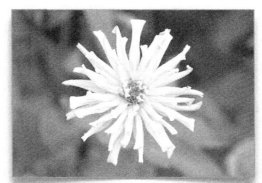

PRIVATE CAREGIVERS

You also have the option to hire a caregiver on your own. You could use a caregiver registry which you can usually find online. There will be a small charge just to use the registry. In addition, you can post with them your add for caregivers and list exactly what kind of caregiver you need. The good thing is that the registry will check the potential caregiver's references, but since you are the direct employer, you need to check their proper education, and address the payroll and state taxes.

> **WHETHER YOU HIRE A CAREGIVER THRU A REGISTRY OR ON YOUR OWN, YOU WILL NEED TO PERFORM A THOROUGH CHECK OF THEIR REFERENCES, ORDER CRIMINAL BACKGROUND CHECK AND INQUIRE ABOUT THEIR QUALIFICATIONS, TRAINING AND CERTIFICATION.**

Since you are the employer, you need to negotiate the pay rate, pay state tax and federal payroll. In addition, it is absolutely advisable to obtain workers compensation insurance. This is just the technical part of what you have to deal with.

UPSIDE OF PRIVATE CAREGIVERS

A private caregiver hourly rate will cost you half less than an agency caregiver. That can make a serious financial difference. You can adjust the schedule directly with the caregiver, without going thru the supervisors and various approval steps that are usually required, each time you wish to clear or adjust a simple hour switch.

DOWN SIDE OF PRIVATE CAREGIVERS

You don't really know who is in your home. Yes, you should do a background check, require a copy of credentials and referrals, but still nobody is guaranteeing you anything. A seemingly lovely and kind person can turn into a nightmare. If they decide to cancel on you, they owe you nothing. So you could be suddenly left empty handed from one day to the next without an explanation or a lame: "I need a break." That is not something you want to hear when you are paying them and not getting a break. There is nothing you can do, but start from scratch which requires time, effort and a lot of energy that you may not have.

> HIRING A CAREGIVER ON YOUR OWN, COULD POTENTIALLY LEAVE YOU STRANDED WITH NO CAREGIVER AT ANY GIVEN TIME.
> THIS CAN BE DETRIMENTALLY STRESSFUL.

You will have to buy insurance for hired help and really watch what's going on. Sudden schedule changes are usually a nightmare. Keep in mind that you will have to find, train and then coordinate at least two caregivers. This way they each have a few days off, however, you could find yourself spending hours trying to figure out how to accommodate their Sunday activities and extra dates, while nobody is paying attention to your needs.

The order of priority will look more like this: caregivers needs, your loved one's needs and at the end of the line - you - the one primary caregiver, who never gets a break and is there every single day and night. When you add to this conundrum the many duties you are obligated to as the employer, you may change your mind. The private caregivers option could quickly become overwhelming, too expensive for what it's worth, and far from an ideal solution.

24 - HOUR CARE

If your budget was limitless, you could hire caregivers generously, every day and night. However, if your loved one lives with you and sleeps through the night, do you really need someone there the entire night? Most likely not. The 24-hour care means that the caregiver is on duty and should be watching over your loved one the entire time. That means, no sleeping for them, they are supposed to be sitting next to the bed in a state of preparedness and ready for action. This is why the fee for this kind of service is considerably higher than a live - in caregiver. This kind of service could make sense in the very late stages of illness, when your loved one requires continuous monitoring and nighttime changes. However, Hospice Services provides such care as part of their services, if they assess your loved one requires it.

UPSIDE OF 24-HOUR CARE

If your financial situation permits this level of service, it can be a great option and a relief not be needed at all times. You will be able to hold a regular job, pay attention to other members of your family, sustain your relationships, live a normal life as far as socializing, going out at any time day or night and still enjoy your life, as much as possible under these circumstances.

DOWNSIDE OF 24-HOUR CARE

No matter how you look at it, this arrangement will cost you a fortune. If you have a cave of gold and riches, you need not worry. Otherwise let me warn you, this illness takes a long, long time. It could very well happen that you underestimate the financial situation, or how much of your loved one's or your own resources will quickly diminish. Then what?

BE INFORMED AND PLAN AHEAD WISELY.
PART OF THIS PROCESS IS READING THIS BOOK.

Other fact is, that you will have a stranger in your house 24/7. I am a very private person and that is difficult for me. Unless you have the luxury of a separate entrance, or a kitchenette where the caregivers can prepare food for themselves, you will have them present in your kitchen, rearranging your fridge contents and often making you feel like they are "taking over your house." That can be overwhelming, stressful and exhausting.

You may find yourself making space for them, adjusting and compromising your own comfort zone, in order to avoid any conflicts and territorial challenges. You will be dealing with minimum two daytime and two nighttime caregivers to accommodate their schedules. That makes for a lot of activity in your house and very difficult to supervise who did what and when. You would be surprised to see how fast a complete stranger can take over your house. If there are four strangers, you may soon feel like leaving altogether.

WITH THIS OPTION, YOU WILL HAVE NO PRIVACY. THIS COULD BECOME ENERGETICALLY AND EMOTIONALLY CHALLENGING FOR YOU.

TWO CAREGIVERS A DAY

Another possibility is to have two caregivers with your loved one thru the entire day. It certainly makes it easier for the caregivers to help each other with various tasks, but more often than not, I have experienced that a caregiver was repeatedly indicating that she needs another helper, when it really wasn't so.

SOME AGENCIES MAY ALSO PUSH THAT SET-UP, AS IT IS OBVIOUSLY TWICE AS LUCRATIVE FOR THEM.

If a caregiver is repeatedly saying that they can't handle your loved one's care on their own, maybe it's time to let them go. If you feel there is a valid point and your loved one is exceptionally difficult to lift, change and bathe with just the help of one caregiver, than you could consider the option of two caregivers a day, at least for a while. But still, be on guard and supervise. You don't want to return home unexpectedly only to find the caregivers having a party, sunbathing or sleeping while your loved one is left unsupervised and alone.

Keep in mind that two caregivers together will be chatting, creating more commotion and this may be quite irritating for your loved one, who requires complete peace and quiet. It is difficult to imagine two caregivers sitting next to each other in silence. After all, the activities that would requite both of them would be limited to bathing, changing and putting to sleep. The other hours would be a waste of two caregivers. And the meter is ticking.

TWO A DAY - UPSIDE

The caregivers will not get burned out so easily. They will support each other and have an easier time with lifting, showering and so on. Depending on the level of attention your loved one needs, this can be a good option for a certain transitioning period of time.

TWO A DAY - DOWNSIDE

This option still presents a very high expense. You must pay attention so that the caregivers don't become a bit too relaxed and chatty with themselves, while paying less attention to your loved one. Also, if there is a territorial thing going on between the two or and alpha dynamic, you must immediately interfere. You must remain in charge and make all decisions about the care. Otherwise, the one that will suffer is your loved one and you.

In addition, keep in mind that in this particular arrangement, you will need at least four caregivers that are well familiar with your loved one's care, in order for the schedule to work for everyone. That is a lot of strangers in your house, which makes it easy for them to blame someone else in case of a mishap. It may feel crowded and the caregivers will overwhelm you in your own home. They each have their unique preferences and approach to care and this may not be an ideal setting for your loved one, who will have increasingly more trouble identifying who is there. It may confuse, frighten, unsettle and agitate them.

LIVE - IN CAREGIVER

In this case the caregiver lives with you. They will require their own room and preferably also their own bathroom. This may be a good option for a certain amount of time. It depends on you needs regarding your schedule and other responsibilities. In reality, you will need at least two live-in caregivers, so they can each get sufficient amount of days off.

UPSIDE OF A LIVE-IN

If you are lucky to get a good caregiver, they become a part of your family. They are there to cover you at all times and it will cost you less than the 24/7 care charging hourly rates.

DOWNSIDE OF A LIVE-IN

You will need to adjust to two different strangers living in your house. The live-in caregivers may easily burn-out and will need regular days off. They will need to respect each other's private belongings left behind, as they interchange their schedule and living quarters. You will need to provide a separate room and preferably a private bath for them. You will also be required to provide all food. That is an added expense and hassle.

THE LIVE-IN CAREGIVER WILL NOT BE THERE FOR YOU 24/7, BECAUSE THE REGULATIONS REQUIRE, THAT THEY GET 8 HOURS OF SLEEP, OR AT LEAST 5 UNINTERRUPTED HOURS OF SLEEP. AS A RESULT, YOU WILL BE DOING THE NIGH-TIME CHANGES ON YOUR OWN. THEY WILL BE SLEEPING, AND YOU WILL BE WORKING.

If you are often absent from home, it will be difficult to supervise. They might be eating your food, washing their own load of laundry and making themselves a bit too comfortable in your home. They can become too familiar with your personal space and easily lose track of boundaries. They may be less helpful, than a caregiver paid by the hour.

On a more personal note, the live-in caregivers can become quite demanding with all the perks they expect and require. From my experience, when I explored the option of a live-in caregiver, she demanded a big-size bed, her own bathroom, her own large TV set and informed me months in advance, that she expected a very generous Christmas gift, specifically - a laptop. She also made known her various preferences in "her house" making it clear she wanted to dominate the entire household, while the rest of us would tiptoe around her rules. Of course she was asked to leave, just as soon as she revealed her unreasonable expectations.

DAYTIME - HOURLY CAREGIVER

This may be a very good option. You will have your days to yourself and privacy in your own home in the evenings. The caregiver is paid by the hour.

UPSIDE OF HOURLY CARE
You can keep a semblance of life during the days and not be completely imprisoned in your challenging situation. Your days are free of hands-on caregiving. You can tend to your career, work, study, and keep having an income. You have some time for your partner, your relationships or children. You can get away for a few hours, meet a friend, go to a movie, or escape into nature and get replenished. You can take time for self-care, get a massage, take a yoga class, or go work out.

This option will cost you less than a 24/7 care or a live-in caregiver. You won't be required to provide meals for the caregiver, since they usually prefer to bring their own snacks for lunch. There will be no strangers in your house through the night, early in the morning and in the evenings. This will give you an opportunity to relax without having to adjust to an outsider in your private environment.

YOU WILL HAVE MORE PRIVACY IN YOUR HOME IN THE EVENINGS, SOME TIME FOR YOURSELF DURING THE DAY AND WILL MAINTAIN A CERTAIN SENSE OF NORMALCY.

Last but not least, you will not worry what is going on with your loved one, how they are and if they are feeling abandoned. You will know they are safe in your home and you will see them every day. This may not seem like much, but it is a huge bonus.

DOWN SIDE OF HOURLY CARE

Once the caregivers shift is over, you are on your own. Since their usual workday is eight to nine hours, that gives you just barely enough time to juggle your workload, all errands and responsibilities during the day. You will have to rush home in time for the caregiver to leave, usually in the late afternoon or early evening around 6pm. After they leave your home, you are left with an all-night shift. If your loved one sleeps like a baby, that's fine. But as that is practically never the case with dementia patients, you could be going thru challenging nights with no sleep and the next day hardly recognize yourself in the mirror. In the morning you will remain on-call until the caregiver arrives, usually at 9am.

Basically with this arrangement your evenings and nights are gone and done for. Your evening social life is over. You nights are spend with the baby monitor statically squeaking away and a good night's sleep will be rare. While the two exchanging daytime caregivers will have days off, you on the other hand will never have an early morning, evening or night totally off. That can often become very challenging.

YOUR TEAM OF CAREGIVERS

The caregivers and you make a team. However, never forget that you are the one in charge. You must make it clear that this is your loved one, your home, your family and your money that you are spending to get the needed services. It is always good to listen to suggestions, but make it clear that the final decision is always yours. The caregivers will be asking you never-ending questions, such as:

- ✺ Do you want this or that?
- ✺ What does your loved one want?
- ✺ What do you want done for your loved one?
- ✺ Should they wash the hair today or not?

There will be a million questions and no matter how fantastic the caregiver, there are many decisions that have to be made with common sense or good intuition.

If your loved one is yelping and the caregiver assumes it is a yelp of hunger, but you clearly see the source of discomfort is a leg cramp, you will need to get involved. You need to be kind, but firm and demand a complete detailed report on any and all changes, or general ongoings.

If you get too familiar or too friendly with the caregivers, you may end up listening to their problems. Just the sight of them settling into a comfy and chatty morning routine will exhaust and irritate you. Once you allow someone to get too comfortable, it is difficult to change that dynamic later. They will take it the wrong way and think you are giving them a cold shoulder, when in fact; you just can't listen to their personal problems. You are paying them to unburden you and not the other way around.

PROFESSIONALISM

Keep the distance with your caregiver. You are paying them for help. They are responsible for the caregiving. That means: no sloppy or missing report notes, dirty dishes or laundry lying around, and or messy closets. Everything has to be in perfect order, otherwise you are going to crash.

They have to come promptly and on time, otherwise they are unreliable and you cannot count on them. I suggest you don't adjust your schedule too many times for any special favors, like early departures they may request. That is unacceptable. Everything has consequences.

If a caregiver wants to get off work half an hour early, it may not seem like such a big deal to them. But it is to your loved one. Since the caregiver spent a few hours just sitting around when your loved one was sleeping, they can now hardly wait to get home. To the caregiver, half an hour is nothing, but it will be disturbing to your loved one and you.

A half an hour too early for their evening routine, might leave them restless and nervous in bed so they won't fall asleep, and the whole night could be ruined. Your loved one and you will suffer in the end.

CHAPTER EIGHT

House Rules for In-home Caregivers

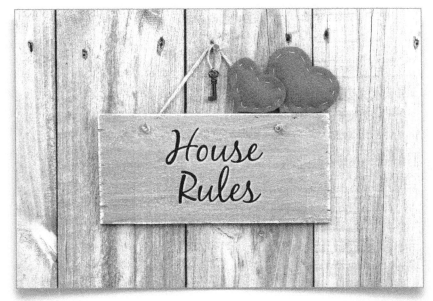

ESTABLISHING THE DO'S AND DON'TS IS ESSENTIAL

ABOUT THE RULES

Your loved one should have a set schedule when they get their evening medication, have their evening bath or go to bed. Reliability and non-compromise go for everything; changing your loved one, preparing proper food and feeding, cleaning the room, doing the laundry and anything else you may need the caregiver to do. You need to set the rules and check daily to assure they are respected.

HARMONY IS A TOP PRIORITY AND MUST BE KEPT AT ALL TIMES.

The caregiver is there to do all the tasks directly connected to the care of your loved one. They are not there to clean your entire house or cook for you. Caregiver needs to be respected, guided and appreciated. Good and clear communication is an absolute must. To make things easier, you can write down the required order of tasks, any special caregiving requests or needs, and your house rules. This way everything is very clear and there are no misunderstandings.

OBSERVATIONS

The truth is that you cannot rely on anyone else but yourself. Your attention and scrutiny, your feelings, intuition and observations are very important. You need to always keep a close eye on your loved one and any changes that occur in their appearance, behavior, communication, functioning and any activities, day and night. Let's also review the dynamic with the caregivers. What you need to pay attention to is your loved one and how they seem to react to the caregiver.

Here are a few observation tips you can use with in-home caregivers:
- Does your loved one seem peaceful in their presence?
- Does your loved one look at the caregiver with a fearful eye?
- Is your loved one agitated and unhappy in caregiver's presence?
- Does your loved one eat when the caregiver attempts to feed them?
- Does your loved one seem relieved when you show up, as if they've suffered alone with the caregiver?
- How is the caregiver's disposition towards your loved one?
- Are they spoon feeding your loved one at the right pace, paying attention to what is comfortable for them and allowing sufficient time to properly swallow?

- ❋ Do they wait until your loved one comfortably finishes swallowing or do they just keep filling them up?
- ❋ Is the caregiver gentle or too rough?
- ❋ Are they strong enough to hold and physically support your loved one?
- ❋ Do they listen and accommodate your requests?
- ❋ Do they behave as if they know everything and insist on doing it their way?
- ❋ Do they speak too loud for your loved one?
- ❋ Do they act as if your loved one cannot hear or understand them?
- ❋ Do they talk about your loved one, as if they were not present in the room?
- ❋ Do they act as if your loved one is a small child?
- ❋ Is the caregiver respectful and gentle with your loved one?
- ❋ Does the caregiver constantly hang on their cell phone?
- ❋ Do they watch TV and ignore your loved one?
- ❋ Do they seem bored and can't wait to go home?
- ❋ Do they avoid changing the pad for your loved one and keep making excuses?
- ❋ Are they keeping the room clean or expect someone else to do it?
- ❋ Are they preoccupied with their own meals?
- ❋ Are you keeping an eye on your supplies and how frugal or amply they use them?
- ❋ Does the caregiver sleep on the job?
- ❋ Do they continuously sigh?
- ❋ Do they scold your loved one?
- ❋ Do they get nervous and reactive, if your loved one screams?
- ❋ Do they wash your loved one properly?
- ❋ Are they rearranging your loved one's room without consulting you first?
- ❋ Are they reading, when they should be tending to your loved one?
- ❋ Are they adjusting your loved one's sitting position to assure their comfort?
- ❋ Are things mysteriously disappearing and appliances breaking down way too fast?
- ❋ Does the caregiver roam around your entire home when you are absent?
- ❋ Has the caregiver expanded into your kitchen way too much?
- ❋ Can they caregiver keep the boundaries you outlined?
- ❋ Do you have to remind the caregiver of the same things over and over again?

These are only a few observation facts that you should pay attention to. If anything is going in this direction, you need to address it right away. If it does not improve immediately, you may want to reconsider about keeping this caregiver. It is time to call the agency and request a more suitable caregiver for your needs.

IMMEDIATE ACTION

When something is not working with your caregiver, you need to address it right away. Do not wait for a better moment. There won't be one. This is it. If you see unacceptable behavior, kindly and diplomatically request and instruct they change their behavior. If they respond favorably and correct the mishap, all is well. If there is no improvement, you will release them sooner or later, so why not chose now.

> **A CAREGIVER'S BAD HABIT, MESSINESS OR MEDIOCRE CARE COULD BE VERY UPSETTING FOR YOUR LOVED ONE AND COULD CREATE A REAL SETBACK FOR YOUR AT - HOME CARE.**

You should follow your instinct and if you feel in some way that something is not right or your loved one is not cared for in the best way, you must take charge immediately.

You worked on finding a solution for your loved one's comfort and care for months. Now you need to maintain a high level of order and work ethic. Only so can you create a truly safe and nurturing healing oasis for your loved one at home.

TRAINING THE CAREGIVERS

No matter how experienced the caregiver is, you will need to teach and guide them. Firstly, house rules need to be set right from the start. You need to have them all sorted, especially any specific boundaries about care, privacy or access to various areas of your home. If you are unprepared, it will be considerably harder to establish new rules later on.

One major challenge is going to be the dynamic in the kitchen. It is not pleasant when a stranger roams in your kitchen and rearranges your food. No matter who is your caregiver, as soon as there is disharmony around the refrigerator, the "romance is over."

An ideal solution is to provide a small size refrigerator for the caregivers. You can place it in the hall, or entry area to your loved one's room. That way the boundaries are absolutely clear. I also recommend a small microwave oven. Now you have eliminated caregivers from coming into your kitchen and disturbing you. This may seem a small adjustment, but will help you keep your privacy at meal times for yourself and rest of the family.

We created a small kitchenette area for my Mom's caregivers in the entry hallway to my Mother's wing of the house. That way the caregivers had their own entrance and space where they could take a break, make a private phone call or prepare a quick meal for themselves. It did not disturb my Mother and it gave them privacy. You can create this space in a small hall, or even the corner of a room.

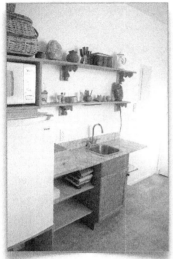

KITCHENETTE

Of course the caregivers are not supposed to be hiding in the kitchenette and sitting on the phone. By providing a mini fridge and small microwave, you have outlined the boundaries very well. You still need to clarify any specifics with explanation and instructions.

Next, you need to make it clear where the caregivers move - about space is. If you don't mind having them all over your home, then go right ahead. I think it is a much better idea, to limit them to your loved one's room and laundry space. They are supposed to be watching and caring for your loved one, not strolling around the house checking your closets. Be clear about what you want done for your loved one, how many times you want them showered, changed, how they need to be dressed and what the basic daily schedule is.

MEALS AND FEEDING TIME

I prepared all the food for my Mother myself. I have tried a few different options and nothing else worked as well. When I prepared meals for her, I could oversee the exact amount and contents, and that way I knew how her digestive system reacted to a certain diet and could make any immediate required adjustments. This was a decisive and crucial aspect of managing her optimal care.

The feeding is another very important matter. As you will see later in this book, diet is extremely decisive. It may need to be adjusted every day according to your loved ones' needs. I suggest you prepare the food yourself and place it in various small bowls. Now all the caregiver has to do, is feed your loved one the amount of food that you already designated.

This way you have eliminated two problems: you prevented someone from cooking in your kitchen and driving your crazy while at it, and you have assured your loved one's diet is ideal for them. If your caregiver was cooking, you would not have such good overview and it would be very difficult to keep track.

I will never forget an occasion, when I was stuck in traffic and came home a bit later than usual. I had failed to prepare the food for my Mom's diner and found the caregiver frying sausages for her - something my Mother would never eat, and in fact could not eat, because of her teeth. Every caregiver will most likely cook the way they like to eat, without an idea that your loved one may not like that food, or may be simply unable to eat it.

As you will see in the chapter on diet, you will be serving the food for you loved one in small cups on a tray. To assure that you have a complete overview of how much your loved one really ate, you need to see any and all leftovers. Only that way will you truly know their food intake. That means the caregiver should rinse clean the small cups that were emptied and leave all the cups with the leftovers, so you can oversee and log proper food intake amount. Make this a non-negotiable rule. You need to keep a daily log on all fluids and food intake to properly track your loved ones hydration and appetite level, food preference, and overall condition.

HYGIENE

The other important area is hygiene. You need to make very clear how and where you want your loved one washed and with what. You would be surprised what some people consider a thorough shower-wash. There is a big difference between just a small rinse, as if testing the waters, or a decent thorough cleansing shower that gets into all the problem areas.

Make it clear what you want your loved one to wear each day and night. Also clarify how much they should be covered if they are in bed. Clarify everything about preventing drafts that could be dangerous and the seemingly most mundane behavioral regulations.

To you, it is logical that there will be no loud blasting TV in the bedroom with disturbing news, and yet a caregiver may want to do precisely that. You may wonder, why have a TV in the room at all? And the answer is: because there are certain nature programs that create a very healing visual environment for your loved one, and they may enjoy watching them immensely, for example ocean waves and forest streams. But the loved one definitely must not be exposed to any kind of disturbing images or news programs.

You will have to explain to the caregiver what is acceptable and unacceptable regarding ambient for your loved one's room. Now here is the bummer. After you have taken the time and effort to train a caregiver and have to later replace them with a new one, you can start with the whole training ordeal right from the beginning. But here is the consolation. It will make you a very good, effective and fast teacher, and you will know right away if you have a winning combo caregiver, or one that won't last even a week.

On final note, my word of advice is, that you create a clear list of house rules, post them in your loved one's room and insist that they are followed. It will save you a ton of precious energy and time, so you won't be repeating the same drill over and over again and discussing later what was said or not. It will all be clearly laid out in the house rules. Here is a sample of House rules I used for my Mother's care:

IMPORTANT GENERAL INSTRUCTIONS
FOR THE CAREGIVER

MORNING
Arrive at 9AM.

WAKING UP AND GOING TO BED SCHEDULE
Let Mom sleep as long as she wants, but no longer than 10 am.
Start preparing for bedtime at 5:30. She needs to be in bed by 6PM.

MEAL TIMES:
BREAKFAST: between 9:30 - 10 am depending on her waking up
LUNCH: between 12:00 - 12:30 If she slept longer, then adjust to 1:00
DINER 4:30   **Very important: never feed her past 5 pm!**

FEEDING:
Liquid intake is extremely important. Feed her slowly, throughout the day. Do not rush. Give her plenty of time to swallow comfortably and completely.

Please be extremely careful that she DOES NOT CHOKE on food or cough.
Make sure her mouth is EMPTY when she is getting sleepy.
NEVER move recliner chair too far backwards when she is eating or drinking or has anything in her mouth
When feeding, offer her different foods, do not feed from one cup until its empty.

CHANGING:

1. First thing in the morning when getting out of bed - Approx. between 9am - 10am

2. After the first nap - before lunch, change her again - Approx. between 12 noon - 12:30pm

3. Following her afternoon nap before diner, change her again - Approx. between 3pm - 3:30pm

Change her approximately 3 times a day (as needed) AND in the evening before bedtime - at Approx. 5:30-6pm

THINGS TO REMEMBER:

She is very **sensitive to noise**, please no loud talking into her ear.

Sensitive to **too much light.**

Sensitive to **cold hands or touch.**

Her right hand and arm are sore.

Give her some privacy, when she is resting, sit out of her range of view.

Always tell her what you are about to do, or what you are feeding her.

If she seems uncomfortable you can ask her the following:

Are you hungry?

Are you thirsty?

Do you have pain in your leg?

Are you hot?

Are you cold?

Are you comfy?

Ask slowly and give her plenty of time for answer.

It requires extreme effort for her to answer or speak.

Maybe she is sitting uncomfortably or has a cramp - usually in her left calf.

Make sure she doesn't slide down too far in the chair and is uncomfortable.

STAYING ON TOP OF THE SITUATION

Once all rules have been made clear and have been fully explained, you still won't be able to avoid oversight and completely relax. You need to keep on top of the situation by daily checking the logbook where everything is documented.

If you hire an agency for caregivers, they will provide you with a basic logbook that will help keep track of basics regarding your loved one's care.

When you are doing the caregiving on your own, you can use any log samples from a wide selection in Chapter *Doctor Care and Home Visits*. You will be measuring blood pressure, checking oxygen level, tracking appetite and food intake, documenting bowel movement, and notating medicine administration. All this valuable and helpful information will be kept in your own log folder. It may seem like an additional task, but it will take you less than a few minutes a day and strongly recommend it. The log is very important and helpful to remember various details. It will be a useful tool and not an extra burden. It will also serve as your documentation of proper care that you provided for your loved one.

If you have caregivers, it will also help you assess which caregiver is properly doing their job. In the log for tracking your loved one's fluid and food intake and appetite, caregivers very often just put an assessment number of 100%, as if your loved one ate 100% of everything that was prepared for them. That may not always be true, however the caregivers will have a tendency to still write 100 %. Why? Partly because they want to make sure it looks as if they feed them really well. Secondly, maybe because they are not able to really assess what percentage was eaten and what was not.

The logging needs to be done truthfully, otherwise you might as well dismiss the whole tracking system. If you count how many cups of food your loved one consumed during the entire day, it will be much easier to track. At the end of each day, keep track of any food that was left over in the cups on the food tray. It will give you perfect oversight on the amount of consumed food. Instruct your caregivers to avoid randomly emptying and washing all the food bowls. You will completely lose track of the actual food intake.

As the illness progresses, the correct food combination will become even more important. Pay attention to every detail. This will help you asses diet changes, adjustments and remedies.

I. SAMPLE OF MORNING INSTRUCTIONS FOR THE CAREGIVER

Arrive 9am. Get the breakfast from the main kitchen and bring to Mom's room. Keep the noise down. Let Mom sleep as long as she wants, but no longer than 10 am.

THINGS TO PREPARE

Place the prepared outfit for the day in the bathroom.

Make sure Mom's lounge chair is covered with protective pad and prepared for her.

GETTING MOM OUT OF BED

Remove the side cushions on the right side of the bed.

Remove two lower bed rails on the right side of the bed.

Place bed rails away from bed.

Gently greet Mom - not too loud.

Ask her if she is ready to get up.

Put her hair in small bun - use hairband so it stays clean, away from her face.

Put on the plastic gloves.

Get a plastic trash bag, wipes and scissors, place them on bed.

Get the laundry basket, place it by the side of the bed.

MORNING CARE

Do not uncover her completely.

Remove only the lower sheet and place it into the laundry basket.

Move basket out of the way.

Take scissors and cut mesh panties on both sides at the hip.

Remove the incontinence diaper/pad and mesh and place them in the trash bag.

Clean her with wipes front to back.

Place trash bag out of the room.

GETING UP

Slowly and carefully slide her feet to the edge of the bed.

Sit her up by gently holding her left hand and her right side of her neck to help her sit up.

Wait a few moments, so she doesn't get dizzy.

Hold her with both hands and help her get up.

Walk her to the bathroom and place her on the toilet seat.

II. SAMPLE OF MORNING INSTRUCTIONS FOR THE CAREGIVER

WASHING AND DRESSING UP

Remove her nightgown.

Wash her back, hips and front with warm soapy washcloth.

Rinse off with warm wet washcloth.

Gently dry off with a towel.

Dress her upper body.

THE FASTEST PART

Use the small cup to quickly wash below, rinse a few times and pat dry.

Put on mesh panties. (do not pull up all the way)

Dress lower body. (do not pull up sweatpants all the way)

Help her get up from toilet.

Guide her a few steps to sink-vanity and help her hold on to handrail.

Right away put blue day-pad in place and finish pulling up mesh panties to hold pad.

Finish pulling up sweatpants. She is dressed and ready for the day.

SLOWLY TO HER SITING AREA

Guide her to her reclining chair by holding her hands & lower arms and walking with her.

Elevate the reclining chair so she can easily sit down.

Once she is sitting, slowly lower the recliner to a comfortable upright sitting position, legs slightly elevated.

If she is very hungry you can do the face care after breakfast, otherwise continue with the following steps:

FACE CARE

Wash her face with a washcloth (use only pink washcloths for face)

Gently pat dry

Very gently put on face cream

Comb her hair

BREAKFAST

Make sure chair is upright position before breakfast

MEDICATION ON AS NEEDED BASIS

I never let a caregiver decide whether my Mom should get a dose of as-needed medication. Take into consideration that the tendency in nursing homes is always to overmedicate the patients, simply because it is less challenging when everyone is calm, quiet and sleeping. But in your case, with loved one in your own home, the positive side is exactly the fact, that you can make sure they are never overmedicated.

A tired caregiver may have the tendency to - at the end of the day - report that your loved one was difficult. Such a caregiver would gladly give a sedative to your loved one, so the problem would go away. You need to be the one to asses the situation very well, before administering any as-needed medicine sedative. Maybe your loved one is just uncomfortable with a simple thing, like a shirt that is not tucked in, a wet diaper, or not sitting comfortably. Being observant will help you rearrange them and regain their comfort zone.

I SUGGEST YOU ALONE PREPARE THE DAILY DOSES OF ANY MEDICINE FOR YOUR LOVED ONE. IF THERE IS A MEDICINE THAT IS TAKEN ON AS - NEEDED BASIS, YOU WILL MAKE THAT DECISION, NOT THE CAREGIVER.

To sum up the caregiver tips, it is my opinion that you need to supervise everything at all times. If you were absent during the day, you need to have a clear report from the caregiver on what happened while you were gone and any and all changes in your loved one's condition. This does not have to be complicated, it is just a simple sentence about the current status and any new developments.

You are the primary caregiver and it is your duty to do everything in your capacity and power to make your loved one comfortable, understood and well cared for. Remaining meticulous will result in your loved one feeling comfortable and in pristine condition. You will enjoy organized order in your house, well-set boundaries and caregivers who will truly help you. Do not burden them with responsibilities that are beyond their capacities.

If you select the caregivers well, they will be your true saviors. It will be pleasant and comforting to know someone is there who respects your loved one, you and your home. If you fail to invest time in training, communication, a clear set of rules and rigorous follow - up reports, the caregivers will unwillingly become a source of stress, aggravation and an unnecessary, expensive, additional challenge.

SHOULD YOU HAVE a MALE or FEMALE CAREGIVER

I have engaged both, male and female caregivers and found them to be equally helpful. We had a male caregiver that was of an incredibly gentle and sweet disposition, very tall and strong, so that despite my Mother's height, he could pick her up like a little girl and tuck her into bed with ease. She enjoyed that. He sat with her quietly for hours and fed her meals with tremendous patience and the kindest temperament.

We also had a male nurse who was very different and struggled with the aspect of physical care. While dealing with the aftermath of shower routine, he let my Mother out of sight and she fell out of her wheelchair. Luckily nothing happened to her, but as a result, he was so stressed, he never came back.

I have known female caregivers who were the gentlest, and others who were completely absent minded and distracted, not paying any attention and rushing through care with frustration. There was also a wonderful female caregiver who was very experienced, tall, strong and of exceptionally cheerful nature. However, when my Mother's illness entered the very last phase, this caregiver did not have the emotional stamina to watch the final difficult process. She disappeared without forewarning and left me alone and stranded when we were at the most difficult point of the journey. She was hired through an agency, but since they knew our need for their services was winding down, they simply didn't care.

**SO YOU SEE, A CAREGIVERS CAN BE
AS DIFFERENT AS THERE ARE PEOPLE IN THIS WORLD,
IT MAKES NO DIFFERENCE WHETHER THEY ARE MALE OR FEMALE.**

**WHAT MATTERS IS THEIR NATURAL ABILITY TO RISE TO THE OCCASION,
THEIR COMPASSIONATE HEART, SKILL-SET, STAMINA,
PATIENCE, INNATE COMMON SENSE,
AND MOST OF ALL, PROFESSIONALISM.**

**A CAREGIVER WITH ALL THESE QUALITIES
IS CERTAINLY EXTREMELY HARD TO FIND.**

LETTING GO OF A CAREGIVER

There may come a time when you will have to let go of a caregiver. Usually you will notice when a caregiver becomes lees patient and kind, that they are close to burning out. It is always difficult when you have to let go of a caregiver that you have trained and gotten used to. It is quite a disruption to let them go and start from scratch. Even if you work with an agency, it will most likely take time before you will feel that you have found a new appropriate caregiver again.

> **IT IS IMPERATIVE THAT THE FEAR OF LETTING GO OF A CAREGIVER
> IS NOT HOLDING YOU BACK.
> WHEN THE CAREGIVER IS BURNED OUT,
> THEY WILL EVENTUALLY LEAVE ON THEIR OWN ANYWAY.**

One day, they just won't show up. So it is better you avoid unnecessary additional stress, remain in control and ahead of the inevitable.

If you work with an agency, I advise you to call the agency as soon as you notice the changes and inform them, that you have noticed the caregiver is tired and you need a backup and different options. Even if the caregiver will insist that they are not tired, it is better to end on a good note. Maybe they can come back later, in a few weeks or months, but most often that will not happen.

If you are hiring the caregivers on your own, then it is better to let go of the caregiver before they unexpectedly depart themselves. It may happen that after they receive the last paycheck, they will inform you, that they are not coming back tomorrow. And that could mean – you are on your own as of NOW. It is much more difficult to be left hanging when you are finding caregivers on your own, since you could suddenly find yourself completely without help. But nevertheless, it is better to remain the one in charge and end on a good note.

Remember, any hard feelings, unhappy situations at the end of a working relationship could be very uncomfortable for you, since the caregiver intimately knows your household and vulnerable family circumstances and dynamics. It is better to be on your own with no help, but in good spirits and take your time in finding the next appropriate caregiver.

In the beginning, whenever I had to let go of a caregiver, I was reluctant. Just the thought of having to train someone new was exhausting. But it is much more tiresome keeping a diplomatic, friendly and peaceful environment when a caregiver is unhappy, tired and just waiting to get the heck out of there. And you never know, the next caregiver may turn out to be better than the one you just let go.

Certainly one thing is clear, the condition of your loved one will be changing all the time and so will the help they need. Maybe in the beginning they require a more high energy person with some physical power, who will be able to pick and lift them with ease and walk with them a few steps, and so on.

At the end of the caregiving journey as the illness progresses, your loved one will be bedbound and will require a caregiver with a very different temperament than before. Now they will need a very peaceful person, who will understand small signs of need and will be able to sit still without creating a big commotion all the time.

Not every caregiver can adjust to these two caregiving extremes. Some are more vivacious and others are very quiet. You will be adjusting caregivers all the time. Especially towards the end of the caregiving journey, your loved one will need sleep and not a rambunctious personality going stir crazy and restlessly vacuuming around the room. So, what that means is, that with time, it will most likely become inevitable to go thru a group of different caregivers, appropriate to your loved one's and your needs.

ON YOUR OWN – NO CAREGIVERS

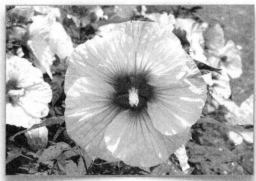

YOU ARE NEVER ALONE...

While this may sound extremely difficult, you would be surprised how many millions of people in this world find themselves in this situation.

THE PURPOSE OF THIS BOOK IS TO HELP YOU THROUGH THIS JOURNEY.

If you cannot, under any circumstances, afford some help from even an occasional caregiver, my heart really goes out to you. You have been dealt a very challenging assignment. But keep the faith in knowing, that you will get through it. Get informed, pace yourself, and always continue to find time for some self-care. Priorities will change, time will take on a whole other meaning, but always make an effort to protect, nurture and love your precious self.

UPSIDE OF NO CAREGIVERS

You are your own boss. You can keep a close eye on everything and have no worries if someone is not doing their job, prancing in your kitchen and invading your privacy. You can retain peace in your home and truly accommodate your loved one even better at sleep times, thru any changes in schedule and ever evolving adjustments. That can be very freeing and positive.

YOUR PRIVACY IS SACRED
AND KEEPING YOUR HOME ENVIRONMENT AS PEACEFUL AS POSSIBLE
WILL HELP YOU NURTURE AND SUSTAIN YOUR TRANQUIL STATE.

By having to pay attention to healthy diet for your loved one, this will present the ideal opportunity to begin eating super healthy yourself as well. Because your schedule will undertake a massive adjustment, this is also a good opportunity to completely change gears and stop rushing and being constantly busy.

Learn to take advantage of times when your loved one is taking a nap and rest as well. I know a million things need to be done, but not everything has to look and be perfect all the time. If you can, get some help with house chores, shopping for supplies or some less important time consuming errands. If you are going through this journey solo, became a master at organizing. You can eliminate many daily tasks by ordering supplies online. Try engaging extended family members with online calls with loved one, even if they can't really communicate and may just participate on sidelines.

ANOTHER VERY POSITIVE FACT IS THAT YOU ARE NOT SPENDING A FORTUNE ON CAREGIVER SERVICES. YOU HAVE MORE FUNDS FOR PROPER SUPPLIES, GOOD HEALTHY FOOD, SUPPLEMENTS AND BASIC LIVING EXPENSES.

Be frugal and plan well. Every state has different rules, but you can inquire about any public financial assistance offered to family caregivers. Become well informed and gather knowledge.

Your primary caregiving journey will also offer an opportunity to form a different and deeper bond with your loved one. This transformation can bring additional new and wonderful experience of unconditional love, peace and harmony to you both. In your final time spend together, you will have fulfilled a promise made long ago. Whether you are a partner or child of loved on with Alzheimer's and dementia, your loyal care will protect and save them from a much more dire passing.

AS A RESULT OF YOUR CAREGIVING EFFORTS, THE SENSE OF INNER PEACE THAT WILL REMAIN WITH YOU FOREVER IS INVALUABLE AND A MOST TREASURED GIFT. IT IS A TREMENDOUS SPIRITUAL OFFERING AND ACCOMPLISHMENT.

DOWNSIDE OF NO CAREGIVERS

I would not be truthful, if I would not mention the extent this assignment will affect all aspects of your life. Once you become a family caregiver for a loved one with Alzheimer's dementia, especially in the late phase of the illness, your life will change and won't ever be the same again. Obviously, your time is no longer truly yours. Everything will revolve around your loved one's needs and that can be an overwhelming circumstance.

If you are a caregiver to your parent, your career and personal partner-relationship may not survive this ordeal. Unless you have an amazing partner or spouse, the priorities will require a major adjustment, which may become too difficult to accept. If your partner can understand this and help you through this period, you are incredibly fortunate. If your partner abandons you, then console yourself with the fact that it would have been impossible to keep them content, while you care for your parent. This would have made your journey considerably more difficult.

If you are a caregiver to your partner or spouse, this illness will challenge you into a forceful restructure of your usual dynamics, which may be quite uncomfortable and difficult. You will experience many deeply emotional transformations, feel challenged out of your comfort zone and tested for your resilience, strength, stamina and patience. One consolation is the fact, that your loved is not abandoned and alone. You are together.

> **MOST OF ALL, YOUR TEST WILL BE ABOUT LOVE.**
> **ARE YOU CAPABLE OF UNCONDITIONAL LOVE?**
> **REST ASSURED, YOU ARE.**

Unless you have hired caregivers that can help you out and free some of your schedule, your social life will basically vanish, except for a few unconditional really good friends that will stand by you, probably mostly per phone.

You will have to be extremely careful not to burn yourself out and suffer from life lasting health consequences. This will require your self-restraint when overdoing, overworking or over managing day to day elements of care.

Unless you work from home, it will become impossible to hold a regular job. Your life will be very restricted; vacations and holidays will be rare or on indefinite hold. Your days and nights, months and years of caregiving will all blend into one.

FINDING YOUR SUPPORT SYSTEM

Under ideal circumstances, your support team would involve your family and friends, if possible. Hopefully they are able to offer you the basic support. They could watch over your loved one a few times a week for a few hours or a weekend, so you can get away for a break. They can help you out by sharing responsibilities, therefore encourage them to visit, so you have a breather. If possible, organize exchange of primary caregiver duties every few months, so you may get away for a bit and thoroughly replenish.

Quite often, this is not the case. Sometimes this illness triggers a dramatic shift in family dynamics and the resulting family conflicts often prevent any kind of communication or help. Other times there simply is no one to call. In such a case, hopefully you have a few friends you can communicate with. Perhaps they are experiencing similar challenges and you can share helpful suggestions and support each other that way.

**CONTACT THE LOCAL ALZHEIMER'S SUPPORT ORGANIZATION.
GET CONNECTED TO SUPPORT GROUPS.**

If there are no family members or friends in your immediate support circle, there are still things you can do in order to get some relief.

There might be a volunteer organization that can relieve you of your caregiving duties for bit, at least a few times a week. That way you can get out and feel free of obligations for a few cherished hours. If you get relief with volunteers, family or friends at least a few times a week, you will be able to manage.

Your support system can also consist of friends and family that may reside long distance. Simple conversations where you can exchange your feelings and concerns are very important. Staying connected with immediate neighbors can be a life saver, especially in case of emergency. Consciously make an effort to establish a circle of support in your immediate environment. This will help you fight feelings of isolation and overwhelm.

Any dear friend who can occasionally visit to keep you company, even if they cannot offer any help with actual caregiving tasks, is a positive influence on your emotional health. Stay engaged, connected and keep communicating. Schedule regular weekly calls with your selected support group team of friends.

YOUR SLEEP

You need to do everything possible to get enough sleep and rest on a regular basis. Nights must be yours, otherwise, it will be physically, mentally and emotionally impossible, to continue this kind of assignment for an indefinite amount of time.

That means that you need to discuss with your loved one's physician all alternative solutions, if your loved one is sleepless and restless at night. In consideration of the entire situation that involves your loved one's care and yourself - the physician will prescribe proper medication for your loved one on a as-needed basis, so that you can sleep at night as much as possible.

There will still be nights where you will have to get up and tend to them, but at least the majority of the nights will be peaceful. It is completely unrealistic to think you can last thru caregiving journey without proper sleep. That is where the line has to be drawn. You simply have to take into consideration that the best care for your loved one will be provided only when you can still function properly.

**IF YOU DO NOT TAKE CARE OF YOURSELF,
YOU ARE ALSO NEGLECTING YOUR LOVED ONE.**

There will be of course major adjustments through the very final weeks and days of your loved one's life. But at that time, you will be able to receive help from Hospice Services and that will make all the difference in the world. You will not be alone.

Read more in Chapter *Self-care for Caregivers.*

ON A FINAL NOTE

Through my Mother's long illness, we found a few great caregivers, but they could only remain with us for a certain period of time. With the progression of her illness, she required another kind of care and a differently dispositioned and experienced caregiver. I explored every possible version: a live-in caregiver, 24-hour caregiver, day-time caregiver, two caregivers, male and female caregivers, agency caregivers, private caregivers, and finally - no caregivers. I have shared with you the pros and cons of every and each of these possible combinations.

> **I TRULY HAVE IMMENSE RESPECT FOR GOOD, KIND AND COMPASSIONATE CAREGIVERS.
> THEY HAVE AMAZING PATIENCE, A LOVING HEART, AND ARE TRULY KIND AND GENTLE SPIRITS.
> THEY ARE RARE INDEED.**

Putting everything aside, no matter how good or bad your experience with professional caregivers is, there is of course that rare, hard to find, special and amazing professional caregiver that exists. They are out there. Working quietly, long hours, days and nights. And if you are lucky, you will find them, or they will find you.

They are strong, trustworthy, inventive in distress, reliable and calm when you're anxious, burned-out and exhausted. Just imagine dealing with this demanding job day and night for years, taking care not of your loved one, but of complete strangers.

A true gem of a caregiver becomes a part of your family, in certain cases, the better part. Those special caregivers who have chosen this profession with a deep desire to lovingly help people in the final years of life before their transition, they are truly the salt of the Earth. If you found one, treat them kindly and let them know how much you appreciate them, as often as you can. They are very special beings.

However, in the big picture of things, the one ever present primary caregiver who will remain with your loved until the end is You. Only you knew your loved one, when they were healthy and fully functioning. Therefore you know their character traits, their life's accomplishments, talents, abilities, their natural dispositions, their good and bad qualities, the likes and dislikes and what makes them feel comfortable, content and peaceful.

AN OUTSIDE HIRED CAREGIVER ONLY SEES YOUR LOVED ONE AT THEIR WEAKEST, MOST VULNERABLE POINT. THEY HAVE NO IDEA OF THE STRENGTH, MAGNITUDE AND LIFE-FORCE THAT YOUR LOVED ONE EXUDED WHEN THEY WERE IN THEIR BEST YEARS.

YOU KNEW THEM AS A WHOLE, BEAUTIFUL AND HEALTHY PERSON.

You still know who they truly are, under the veil of this illness and the vulnerable state they are in now. Nobody can replace that kind of familiarity. Therefore the care you offer them, will provide most comfort and ease of functioning, while they are forced to tolerate the restrictive conditions.

Just imagine, if you were ill and could not say or do whatever you wanted. Would you prefer to have someone care for you that knows you, understands you for who you really are?

As a family caregiver you will always hold that advantage. You are family.

YOUR PRESENCE IN YOUR LOVED ONE'S LIFE IS ACTUALLY QUITE IRREPLACEABLE. EVEN IF THEY ARE NOT ABLE TO VOICE THIS TRUTH, ALWAYS REMEMBER AND KNOW IN YOUR HEART, THAT IT IS SO.

CHAPTER NINE

Holistic Caregiving Remedies

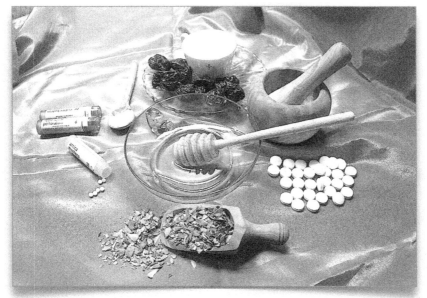

A WELL SUPPLIED HOME APOTHECARY IS INVALUABLE

ALWAYS CONSULT WITH YOUR HEALTH PROFESSIONAL BEFORE CHANGING OR ADMINISTERING ANY NEW SUPPLEMENTS TO YOUR LOVED ONE.

YOUR MEDICAL CABINET

Every household usually has a home medicine cabinet with a few essential or at least a first aid kit. When you are a caregiver, it is time to expand this home apothecary and gather some important basic supplies for preparedness. Obviously you will have all the prescription medicine your loved one may require. In addition, your medicine cabinet should have some Natural home Remedies you need to help relieve basic issues of discomfort and every day caregiving needs. This is where you will organize herbs, natural remedies and supplements.

This is your essential First Aid Kit.

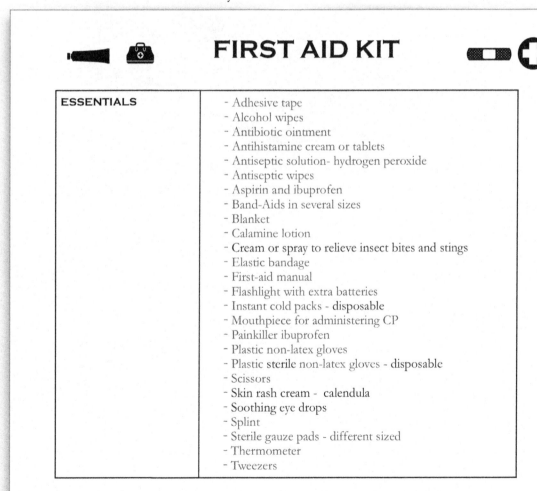

FIRST AID KIT

ESSENTIALS	
	- Adhesive tape
	- Alcohol wipes
	- Antibiotic ointment
	- Antihistamine cream or tablets
	- Antiseptic solution- hydrogen peroxide
	- Antiseptic wipes
	- Aspirin and ibuprofen
	- Band-Aids in several sizes
	- Blanket
	- Calamine lotion
	- Cream or spray to relieve insect bites and stings
	- Elastic bandage
	- First-aid manual
	- Flashlight with extra batteries
	- Instant cold packs - disposable
	- Mouthpiece for administering CP
	- Painkiller ibuprofen
	- Plastic non-latex gloves
	- Plastic sterile non-latex gloves - disposable
	- Scissors
	- Skin rash cream - calendula
	- Soothing eye drops
	- Splint
	- Sterile gauze pads - different sized
	- Thermometer
	- Tweezers

MUST HAVE INSTRUMENTS

PULSE OXYMETER

This is a small, noninvasive lightweight device used to monitor the amount of oxygen 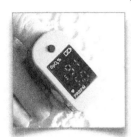 carried in the body along with your pulse rate. It attaches painlessly to your loved one's fingertip, and is very easy to use. This is an excellent device to help you monitor oxygen saturation and alert you of dangerously low oxygen levels caused by numerous factors, including obstructed breathing or other respiratory conditions. Normal oxygen saturation levels are between 95 and 100 percent. A normal pulse rate values for adults range from 60 to 100 beats per minute (bpm).

BLOOD PRESSURE MONITOR

This is a device used to measure blood pressure. It is good to have, especially if your loved one suffers from blood pressure disorders. Keep a daily log on their blood pressure 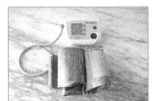 fluctuations. This will help remedy any imbalances and keep your doctor well informed of any changes. The American College of Cardiology (ACC) and the American Heart Association (AHA) updated their guidelines in 2017 to recommend men and women who are 65 or older, aim for a blood pressure lower than 130/80 mm Hg.

NOSE ASPIRATOR

This device will help you keep your loved one's breathing passageway clear by cleaning the nasal cavity. Usually you can find it in the baby section at the drugstore. The newest versions of nasal aspirator use disposable reservoir nozzles. The disposable tips have been specially designed to eliminate bacteria build-up inside the mechanism, to safeguard users from potentially harmful germs. With standard nasal bulb syringes, germs get trapped and can remain inside the syringe after use, even after they are rinsed. With the nose aspirator all you need to do is simply replace the disposable, flexible silicone reservoir nozzle tips after use.

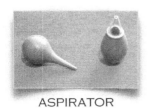

ASPIRATOR

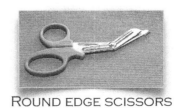

ROUND EDGE SCISSORS

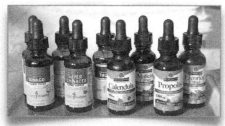

HERBAL TINCTURES

HERBAL TINCTURES

Concentrated herbal tinctures are made by soaking plants bark, berries, leaves, or roots. They carry many healing properties and can help ease various ailments and discomforts. Before adding any herbal tinctures to the health regimen, always consult a qualified physician.

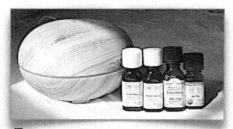

ESSENTIAL OILS AND DIFFUSER

ESSENTIAL OILS

High quality pure essential oils are used in Aromatherapy for awakening the person's vital energies, magnifying their self-healing capacities and restoring balance. Use them in a diffuser, by adding between 3 to 5 drops to 100 ml. Diffuse intermittently in 30 or 60 min intervals, only in well ventilated areas.

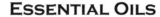

HOMEOPATHIC REMEDIES

Homeopathy assesses the whole person as an individual, with unique symptoms and manifestations of an ailment, based on their natural dispositions, weaknesses and strengths. There are numerous very effective natural homeopathic remedies that can greatly benefit your loved one as well as the caregiver. Before use, I suggest you seek guidance from a qualified Homeopathic practitioner or a Homeopathic medical doctor.

HOMEOPATHIC REMEDIES

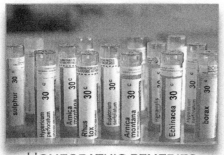

CHERRY PLUM BLOSSOMS

BACH FLOWER REMEDIES

These remedies contain extreme dilution of flower essences and are excellent for supporting everyday emotional wellness. They are safe to use and can be easily obtained in health food stores. Your loved one may benefit from Rescue Remedy, a blend of five flower essences, that can help alleviate stress and anxiety while promoting calmness.

NATURAL REMEDIES
FOR YOUR AT HOME APOTHECARY

 ## HERBAL REMEDY TEAS

CHAMOMILE TEA	Reduces inflammation and pain, help with sleep and relaxation, calming, easing cold symptoms and sore throats
CINNAMON TEA	Reduces inflammation and blood sugar levels, improved heart health, weight loss, fights off infections
DANDELION ROOT TEA	Improves digestion and promotes hormonal balance.
ECHINACEA TEA	Strengthens the immune system during cold and flu season.
ELDERBERRY TEA	For cold and flu, anti-viral actions, rich in vitamin C, A, flavanoids, highly nutritive, excellent for overall well-being.
GINGER TEA	Antioxidant, anti-inflammatory, for nausea, digestive discomfort, high blood pressure, aids weight loss, eases headaches, migraines
🌸 GREEN TEA	Antioxidant - prevents dementia, fights cancer, type 2 diabetes, anti aging, improves brain function, cardiovascular disease, cavities, improves energy & focus, lowers cholesterol, antiviral, detoxifies
HOLY BASIL TEA	Anti-inflammatory, antioxidant, helps stress, anxiety, arthritis & fibromyalgia
JASMINE TEA	Same health benefits as green tea. Used for liver disease, liver pain due to cirrhosis, and abdominal pain due to severe diarrhea, cancer treatment, great for relaxation
LEMON VERBENA TEA	For indigestion, gas, colic, diarrhea, and constipation. Also for agitation, joint pain, trouble sleeping, asthma, colds, fever, hemorrhoids, varicose veins, skin conditions, and chills
🌸 MILK THISTLE TEA	Helps reduce liver inflammation& damage, prevents decline in brain function, protects bones, improves cancer treatment
NETTLE TEA	Anti-inflammatory, aids adrenals & kidneys, lowers sugar
PASSION FLOWER TEA	Relaxing, for anxiety, insomnia, pain relief, heart rhythm problems menopausal symptoms, hyperactivity
PEPPERMINT TEA	Soothing, calming, relaxing, calms digestive system, nutritive with
🌸 ROSEMARY TEA	Antioxidant, anti-inflammatory, boost immune system, circulation, memory, alertness, intelligence, focus, cognitive stimulant,
ST JOHN'S WORTH TEA	For depression, anxiety, tiredness, appetite loss a& trouble sleeping.
VALERIAN TEA	Promotes relaxation and restful sleep.
YARROW TEA	Depression, anxiety, fever, cold, hay fever, diarrhea, appetite loss, gastrointestinal issues, skin & liver inflammation, wound healing

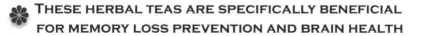

🌸 **THESE HERBAL TEAS ARE SPECIFICALLY BENEFICIAL FOR MEMORY LOSS PREVENTION AND BRAIN HEALTH**

HEALING HERBS
FOR USE IN COOKING

APPLE CIDER VINEGAR Natural Antibiotic	Eliminates harmful bacteria, lowers blood sugar levels, helps manage diabetes, improves heart health, boost skin health.
CINNAMON Natural Antibiotic	Anti-viral, anti-bacterial, anti-fungal, antioxidant, anti-inflammatory, prebiotic properties improve gut health, reduces blood pressure, blood sugar & type 2 diabetes, digestive remedy
CLOVES Natural Antibiotic	High in antioxidants, protects against cancer, kills bacteria, improves liver health, regulates blood sugar, promotes bone health, reduces stomach ulcers.
✹ **CURCUMIN - TUMERIC**	Anti-inflammatory, protects against heart disease, cancer, eases osteoarthritis, prevents diabetes, delays or reverses Alzheimer's, depression, rheumatoid arthritis, skin, protects from free radicals, prevents eye degeneration
✹ **GARLIC** Natural Antibiotic	Reduces blood pressure, risk of heart disease, lowers cholesterol, combats cold and flu, antioxidant helps prevent Alzheimer's & dementia, longevity, athletic performance, detox heavy metals, bone health, improves memory and skin
✹ **GINGER** Natural Antibiotic	Nausea, weight loss, osteoarthritis, lower blood sugars, heart disease, chronic indigestion, lower cholesterol, pain reducer, prevent cancer, healthy brain function, protect from Alzheimer's disease, help fight infections
HONEY Natural Antibiotic	Antioxidant, antibacterial and anti-fungal properties, heals wounds, phytonutrient, digestive issues, soothes sore throat
MINT LEAVES	Rich in nutrients, improves irritable bowel syndrome, helps relieve indigestion, improves brain function, cold symptoms.
NUTMEG	Relieves pain, indigestion, strengthens cognitive function, detoxifies the body, skin health, insomnia, increases immune system function, prevents leukemia, improves blood circulation.
OREGANO Natural Antibiotic	Natural antibiotic, lowers cholesterol, antioxidant, yeast inf., gut health, anti-inflammatory, pain relief, cancer-fighting
✹ **ROSEMARY**	Antioxidant, anti-inflammatory, improving digestion, enhancing memory and concentration, neurological protection, prevents brain aging, cancer, protection against macular degeneration
SAFRON	Powerful antioxidant, improves mood & depressive symptoms, fights cancer, reduces appetite, weight loss aid
✹ **SAGE**	Anti-inflammatory, helps with hot flashes, cold sores, sore throat, fatigue, memory brain health, prevents cancer, improves cholesterol, reduces blood sugar levels, alleviates sunburn

✹ **THESE HERBS ARE SPECIFICALLY BENEFICIAL**
FOR MEMORY LOSS PREVENTION AND BRAIN HEALTH

HERBS WITH ANTI-INFLAMMATORY QUALITIES
ARE ALSO VERY BENEFICIAL FOR PROTECTING MEMORY HEALTH.

ESSENTIAL OILS
FOR SENIORS
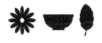

BERGAMOT	Calms the nerves, improves mood, eases pain, helps with depression and anxiety
CHAMOMILE	Calming support of the nervous system, soothes occasional anxiety, relives pain, decreases irritability, balances mood
EUCALYPTUS	Relaxing, calms the nervous system, mind and occasional anxiety, relieves mental exhaustion, clears nasal passages, eliminates harmful airborne bacteria.
GARDENIA	Anti inflammatory, when diluted and blended for massage, it helps with arthritis pain, helps improve digestion
GERANIUM	Helps with anxiety, depression, infection, and pain management, antibacterial, antioxidant, and anti-inflammatory properties
GINGER	Anti- inflammatory, balancing, grounding, energy boost, helps with loss of appetite, constipation, eases nausea,
LAVENDER	Soothes nerves, calming relaxing, fights insomnia, decreases feelings of anger, regulates sleep patterns
LEMON BALM	Energizing, decreases fatigue, boosts memory, relieves anxiety, improves digestion, promotes appetite, fights depression and feelings of loneliness
MARJORAM	Calming, relieves headache, pain, muscle ache
ORANGE	Uplifting, helps with depression and anxiety, helps improve digestion, eliminates bad room odors
PEPPERMINT	Calms anxiety, and nerves, helps mental abilities, increases energy, eases nausea, relieves tension and pain
ROSE	Reduces anxiety, stress, depression, pain and protect against harmful bacteria and fungi. It is expensive, but rose flowers offer somewhat similar benefits
ROSEMARY	Improves memory, relieves inflammation, enhances cognitive functions
TEA TREE	When applied it is antibacterial and helps treat nail fungus and insect bites. With a diffuser, it boosts immunity, fights infections, reduces anxiety, and relieves insomnia as well as congestion
YLANG YLANG	Improves sleep, promotes relaxation, kills bacteria, lowers blood pressure, benefits memory and improves thinking skills.

USE ESSENTIAL OILS IN A DIFFUSER; ADD BETWEEN 3 TO 5 DROPS
OF AN ESSENTIAL OIL INTO A 100 ML DIFFUSER.
USE IT ONLY IN WELL VENTILATED AREAS.
DIFFUSE INTERMITTENTLY IN 30 OR 60 MIN INTERVALS.
Keep essential oils out of reach of children and pets.

HERBAL TINCTURES I.

ADRENAL SUPPORT	Supports healthy function of the adrenal glands endocrine system. Essential for Caregiver to help prevent burn out.
ANDROGRAPHIS	Supports immune system, treats cold and flu symptoms
ANXIETY SOOTHER HOLY BASIL	Supports body's response to mild anxiety, protects against infection, lowers your blood sugar and cholesterol, eases joint pain, protects your stomach health
ARNICA	Anti-inflammatory, promotes healing after bruising, swelling or surgery, pain, post-shingles neuralgia, Diabetic neuropathy
ASTRALAGUS	Immune system support
ASHWAGANDHA	Balanced response to stress
BRAIN MEMORY	Supports healthy brain function, memory, and concentration
CBD OIL	Could be useful for managing pain, agitation and anxiety
DANDELION	Support the body's cleansing and detoxification process.
GASTRO CALM	Supports the gastrointestinal system, digestive comfort for occasional gas & bloating.
ENCHINACEA	Helps immune system combat infections and viruses, which could help you recover faster from illness
ST JOHN'S WORTH	For depression, anxiety, tiredness, appetite loss a& trouble sleeping.
GINGER	Promotes circulatory warming and alleviates occasional nausea
GINKGO BILOBA	Promotes good blood circulation and enhances memory and concentration.
GOLDENSEAL	Traditional support for the respiratory and digestive system.
HOLY BASIL	Anxiety soother Ayurvedic herb to support calm, focused energy, balanced response to stress & support mental concentration.
LICORICE	Support for the digestive system and the adrenal glands & endocrine system.
MILK THISTLE	Promotes healthy liver function.
NERVOUS SYSTEM TONIC	Herb Pharm supports, strengthens and calm the nervous system
OREGANO	Supports the immune system.

ALWAYS CONSULT A QUALIFIED PHYSICIAN BEFORE TAKING OR MAKING ANY ADJUSTMENTS WITH REMEDIES OR MEDICATION.

 # HERBAL TINCTURES II.

PASSION FLOWER	Promotes calm and relaxation, support for mild & occasional anxiety and insomnia
PROPOLIS	Supports the immune System
PROSTATE HEALTH	Includes Saw Palmetto berry, Stinging Nettle etc. for men
REISHI	Supports the immune system, liver health
RHODIOLA	Supports stress response, promotes energy, endurance and stamina.
SAGE	Helps with digestive problems, including loss of appetite, gas, stomach pain (gastritis), diarrhea, bloating, and heartburn. Reduces depression, memory loss, and Alzheimer's disease.
SAW PALMETTO	Helps enlarged prostate, urinary function, reduces inflammation.
SKULLCAP	Relaxing, calms your mind & support the nervous system
SOOTHING THROAT SPRAY	Propolis - relief of minor throat irritation, immune system Support
STONE BREAKER	Supports the urinary system
STRESS MANAGER	Heb Pharm-Supports tincture for healthy response to long term stress, promotes optimal energy, strength and endurance, contaons Reishi mushroom, holy basil, Rhodiola. Supports adrenal function.
THYME	Supports the respiratory system
THYROID CALMING	Support for the endocrine system
THYROID LIFTER	Support for the endocrine system
TRAUMA DROPS	Support for the nervous system during minor, occasional pain (contains Calendula, St. John's Wort, Arnica)
TURMERIC	Anti inflammatory - promotes healthy liver, digestive function
URINARY SYSTEM SUPPORT	Support for healthy kidney & bladder function
VALERIAN	Promotes relaxation and restful sleep.
WILLOW BARK	For pain, headache, muscle or joint pain, menstrual cramps, rheumatoid arthritis, osteoarthritis, gout
WITCH HAZEL	Relief from itching, pain & swelling, inflammation, skin injury, hemorrhoids, bruises, insect bites, minor burns, acne, sensitive scalp, and other skin irritations.
WOMEN'S COLLECTION	Herb Pharm - four herbal blends formulated especially for women. (for women caregivers)

ALWAYS CONSULT A QUALIFIED PHYSICIAN BEFORE TAKING OR MAKING ANY ADJUSTMENTS WITH REMEDIES OR MEDICATION.

MEDICINAL CREAMS & SOLUTIONS

 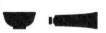

ALOE VERA CREAM	Boost healing of wounds, burns, sunburn, small abrasions, cuts, dry skin, cold sores and eczema
ANTIBIOTIC OINTMENT	For treatment of minor wounds, cuts, scrapes, burns and mild skin infections
ARNICA CREAM	Anti-inflammatory, promotes healing after bruising, swelling or surgery, pain, post-shingles neuralgia, Diabetic neuropathy
COCONUT OIL OR CREAM	Reduces inflammation, moisturizes and helps heal wounds. It has antimicrobial properties that help protect the skin from harmful bacteria.
VITAMIN E 12,000 IU CREAM BY DERMA - E	Replenishes moisture, softens and soothes, natural moisturizer, antioxidant, ideal for the face, elbows, heels, knees and hands, or anywhere skin is in need of nutrient-rich moisture.
VITAMIN E OIL	Nourishes the skin, cures muscle spasms, treats sunburns, cleansing agent, treats chapped lips
CALENDULA CREAM	Soothes and heals minor burns, scrapes, skin irritations, sunburn, and chafing, first aid
NAIL FUNGUS OIL BY ZETA CLEAR	Powerful anti-fungal solution made of soothing, healing natural oils derived from plants and herbs enable healthy nails in looks as well as in essence. It seeps deep down into the nail bed to where the fungus has started growing roots. It takes between 3-6 months of disciplined daily applications to successfully eliminate nail fungus.
RUBBING ALCOHOL	Wound disinfectant, First Aid
CA- REZZ CREAM TO HELP PREVENT AND HEAL BED-SORES	CA-REZZ Norisc Cream is Incontinent Skin Care System that provides the toughest antibacterial barrier against today's complex pathogen. Non-greasy antibacterial cream especially formulated to soothe skin tissue. Ideal for irritated skin and preventing bed sores and diaper rash. Reduces germs that cause rashes, ensures the maximum level of protection against the bacteria, fungi and yeasts that cause skin breakdown and infection. It comes with vitamin A, D, E and Allantonin.
CA- REZZ ORIGINAL WASH	A rinse-less, antimicrobial spray that removes infectious microorganisms and reduces odor. Provide the extra level of protection for today's increased health risks. Intended for frequent daily use. Stops odors. Reduces risk of cross contamination. This advanced skin sanitizer is effective against many of today's complex pathogens. FOR CAREGIVER
BADGER & Co. NATURAL BUG REPELLENT SPRAY	Botanical or plant-based spray for repelling and preventing insect bites

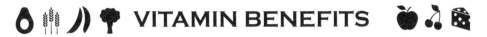 VITAMIN BENEFITS

VITAMIN A	Protects eyes from age-related decline, lowers risk of cancers, supports immune system & bone health, healthy growth
VITAMIN B 12	Helps form red blood cells, prevents dementia, improves mood & symptoms of depression, boosts metabolism, immune system, cognitive function, healthy skin & nails
VITAMIN B COMPLEX	Improves energy levels, brain function, and cell metabolism. Helps prevent infections and supports & promotes cell health
VITAMIN C	Reduces risk of chronic disease, high blood pressure, risk of heart disease, reduces blood uric acid levels, prevents gout attacks, iron deficiency, boosts immunity, protects your memory and thinking
VITAMIN D	Promotes healthy bones and teeth, supports immune system, brain, nervous system health, regulates insulin levels, supports diabetes management, lung function and cardiovascular health
VITAMIN E	Prevents coronary heart disease, supports immune function, prevents inflammation, promotes eye health, lowers risk of cancer.
VITAMIN K	Promotes blood clotting, prevents osteoporosis, support strong bones, improves memory, lowers blood pressure, cardio. disease
PROBIOTICS	Healthy balance of gut bacteria, digestive health, immune function, prevent & treat urinary tract infections, helps Lactose intolerance, improve skin conditions, treat stomach and respiratory infections
CALCIUM	Keeps bones healthy & strong, prevents blood clots, cancer, diabetes, high blood pressure, healthy heart, muscles and nerves
CHARCOAL ACTIVATED CHARCOAL TABLETS	Improves digestive function and growth of good bacteria, removes heavy metals, viruses and parasites, assists kidney function, filters out undigested toxins and drugs, reduces intestinal gas and diarrhea, emergency treatment of poisoning
IRON	Treats anemia, boosts hemoglobin, reduces fatigue, boosts immunity, improves concentration, respires sleep
MAGNESIUM	Boosts exercise performance, fights depression, benefits against type 2 Diabetes, lowers blood pressure, anti-inflammatory
MAX 3 FORTE INOSITOL & MAITAKE & CAT'S CLAW	Superior support for immune system, supports natural killer-cell activity, anticancer and anti-angiogenic effects
RESVERATROL	Antioxidant, anti-inflammatory, protects brain function and lowers blood pressure, eases joint pain, suppresses cancer cells, fight fungal infection, ultraviolet radiation and stress

ALWAYS CONSULT A QUALIFIED PHYSICIAN BEFORE TAKING OR MAKING ANY ADJUSTMENTS WITH SUPPLEMENTS, REMEDIES OR MEDICATION.

VITAMINS IN FOOD

VITAMIN A	Cantaloupe, Pink grapefruit, Apricots, Carrots, Pumpkin, Sweet potatoes, Winter squash, Dark green, leafy vegetables, Broccoli
VITAMIN B 12	Beef, liver, and chicken, Fish and shellfish such as trout, salmon, tuna fish, and clams, Fortified breakfast cereal, Low-fat milk, yogurt, and cheese, Eggs.
VITAMIN B COMPLEX	Salmon, Leafy Greens, Liver and Other Organ Meats, Eggs, Milk, Oysters, Clams and Mussels, Legumes.
VITAMIN C	Citrus fruit, such as oranges and orange juice, peppers, strawberries, blackcurrants, broccoli, Brussel sprouts.
VITAMIN D	Salmon, sardines, herring and mackerel., red meat, liver, egg yolks.
VITAMIN E	Wheat germ oil, Sunflower, safflower, soybean oil, Sunflower seeds, Almonds, Peanuts, peanut butter, Beet greens, collard greens, spinach, Pumpkin, Red bell pepper
VITAMIN K	Green leafy vegetables, kale, spinach, turnip & mustard greens, collards, Swiss chard, parsley, romaine, green leaf lettuce, Brussels sprouts, broccoli, cauliflower, cabbage, Fish, liver, meat, eggs
PROBIOTICS	Yogurt, kefir, kombucha, sauerkraut, pickles, miso, tempeh, kimchi, sourdough bread and some cheeses. Should be kept in refrigerator.
CALCIUM	Milk, cheese and other dairy foods, green leafy vegetables – such as curly kale, okra and spinach, soya drinks with added calcium, bread and anything made with fortified flour, fish where you eat the bones – such as sardines and pilchards.
CHARCOAL ACTIVATED CHARCOAL TABLETS	Improve digestive function and immunity by helping remove heavy metals, viruses and parasites from the gut. Encourages growth of good bacteria. Assists kidney function, filters out undigested toxins and drugs, reduces intestinal gas and diarrhea. Used in emergency treatment of certain kinds of poisoning, helps prevent the poison from being absorbed from the stomach into the body.
IRON	Shellfish, Spinach. Share on Pinterest, Liver and other organ meats,Legumes, Red meat, Pumpkin seeds, Turkey, Quinoa
MAGNESIUM	Pumpkin seed, Almonds, Spinach, Cashews, Peanuts
INOSITOL	Cantaloupe, citrus fruit, and many fiber-rich foods - beans, brown rice, corn, sesame seeds, and wheat bran
RESVERATROL	Peanuts, pistachios, grapes, red and white wine, blueberries, cranberries, and even cocoa and dark chocolate

USE THIS LIST WITH MENU AND DIET SUGGESTIONS IN DIET CHAPTER.

NATURAL REMEDIES FOR
COMMON AILMENTS

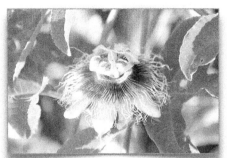

PASSION FLOWER HELPS RELIEVE ANXIETY

In this section we will learn about most common ailments that you need to be familiar with as a caregiver. Most of them are preventable or can be remedied with proper diet, good and attentive care, in addition to watchful observation. Ideally, you will be able to prevent and address a seemingly small issue before it becomes problematic.

NERVOUS CONDITIONS

AGITATION, ANXIETY, NERVOUSNESS

There are numerous natural remedies to help reduce these conditions. You can use various teas such as Passion Flower, Holy Basil, Lemon verbena, Peppermint, St. Johns Worth and Yarrow. Many of these herbs come in tinctures as well. Always consult with your doctor before implementing any natural tincture remedies.

IN SEVERE CASE OF ANXIETY, YOUR LOVED ONE WILL NEED MEDICATION. THE GOAL IS TO ASSURE THEM A COMFORTABLE, PEACEFUL AND CALM STATE.

If your loved one suffers from occasional episodes of agitation, nervousness, mood changes or has a challenging demeanor during daily hygiene routines, it is important to keep track of those occurrences. You can simplify your notes by assessing their morning, daytime, evening and nigh time disposition. Use categories like: sleeping, calm, agitated, severely agitated, aggressive, passive, communicative and non-verbal. The notes are critical for your doctor's management of any calming sedative to help successfully reduce it to a minimum or all together discontinue. For more suggestions on how to find the cause of agitation go to Chapter *The Mind - Communication.*

INSOMNIA

If your loved one suffers from insomnia, keep a thorough log on the details, such as:

※ Do they fall asleep easily, but wake up later in the middle fo the night?
※ Do they struggle falling asleep until wee hours?
※ Do they easily fall asleep, but wake up at early dawn?

Possible reasons and solutions for insomnia or night-time waking up:

※ **PROBLEM:** they are soiled and need a change of their incontinence pad
※ **SOLUTION:** change the pad, give less liquids right before bed, no food after 5pm

※ **PROBLEM:** they ate too late or had sugar or coffee which did not agree with them
※ **SOLUTION:** eliminate sugar and coffee

※ **PROBLEM:** they suffer from nighttime anxiety, or their nervous system is most sensitive at night
※ **SOLUTION:** they may require a calming remedy

※ **PROBLEM:** their schedule is upside down, they sleep through the day and are awake at night
※ **SOLUTION:** make adjustments with daily schedule, keep them awake in the afternoon, so they are sleepy in the evening

※ **PROBLEM:** leg cramp
※ **SOLUTION:** massage, support pillow for comfort, heating pad, supplements

※ **PROBLEM:** too hot or cold
※ **SOLUTION:** adjust room temperature, clothing or bedding

※ **PROBLEM:** night sweats
※ **SOLUTION:** change nightgown immediately, if sheets are wet, place a dry sheet on top until a full bed-change in the morning

※ **PROBLEM:** uncomfortable while lying on their back with a crumpled nightgown
※ **SOLUTION:** gently straighten the sleepwear clothing underneath them

- ❋ **PROBLEM:** bad dreams, nightmares
- ❋ **SOLUTION:** talk to them softy and explain you are here and all is well

- ❋ **PROBLEM:** fear, disorientation and confusion about their whereabouts
- ❋ **SOLUTION:** explain they are home, safe with you and they have nothing to worry about or fear. Assure them that you will not abandon them.

WRITE DOWN VERY PRECISELY:
- ❋ When did they wake up?
- ❋ What was the situation?
- ❋ Did they need an incontinence pad change ?
- ❋ Were they too hot, sweating or cold?
- ❋ Were they in pain?
- ❋ Did they suffer from a leg cramp?
- ❋ Were they calling for you or someone else?

It will be incredibly helpful to actually find the source of their discomfort. Perhaps it could be easily resolved with a change of incontinence pad. Find a solution, first exploring practical care adjustments, natural remedies, such as a cup of Passion flower tea or a droplet of tincture at bedtime, valerian tea and other natural calming remedies. Keep in mind that if this continues, you will quickly suffer from severe sleep deprivation, as it will be an impossible schedule to keep up. You loved one can catch up on sleep any time during the day, whereas you can't. Consult your doctor immediately and protect yourself from severe burn out. The longer you wait, the longer you will need to recover. If no natural remedy helps and the problem persists, your loved one will need a sleeping aid to regulate their sleeping pattern.

> **ALWAYS CONSULT THE DOCTOR BEFORE MAKING ANY ADJUSTMENTS WITH REMEDIES OR MEDICATION. MOST LIKELY THE DOCTOR WILL PRESCRIBE A MEDICATION THAT CAN BE TAKEN ON A AS - NEEDED BASIS.**

This way, if you loved one sleeps through the night, they don't need the medicine, and if they wake up, and care restless and anxious, you can give them the medicine to help them calm down.

RESTLESS LEG SYNDROME - RLS

This is a neurological disorder that triggers an urge to move the legs. This is more prevalent when sitting or lying in bed for long periods of time. It can be caused by numerous factors including side effects of various medications. Usually the discomfort improves with movement, however in elderly chair-bound or bed-bound patients that is often not possible.

THE BEST REMEDIES ARE:

- ✻ a healthy diet with no alcohol tobacco, sugar or caffeine
- ✻ daily movement therapy - with your help apply gentle circular movements to your loved one's ankles, gently stretch and bend their knees, never force or push any movements
- ✻ gentle muscle massage of the leg muscles, using elongated stroking movements, this can be done at bedtime or whenever needed
- ✻ apply compress or washcloth dipped in lukewarm water as a gentle compress to calm the nerves in the affected area
- ✻ use calming stress-relief lotion with aromas such as lavender, chamomile, rose for application and soft massage

TARDIVE DYSKINESIA - TD

This is a neuromuscular symptom that causes involuntary movement of the body. It could lead to blinking of the eyes, grimacing the face, opening the mouth, but no sound or words emerge, ongoing chewing motion, waving arms, or any number of other physical movements. TD is a side effect of psychotic drugs that are commonly used in elderly who suffer from Alzheimer's dementia. Helpful supplements:

- ✻ vitamin E
- ✻ melatonin
- ✻ Ginkgo biloba
- ✻ Vitamin B6

Never change the dosage amount or stop your loved one's medications or take a supplement without the advice and supervision of your medical professional.

IF THESE SIDE EFFECTS ARE IDENTIFIED EARLY ON, THE MEDICATION CAN BE REDUCED AND ELIMINATED, AND THE SYMPTOMS MAY GO AWAY WITH TIME. THIS SHOULD BE DONE ONLY UNDER THE ADVICE AND SUPERVISION OF YOUR MEDICAL PROFESSIONAL.

PAIN MANAGEMENT

PAIN

The main source of chronic pain in elderly is caused by musculoskeletal disorders, such as degenerative spine and arthritic conditions, neuropathic pain and neck or jaw pain caused by ischemia.

Helpful suggestions are a gentle massage of the affected area, long and slow breathing through the nose, warm or cold compress, heating pad, or application of Arnica cream, that is beneficial for its anti-inflammatory properties. Implement a healthy diet that includes anti-inflammatory food, use herbs such as Tumeric and cloves. Use a wet compress with diluted essential oils such as: lavender, chamomile, rosemary and yarrow. For neuropathic pain use remedies such as Passion flower drops, or various teas to help calm the nervous system.

PAIN FROM FALL OR INJURY

Elders are extremely vulnerable to falling and bruising. Practice extreme caution and never leave them alone. If your loved one suffers from pain caused by minor injury or bruising, apply Arnica cream and a cool compress to help reduce any swelling. In case of serious injury or fall, immediately call your doctor and emergency for help.

BACK PAIN AND POSTURE

The posture and general condition of your loved one's back will change and decline with the progress of the illness. Spending most of their days in a sitting or later lying bed-bound position, will weaken the spine and atrophy the back as well as stomach muscles. If your loved one suffers from additional spine challenges such as disk degeneration, osteoporosis, arthritis, hyperkyphosis (excessive curvature of the spine) it could make keeping a straight back or good posture even more challenging. The illness often robs one of the needed strength to hold themselves up. As a result, your loved one may seem to be dwindling down in size. Sitting in a reclining chair all day will make the situation worse and could become very painful.

IF YOUR LOVED ONE HAS WEAK NECK MUSCLES AND CANNOT SUPPORT THEIR HEAD IN AN UPRIGHT POSITION, YOU MUST PAY IMMEDIATE ATTENTION AND PROP THEM UP.

If they are left just a few hours with their head hanging unsupported off to one side, while resting it on their shoulder, imagine the strain on their neck muscles! They become overstretched on one side of the neck and very tight on the other. This can cause extreme discomfort and pain. Do everything you can to keep your loved one's neck straight and positioned as natural and comfortable as possible. You can accomplish this by continuously and attentively rearranging and propping a small pillow, a specialized neck pillow, or a cradling pillow in every possible way, to assure your loved one retains a good straight posture with their head properly aligned. If you fail to do so, their back and neck will become twisted, cramped and they will suffer tremendously. Find more information on the importance of proper sitting in the Chapter *Body Care - Physical Movement*.

LEG CRAMPS

This is a big challenge, especially when your loved one is agitated and has involuntary leg movement syndrome. Leg cramps can cause much suffering. Here are some helpful suggestions:

MASSAGE strokes. Gently massage the contracted muscle with smooth, long moves.

MOIST HEATING PADS will also do wonders. Apply warm moist electric pad compress. Be careful not to set the temperature too high, as it can quickly cause a burn. Never leave heating pad on high temperature or in same position, keep it a low medium level.

REPOSITION THE LEG while propping it up with small support or leg elevation pillow.

ADD B-COMPLEX AND MAGNESIUM to the diet. Unless BM is soft, add 1000 mg of Magnesium for 2 days if cramping is severe, then lower to 300 mg. In case of diarrhea, discontinue. If cramps persists, inform the doctor and check for Uric Acid levels in blood.

DIET, nutrition and supplements can also help prevent leg cramps. Recommended are foods rich in Potassium, which is a mineral and type of electrolyte that helps the nerves and muscles. Serve meals that contain bananas, oranges, cantaloupe, honeydew, apricots, grapefruit, cooked spinach, broccoli, sweet potatoes, peas and cucumbers.

REGULAR MOVEMENT will help and prevent legs for cramping. When your loved one is chair or bed bound, that is a challenge. Provide some movement for their legs by gently and slowly moving their legs as if peddling a bike. Repeat this at various times of the day, to help break up extended sitting periods. If they are chair bound or bed bound make sure the skin on their tailbone does not get rubbed when moving. It could cause a bedsore.

DIGESTIVE HEALTH

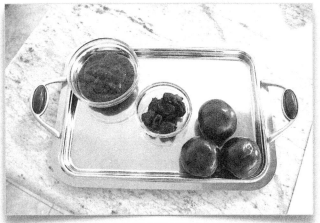

ADDING PRUNES TO DAILY DIET
WILL AVOID CONSTIPATION

HEALTHY DIGESTION

A healthy digestive system is a key component of your overall health. It contributes to a strong immune system, a healthy heart, good sleep and regeneration, and helps prevent cancer and autoimmune diseases. The major neural connection between your gut and your brain is called the vagus nerve. It connects the brain to the gut and other vital organs. Slow, deep breathing, healthy diet and gargling can be helpful in strengthening your vagus nerve.

A HEALTHY GUT ALSO HELPS MAINTAIN A HEALTHY BRAIN FUNCTION.

Stress, unhealthy diet and common food allergies to wheat, gluten, dairy and the presence of synthetic chemicals such as fertilizers, pesticides, antibiotics, hormones or genetically modified organisms regularly present in non-organic foods, can cause a chronic inflammation of your intestinal tract. This condition has been linked to several mental illnesses including anxiety and depression. This is very important information also for you as a caregiver that is under continuous long term stress. To learn about various caregiver stress management tools, go to Chapter *Self-Care for Caregivers.*

To summarize, intestinal inflammation adversely affects a healthy brain function and every aspect of your physical and mental health. I cannot stress enough how very important it is to keep the digestive system at its optimal capacity. To assure a digestive system free of inflammation, you need to follow a healthy diet and be familiar with any food allergies that are present in the system.

Keep in mind, that whatever eating habits and digestive issues your loved one had before the onset of illness, have most likely contributed to their poor brain health. It is very likely that previous digestive imbalances; such as constipation, irritable bowel syndrome or bouts of diarrhea, will increase and magnify. In other words, they will not disappear, but worsen with time. Thankfully this is preventable, especially since now you have the opportunity to directly oversee the quality of your loved one's diet and food intake.

> ## IT IS IMPERATIVE THAT YOU KEEP A VERY CLOSE WATCH
> ## ON YOUR LOVED ONE'S OVERALL DIGESTION
> ## AS WELL AS ELIMINATION.

In the Chapter *Healthy Diet*, I share with you the basics of making healthy food choices. When any changes or challenges with your loved one's digestive functions occur, you can make certain diet adjustments to help and quickly improve the situation. In addition, below you will also find natural remedies that can be very helpful.

ELIMINATION - REGULAR BOWEL MOVEMENT

There is no set rule of what is the optimal bowel movement schedule. Common belief is that between three times a day to three times a week is acceptable. That is certainly a very wide and quite inappropriate margin. Perhaps it simply indicates the general avoidance of such an important subject that concerns the state of wellness of every human being.

To begin understanding and finding remedies for challenges in this area, you need to have a general idea of your loved one's usual elimination schedule before they were ill, so you get an idea of what was their normal digestive functions pattern.

> ## IT IS A FACT, THAT CHRONIC CONSTIPATION
> ## EVENTUALLY CONTRIBUTES TO DECLINE IN HEALTH
> ## AS WELL AS MENTAL FUNCTIONING.

The toxins that linger in the body for days at a time are in no way beneficial, but very unhealthy. If one's usual bowel movement schedule was to eliminate once a day, consider this as their optimal timetable. In such case, when there is no bowel movement for longer than a day, or if there is bowel movement too many times each day, something is probably off balance. You can immediately take proper action, for if you do nothing, the issue can quickly escalate and cause unnecessary discomfort.

If one suffered from chronic diarrhea in the past, the body was continuously deprived of important nutrients. Take this into consideration as well. People avoid discussing the topic of bowel movements despite the fact that elimination is a part of everyone's life and in fact plays a crucial role in overall health. When you are a caregiver, you need to pay attention to your loved one's elimination, as this is a crucial contributor to their level of functioning and overall comfort. I can assure you that by managing your loved one's healthy digestion, you will reduce caregiver stress by 50%.

It is a fact, that families often simply become overwhelmed by one significant and dramatic mishap - a bowel incontinence disaster. As a consequence, this often results in moving the loved one into a facility. Bowel incontinence is very difficult to manage as it is. But to have an unpredictable factor such as diarrhea, or difficulty with elimination, this usually sends family members over the edge.

In a nursing home, the digestive issue will be managed with either a laxative or an anti-diarrheal medicine. But the cause of the issue itself, will most likely not be permanently resolved. Once the urgent issue is managed, it will be impossible to further manage individual digestive issues. Why? Simply because in a facility the diet cannot be adjusted to one's individual needs. As a result, the majority of seniors in nursing facilities are continuously given laxatives. Considering that very often constipation in elderly is caused by high dosages of sedatives, this becomes a worrisome never-ending circle.

IF THE DIGESTIVE AND ELIMINATION ISSUE CONTINUES, IT WILL EVENTUALLY WORSEN AND COULD BE ONE OF THE MAIN CONTRIBUTING FACTORS TO YOUR LOVED ONE'S OVERALL RAPID DECLINE AND EVEN DEMISE.

Keeping track of bowel movement frequency and consistency is simply part of good care. The optimal times for bowel movement are soon after waking up and after meals, when normal colon focuses its attention on motor activity.

Paying attention to the natural urge to have bowel movement is also important. Communicate with your loved one and inquire, if they feel the urge to use the bathroom. This could help you place them on the toilet in time, which will be considerably more comfortable for everyone, instead of remaining passive, using incontinence pad and then facing a prolonged and tedious clean up, which is demoralizing for your loved one and exhausting for the caregiver.

You also need to be aware of the consistency of stool, is it hard, soft, or if they struggle with constipation or diarrhea. Keep in mind, if there is no proper elimination, the entire system is literally being poisoned, by all the toxins that are not eliminated. A sensitive and delicate elderly person is quite vulnerable to an excess of toxins in their system, especially if this persists for any length of time. It can quickly cause a negative reaction of the entire system.

CONSTIPATION REMEDIES

Constipation is a very common problem with elderly patients with a reported prevalence of up to 70 % in nursing-home residents. The main contributors that slow down the food transit movement and cause a sluggish digestion are:

- Prescriptions of opiates and pain medications
- Sedentary lifestyle
- Reduced water intake
- Insufficient fiber in diet
- Ignoring the urge to defecate
- Anal fissures or hemorrhoids that cause pain and make one resist urge to pass stool

Constipation can present a persistent problem. Diet adjustments will help. However, daily use of prescribed stimulant laxatives will slow down the natural movements even more and the struggle with constipation evacuations will most likely continue.

This is going to be your daily concern when your loved one is in late stage of dementia. The entire system is slowing down and the most obvious sign is the digestive issue of constipation. If this is not immediately remedied, you could see a fast decline within days.

It is easy to understand that the consequences of retaining toxins is damaging. But with a delicate system like your elderly loved one, you need to be swift and quick to act.

REMEDIES:

* Work with your loved one's medical professional to help reduce the amount of any unnecessary prescriptions. Often the constitution of an elderly person can become overwhelmed with the amount of prescriptions they consume and the many side effects that require more medication. Even a small adjustment could be very helpful. Never reduce or eliminate a medication on your own or without the approval and under advice of a medical doctor.
* Healthy diet with plenty of fiber. Ground flaxseed meal is your best friend. It can be added to practically any food. Gradually increase fibers and pay attention to physical response.
* Increase fluid intake. The diet needs to be as liquid as possible and easily digestible. If your loved one eats very little, it is even more important to give them plenty of liquids, even if it takes a while to tea spoon-feed them a cup of herbal tea.
* Regular elimination. Be rigorous and alert to make sure you have done everything to help them with a regular bowel movement.
* Probiotics taken as part of a daily regimen will shorten bowel transit and soften stools
* Swiss Kriss is a 100% natural herbal laxative that is available in capsules or flake form. It consists of sun-dried leaves, herbs and flowers for easy mixing with food.
* A teaspoon of Coconut butter a day may be very helpful

DIARRHEA REMEDIES

Ongoing diarrhea can quickly cause severe dehydration and electrolyte loss, serious nutritional deficiencies and even **death**. It can be caused by a variety of health conditions, such as celiac disease, inflammatory bowel disease, colitis as well as unhealthy diet. Sugar, caffeine, gluten, very spicy food, as well as food high in fat may be too much for sensitive digestive system, especially in and elderly person.

REMEDIES:

* BRAT diet - a most effective diet that consists of bananas, rice, applesauce, and gluten-free toast
* Foods that are low in fat, starchy and help bulk up the stool.
* Avoid all fried, greasy, fatty or spicy foods, milk and dairy products, pork, veal, raw vegetables, salads and sugar for at least a few days or longer, if the problem persists.

FECAL IMPACTION

This condition occurs due to chronic constipation, when a hardened stool is stuck in the rectum. No bowel movement for three consecutive days, cramping, bloating and stool leakage are clear indicators. The most effective treatment is an enema, administered by a doctor who inserts a special fluid into the rectum to soften the stool.

IF LEFT UNTREATED, IT CAN CAUSE SEVERE DAMAGE OR EVEN DEATH. IF YOU CANNOT ADMINISTER ENEMA TO YOUR LOVED ONE, SEEK MEDICAL ASSISTANCE AS SOON AS POSSIBLE.

The best cure is prevention. If you are paying daily attention to regular elimination, you will prevent this from occurring. Keep in mind that remedies like extra fluid intake, fiber or even Swiss Kriss, will require at least a few hours to work.

HEMORRHOIDS

The elderly are more vulnerable and prone to this conditions for various reasons. A healthy digestion is the key to keeping your loved one healthy and avoiding this painful condition altogether.

THE BEST PREVENTATIVE MEASURE IS A HEALTHY DIET RICH IN FIBERS, WITH A WIDE SELECTION OF FRUITS AND VEGETABLES.

If your loved one already suffers from hemorrhoids, you can use soothing compresses infused with the herb Witch Hazel for help in reducing pain, itching and bleeding. The cooling effects of Aloe Vera gel may also be very helpful and offer some relief. Apply these natural remedies each time after washing or going to the bathroom.

A Sitz Bath - sitting bath - is also very soothing and effective. This can be managed with the help of a small Sitz Bath Tub, that can be placed on the toilet. This is excellent for hemorrhoids care. Make sure the water temperature is comfortable and add a small amount of Epsom salt to the water. Always consult with your doctor before beginning any treatment.

SKIN

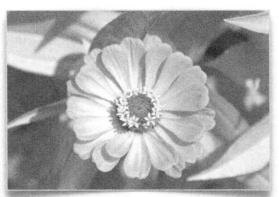

HEALTHY SKIN PROTECTS THE BODY FROM GERMS
AND IMPROVES THE OVERALL SENSE OF WELLBEING

When my Mother was bed bound at the end of her life, she was facing the real danger of getting bed sores. I set my alarm clock and woke up every few hours to make sure we prevented this from occurring. I went on a warpath against bed sores, and it was well worth it.

I changed my Mother's night gown every morning after shower and again in the evening before she went to sleep. In her last months during night sweats, I would change her additionally at least once, sometimes twice during the day or night, to assure she was always in pristine dry clothing and bedding. Until the end, she never suffered from a single bed sore. I encourage you to stay diligent with this, as it will eliminate so much unnecessary pain and suffering.

SKINCARE

Skin is the largest organ of our body and therefore requires special care. Your loved one's skin is especially vulnerable and more sensitive, since they are older and their thinner skin has lost elasticity and is easily punctured. Daily application of gentle natural or organic lotion, immediately after bath time and in the evening, will help maintain its elasticity. Applications of creams and lotions offer also a wonderful opportunity for a gentle massage of face, hands and feet. Create a special evening routine that includes this element of healing touch and observe the response from your loved one. If they enjoy it, you can use this at any time during the day, when they suffer from anxiety and need to calm down.

BED SORES

Bedsores or pressure sores are one of the most difficult health challenges for a chair-bound or bed-bound person. They can develop and progress very rapidly and are usually very difficult to heal. The moment an area becomes excessively reddish, pinkish and super thin skinned, you need to become a "skin watchdog." Once a bed sore occurs, it becomes a challenge to cure. If you are tedious, and really watch and tend to it, you will manage to heal it. But the better option is that you prevent it from forming in the first place. And that is definitely possible.

The causes for a bed sore manifestation are many; loss of blood supply to an area for two to three hours, poor skin elasticity and thinness due to old age, weight pressure in a specific area, natural thinness and loss of cushion to your bones, bad incontinence care, excessive wetness and general bad senior care hygiene. Bed sores tend to form on areas that are less padded with fat or muscle and are close to the bones. Usually they can appear on the spine, tailbone, shoulder blades, hips, elbows, head and even heels.

When the skin in a vulnerable area dies, it turns red, painful and eventually turns purple. The area breaks open and a sore forms, which can get infected if left unattended. If your loved one is suffering from bed sores, you need to seek immediate medical attention.

**ALL CARE MUST BE ENGAGED
TO PREVENT A BED SORE FROM INFECTING
AND RAPIDLY BECOMING WORSE.
A BEDSORE CAN DEVELOP IN A MATTER OF HOURS.**

BED SORE PREVENTION

To prevent bedsores from occurring in the first place, you can do the following:
* Maintain impeccably scrupulous incontinence care and body hygiene,
* Have your loved one sleep on medical sheepskin,
* Use soft specialty supportive devices that you can get in any medical supplies store,
* Never let your loved one lie in sweaty clothing for any length of time,
* Practice daily careful skin inspections,
* Be disciplined and insistent about implementing a daily healthy diet

No matter how exhausted you are and what ever else is going on, your loved one needs to be dry and clean at all times. Sloppy, slow and inconsistent incontinence care can cause tremendous suffering. If your loved one is wet, you need to change them immediately, do not wait. Every minute counts.

It is common knowledge, that a bed bound loved one in the late stage of illness is at a very high risk for developing bed sores. They need to be moved or repositioned every two hours. That is one tough assignment. First of all, if you are the only caregiver, that is difficult to endure on an ongoing basis during the night. Secondly, you loved one may not feel comfortable, when you reposition them to lying on the side. In that case, change the pad, and reposition them in the position where they are most comfortable, but with a slight variation, so the body weight is not pressing on the identical pressure points.

If you keep them impeccably dry at all times, it might be all right that they are not changing positions too much. Their comfort comes first. When you reposition them, make sure there are no clothing wrinkles, or bunched up sheets under their body. Check for any uncomfortable undergarment fabric or the edge of the pad, that may create a crease or indentation on the skin. Such attention to detail will help you prevent a bedsore.

Avoid having them lie directly on their hipbones and place support pillows for their optimal comfort under their knees, feet and elbows. Prevent knees and ankles from close contact of touching. Place a pillow in between knees. The head of the bed should not be elevated higher than a 30 degree angle, unless you are feeding them. If the head of the bed is too high, your loved one will be sliding down and putting more weight on the tailbone area. This will create the risk of friction on sensitive thin skin in backside-hip regions and very uncomfortable additional pressure on their tailbone. Always readjust their position on recliner or bed after a meal.

**ANOTHER EXCELLENT PREVENTATIVE MEASURE
FOR BED SORES IS MEDICAL SHEEPSKIN.**

The air flows through the natural wool fibers of medical sheepskin, so they can move with the body and provide a comfortable air cushion. Sheepskin will also help if your loved one suffers from backache, arthritis or rheumatism.

Place medical sheepskin directly on the bedsheet and under your loved one's back to assure good air access. Medical sheepskin will keep them warm in the winter, and help cool them down in the summer. It will prevent skin damage, that can easily and quickly occur thru excessive perspiration. You can order medical sheepskin thru any medical supplies stores. It is ideal to get at least two medical sheepskin pieces, one to be placed under the body and another one under legs. That way you also have the option of washing one if necessary, while you still have one left. Or you may get one long sheepskin piece that reaches from top to the bottom of your loved one's body. That way, their legs can also rest on sheepskin and provide them with optimal comfort. In either case, you need two sets of sheepskin, so that you may wash one and have a second set ready right away.

NO MATTER WHAT, NEVER ALLOW YOUR LOVED ONE TO LIE IN A SWEATY, MOIST NIGHTGOWN FOR ANY LENGTH OF TIME.

It doesn't matter what time of day or night it is or how inconvenient it may be. If your loved one is perspiring, immediately change their clothing and replace any and all moist sheets, pillow covers and bedding. They need to be in a nice dry bed with dry and soft clothing at all times.

When you loved one is in their final stage of life, these nightgown changes are much more frequent, sometimes every hour. This way you will successfully prevent bedsores and spare your loved one from unnecessary pain and suffering. Please see the special details for late stage care in Chapter *Final Weeks and Days*.

BED SORE REMEDIES

If your loved one is chair bound or bed bound, bed sores present real danger. Even if you are diligent about your loved one's hygiene, eventually you might notice a small, darker pinkish spot in an area. That is the beginning of a bed sore. It can occur in a matter of a few hours and if not treated right away, a bed sore can spread, expand and quickly burst creating a painful open wound.

As a preventative measure, at the first onset of redness, you need to immediately apply protective cream. I highly recommend CA- REZZ Cream which is available online or in health supply stores. Make sure you always have a few extra jars on hand. In addition to cream application, you need to change the incontinence pads or diapers at least every two to three hours around the clock. If you can prevent a sore and overcome this dangerous phase, you will avoid a very painful condition.

As fast as the beginning redness of a possible bedsore can appear, if preventative measures are taken immediately, the redness can also just as quickly disappear. You may need to watch out for them a night or two, but if you react right away, the sensitive darker pink spot will disappear.

IF YOU HAVE SUCCESSFULLY PREVENTED A BED SORE, YOU CAN LENGTHEN THE NIGHTTIME CHANGES TO EVERY FIVE HOURS. STICK WITH A THREE HOUR INCONTINENCE CHANGE SCHEDULE FOR ALL OTHER HOURS OF THE DAY.

If the bedsores persist and you cannot manage to do the increased nightly changes, there is a patch that your Hospice nurse can provide. It is a medicated plaster that you place over the bedsore to help keep it clean, while it heals. You can leave it on for up to 72 hours. So you do have options, but nothing will work better than making sure bed sores don't happen in the first place. Trust me, it is considerably easier to prevent a bed sore that get rid of it.

DRY SKIN

Elderly are especially prone to dry skin, therefore your choice of cream and lotion is very important. Select natural and organic products that are light and absorb easily. Keep in mind the skin is most absorbent when still moist immediately after washing, so apply it right away. If the skin is exceptionally dry in certain areas, use additional vitamin E hydrating creams, that will help heal any extra vulnerable dry spots. In addition, make sure your loved one's diet contains sufficient healthy fats that can be found in wild caught salmon, chia seeds, nuts, organic cheese, avocados, olive oil, coconut oil and flaxseed oil.

DRY FLAKY SCALP

It is quite common that your loved one may get extra flaky and scaly skin on their scalp. This could be the result of declining immune system, that is unable to prevent the spread of fungal growth over scalp. It may also be caused by insufficient rinsing after washing hair, an allergy to a harsh shampoo, or an eczema. First and foremost, use only extra mild hypoallergenic shampoo and make sure that you thoroughly rinse their hair after soaping up. Left-over residue of shampoo can quickly irritate the sensitive skin on the scalp. Next, after washing hair, apply a very small amount of Vitamin E oil to the still-most skin of the affected area and reapply regularly or at least once a day, until the flakiness disappears.

> THE HYPOALLERGENIC ECZEMA RELIEF CREAM FROM DERMAE HELPS RELIEVE FLAKY, SCALY AND ITCHY DRY SKIN ASSOCIATED WITH ECZEMA.

HYPERSENSITIVITY TO TOUCH

When your loved one is suffering from a cognitive condition called Agnosia, they can no longer identify different sensations. This may cause them great confusion, especially in every day situations such as bathing or toileting. They struggle with sensing the difference between hot and cold water on their skin, which can cause them to feel frightened and agitated. As a result, they may become resistant or difficult during basics body hygiene routines, showering and washing.

The best way to manage this problem is to use the communication skills as described in Chapter *The Mind communication*. Always inform them what you are about to do, ahead of every step. Approach them from the front, so they can see you and you can assure them with your very calm and steady voice and presence. It is imperative that you become well capable and swift in their physical care, especially when exposing their skin to water.

Minimize and expedite any activities that involve touching, such as undressing, washing, drying and applying cream. Touch them with high attention to their condition and be very gentle. Your hands must be warm and never cold. Accomplish the task swiftly and with confidence. Hold them firmly so they will not slip out of your hands, if acting defensively. Comfort them and encourage them, always describing what you intend to do or are doing. Immediately after bathing and dressing, place them in the recliner or bed and comfort them with their favorite small snack or a sip of tea, to help them calm down.

HANDS AND FEET

Elderly often suffer from cold, tingling or numbness in hands or feet. If their feet are swollen, it may be sign of edema. Many of these ailments can be caused by variety of factors including poor circulation.

THE BEST REMEDIES ARE:
- **Light, gentle movement**
- **Gentle massage**
- **Elevate the legs**
- **Compression socks**
- **Changes to diet by adding: ginger, pomegranate juice, cinnamon, fatty fish, beets, tumeric, leafy greens, citrus fruits, tomatoes and berries**
- **Eliminate all inflammatory foods, such a sugar or gluten**

FEET

Feet are often a source of discomfort. Your loved one could be experiencing leg cramps that extend all the way down to their toes. I suggest that you bathe their feet in a small sized lightweight plastic bucket, filled with room temperature warm water. Add a half a cup of pure apple cider vinegar. It will prevent any fungus from infesting the feet and will also heal many nail problems.

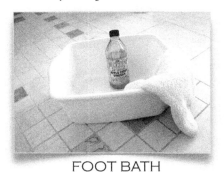

FOOT BATH   NAIL CARE TOOLS

NAIL FUNGUS

Many people, especially the elderly, often suffer from nail fungus. Everybody pretends they don't see it and women try to cover it up with a nail polish. That makes matters even worse. Nail fungus, like any other fungus, thrives in an acidic environment. That is why organic apple cider vinegar, which is alkaline, neutralizes and seriously impacts the spreading of nail fungus. If your loved one suffers from a long ignored nail fungus, do the following:

Soak their feet for at least three minutes in a mix of 1/2 cup organic apple cider vinegar and warm water foot bath. Next, clip the nails and gently file away as much of the top layer of the diseased dead nail as possible. Then apply a remedy solution made of Tea tree oil called ZETACLEAR - nail fungus treatment. It can be easily found in natural health food stores or online. You have to be rigorous and disciplined with this routine.

The toe nail clipping is done just once a week, but the fungus-removing maintenance program needs to be followed daily. That means; every day soak the feet in vinegar/water foot bath for a couple of minutes, and follow with the application of the remedy. Then continue with this regimen: once a week, clip the toe nails and file away the diseased top nail layer, followed by daily vinegar foot bath and daily application of the tincture.

Within approximately one month you will see a definite improvement and in about six months your loved one could have completely clear and healthy nails. Everyone's nails grow at a different pace, but eventually they do grow out. You will feel really proud that you have eliminated this pestering and ugly issue and your loved one's feet will be nice and healthy. This is another reminder that despite your loved one's extremely difficult illness, they can be otherwise exceptionally well maintained and optimally comfortable. This will make a decisive difference in their overall quality of life. And that is the ever important point!

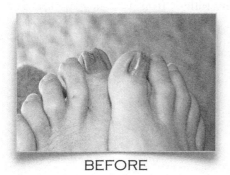

BEFORE

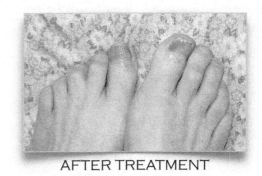

AFTER TREATMENT

CHAPTER TEN

Body Care

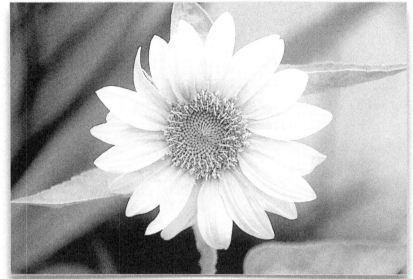

A BODY IS A GIFT THAT SHOULD BE LOVINGLY
CARED FOR, REGARDLESS OF AGE

*C*aring for my Mother was a task I performed with joy. She didn't much care for bathing and daily routine, so I tried to be as quick as possible, always talking to her and explaining everything that was going on, as we went along. I felt her frustration of having to depend on someone's help for her basic physical needs.

Whenever I let her know, that I understood her ridiculous predicament and was doing everything to make it quick, she calmed down. It made a difference to her, knowing that her evident frustration was understood.

At the end of each day when she was placed into her crisp clean, comfortable bed and I gently massaged her scalp, she looked completely serene and content. To me, she was the most beautiful person in the world. She had a perfect complexion and gorgeous hazel eyes.

Later, when I dimmed the lights and was about to leave her room, I always asked her is she was comfortable. She looked at me with a slightest smile she could muster up, made a tiny nod and whispered,"Yes."

I cherished those moments. They are forever engraved in my memory.

HYGIENE

One of the key elements to help maintain your loved one in an optimal condition, is good personal hygiene. In the beginning phases of this illness, the daily personal hygiene routine is often the biggest challenge. You loved one may resist you with all their might, so it will be a challenge to get anything accomplished. Now, while they are in the last phase and at home with you, this can become a more positive experience. You can manage to keep them very clean and fresh.

If your loved one or the room where they reside smells bad, it is a direct reflection of your poor hygiene and care. It indicates mediocre caregiving. Therefore, mastering the task of personal hygiene is an absolute priority. It is definitely possible to eliminate any and all foul odors with a completely incontinent person, if you remain diligent. I have often heard caregivers make ridiculous excuses why they don't want to wash someone thoroughly, their excuse being "because they smell bad." Can you believe this? It is the caregiver's duty to make sure the patient never smells bad!

MAKE IT VERY CLEAR TO YOUR CAREGIVERS THAT YOUR LOVED ONE NEEDS A GOOD WASH IN ALL REGIONS, ESPECIALLY AND OBVIOUSLY THE GROIN AREA. IF YOU ARE THE CAREGIVER, THIS IS YOUR FOREMOST PRIORITY.

My suggestion is, that you give your loved one a shower once a day. A normal person needs that and so does your loved one. Especially if they are incontinent. If your loved one is too weak to be moved to the bathroom and back, you may have to settle for a sponge bath in bed. I have never been fond of sponge baths, just because I know that the cleansing, relaxing and soothing effect a shower cannot compare to a sponge bath. But under certain circumstances, such as the last stage of life, a sponge bath is your best and only option.

Otherwise, shower your loved one in the morning, and if the day is without any major incontinence mishaps, you can just freshen them up in the evening before sleep time. Once your loved one is bedridden, they will mostly be sleeping anyway. It is better not to disturb them before nighttime, especially if they seem comfortable. Mornings are different and really require a good wash. If your loved one is bed ridden, but can still sit in the shower chair, give them a daily shower. Once your loved one is too weak to sit in the shower chair, you can clean them with a thorough sponge bath. See detailed instructions on how to give a sponge bath in Chapter *Final Weeks and Days - Body Care in The Last Stage.*

PREPARING THE BATHROOM

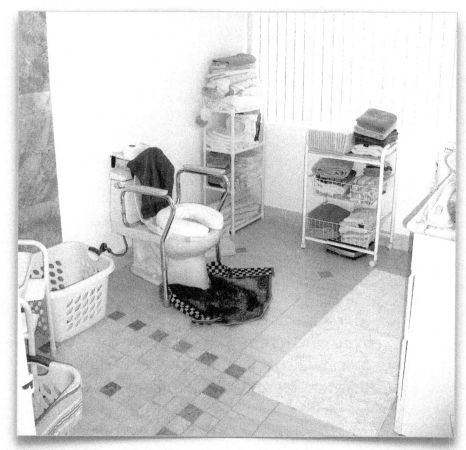

A WELL PREPARED BATHROOM WILL SIGNIFICANTLY EASE YOUR DAILY CARE

Take the time to get ready and have all the supplies in place. As you see in the picture, the toilet is prepared with toilet seat safety handles, so your loved one cannot fall off. There is a soft toilet seat cushion on top of the regular toilet seat, to make them more comfortable. There is a medium size towel covering the opened toilet seat cover, so the loved one's back does not get cold when they lean on it, or their fragile skin does not get bruised or punctured on the edge of the toilet seat cover. A towel on the floor around the toilet is there to catch any spillage, when washing the groin area with a small cup, which would be the case when you are not giving them a full shower. The bath has plenty of extra towels, two laundry baskets and a good supply of incontinence pads. When you have all this in place, you are ready to proceed effectively and swiftly.

HOW TO GIVE A MORNING SHOWER

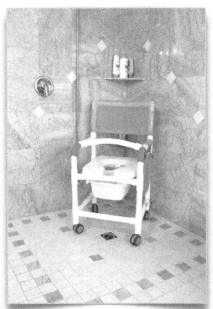

A GOOD QUALITY SHOWER CHAIR IS A NECESSITY

WHAT YOU NEED:

- 3 large bath towels
- face washcloth - pink color
- body washcloth - blue color
- hypoallergenic mild shower gel
- hypoallergenic body cream
- new incontinence pad
- clean incontinence mesh panties, if that is what you use
- fresh undergarments or first layer of clothes
- plastic gloves
- plastic trash bag for soiled incontinence pad
- bed sore prevention cream
- 2 smaller towels

WEAR APPROPRIATE CLOTHING AND NON-SLIPPERY RUBBER SHOES.
YOU WILL GET PARTIALLY DRENCHED.

PREPARE THE BATHROOM

✳ Prepare a small and a large towel and special bed sore preventing cream within easy reach after the showering is complete.

✳ All supplies are laid out in the bathroom easily accessible.

✳ Make sure the room and bathroom are at a comfortable temperature.

✳ No Air Conditioner turned on high or fans blowing directly on loved one.

✳ Put on the plastic gloves.

✳ Clean the loved one by removing the incontinence pad as described in the Chapter *Incontinence care*

IMPORTANT - SORE PREVENTION ON SHOWER CHAIR

Your loved one's skin is exceptionally vulnerable and can be easily bruised if you are not careful. Pay extra attention to this, as they can quickly get a sore by simply sitting on a hard toilet seat with rough edges, or leaning with full weight on the edge of the open toilet sit cover. Make sure they sit on an extra soft toilet seat cushion, and place soft towels on hard surfaces they may touch or lean on. A small wound, bruise or indentation can quickly turn into a big bedsore. If your loved one is frail and thin, you may need to place an additional cushion seat on the existing soft cushion of the shower chair. That way you will assure their optimal comfort and prevent any skin puncturing.

GETTING OUT OF BED AND PREPARING FOR SHOWER

Follow these steps:

✳ Place the shower chair alongside the bed and secure the wheels with safety brake locks.

✳ Slowly lift the upper body of your loved one into a sitting position on the bed, while supporting their back and neck.

✳ Gently turn them towards you, so both of their legs are off the bed.

✳ Stand sturdily with both of your feet firmly planted on the ground.

✳ Wait a few moments before transferring them with one calm and firm move onto the shower chair.

✳ Once they are sitting on the shower chair, secure them by closing the safety rail to prevent a fall.

✳ Now unblock the wheels and roll them into the bathroom where you have prepared all your supplies: plenty of fresh towels, soap, body cream, new pads and all fresh clothing for the new day.

- Place the shower chair with the back of the chair against the corner of the shower, so that your loved one is facing you.
- Now secure the chair's safety brake locks again. That will help assure stability and will ease your access to perform the shower.
- Place a non-slip rubber bathroom mat below your feet.
- Remove the loved one's nightgown or nightshirt.
- Place a small towel onto the back railing of the shower chair to assure soft comfort for their back. The slightest pressure of a hard backseat surface could easily bruise their frail back.
- Take the shower handle in your hand and turn on the water, while directing it away from your loved one.
- Test the water temperature on your upper hand. When proper water temperature is adjusted, you may begin with the shower.

THE SHOWER

Remember, this is not going to be a long episode. It must be performed gently but confidently, quickly and effectively.

- Begin by a quick rinse of the entire body.
- Then place the handheld shower into the side pocked of the shower chair. Do not turn the shower off until you are completely done. If you do, you would have to find and readjust the perfect temperature again, while your loved one sits waiting in the chair, getting cold. You would also waste more water by continuously searching for the perfect water temperature. By placing the shower head into the back net-pocket of the chair, you are also preventing an out of control shower head "attack" in your direction. It would be too bad if you end up just as wet as your loved one, while you're fully dressed.
- Next, quickly and gently soap up the body all over, especially under arms and in the lower region. You may use a natural sponge or small washcloth.
- Do not put soap on the perineum - the region between the thighs.
- Right away rinse off the soap very thoroughly and make sure you reach and rinse especially well.
- For the perineum/groin region you may use a gentle shower handle stream.
- Do not forget to slightly lean the loved one forward while you securely hold them, and thoroughly rinse the back of their body.
- Do not spend long time in one area of the body, while they get cold in other parts.

- Keep moving the shower handle to assure they are continuously kept warm.
- Before you finish, quickly rinse a once over so the entire body feels nice and warm.
- When the shower is over, you can open the front safety rail bar on the chair.
- Now you are ready to towel dry.
- Never rub the skin, instead only gently pat dry.
- Immediately apply skin lotion while skin is still moist for optimal absorbency.
- Wipe off any wetness on shower chair to assure the entire body is nice and dry.
- Remove the small wet towel from the back of the seat.
- The only wet area now remains the seat and under the buttocks.

DRESSING

You are now ready to dress your loved one into a new set of fresh clothes for the day.
- Begin by dressing the upper area of the body, so that they don't feel exposed for too long, and are kept nice and warm.
- Now place the mesh undergarment that holds the incontinence pad in place thru both feet and pull it up above the knees, onto the mid-thigh area.
- Prepare the pad and place it between legs while the loved one is still sitting.
- Reach for the small and a large towel and the special bed sore preventing cream for the backside - buttocks.
- Stand in front of the chair and place both your loved one's feet on the floor.
- Carefully but firmly place your hands under their arms and lift them up into a standing position.
- You are continuously holding them in an embrace.
- They are facing you.
- Quickly take the prepared small towel and very gently pat - dry their backside.
- Apply a small amount of sore prevention cream on the buttocks.
- Pull up the prepared undergarment with incontinence pad in place.
- Place the larger dry towel on the seat of the chair.
- Now gently lower them back onto the shower chair.
- They are now ready for transfer to the recliner where you can easily finish dressing them into comfortable day clothing — sweat pants, or if they are in bed, a nightgown or a nightshirt.

CHAIR BOUND VERSION

If this version of standing them up seems too difficult or cannot be done, then use a different approach:

- ❋ Prepare a regular wheelchair next to the shower chair.
- ❋ Place a soft cushion onto the wheelchair seat for better comfort.
- ❋ Transfer them onto the wheelchair.
- ❋ While you are transferring them from shower chair to wheel chair, gently but quickly pat dry the behind.
- ❋ Apply sore preventing cream to their buttocks.
- ❋ Pull up the mesh undergarment with pad properly in place.

You can also apply a small amount of protective bedsore cream directly onto the pad before you dress them. Spread it thinly in the area that touches the most delicate and vulnerable part of the buttocks, where a sore could most likely appear. That way, you have saved yourself and them some standing time, when you would be applying the cream to their buttocks. In these situations, every second counts. After you are done, roll them to the recliner for their breakfast.

BED BOUND VERSION

If they are bed bound, use this approach:

- ❋ Move them on the rolling shower chair to the bed
- ❋ Place a disposable bed pad on the bed for protection.
- ❋ Transfer them back onto the bed
- ❋ Do the entire change of diaper or pad while they are lying down on the bed.

CAREFULLY CHOOSE THE VERSION THAT IS SAFEST AND MOST COMFORTABLE FOR YOUR LOVED ONE AND EASIEST FOR YOU.

IMPORTANT - PREVENTING IMMEDIATE INCONTINENCE MISHAP!

Keep in mind, the most challenging part is when you are drying their buttocks, applying cream and pulling the incontinence pad properly in its place. If you are too slow, they could have an immediate incontinence accident. In such a case, you would need to use a washcloth to rinse the soiled area again, and then proceed with applying cream and again securing a new clean incontinence pad into proper position. I suggest you tackle this part right away after the shower while they are still in the shower chair. This way a chance of an immediate accident is least possible.

HOW TO PLACE LOVED ONE ON THE TOILET

This is an important order to follow:
* Place handrails on the side of the toilet for safety.
* Place a towel around the base of the toilet for spillage.
* Place a smaller towel on the open toilet seat cover, to protect loved one's bare skin.
* Place toilet seat cushion on top of the regular toilet seat.
* Place your loved one on the toilet seat.
* Be very gentle when wiping.
* Always wipe them front to back.
* Check for hemorrhoids regularly. If that is an issue, read the Chapter *Remedies for Common Ailments.*

NO SHOWER - PARTIAL BODY WASH

If you do not feel the need to give your loved one a full body shower every day, you may wash various areas of their body with a washcloth.

IMPORTANT:
These are the steps for washing your loved one's groin area without taking a full shower:
* Place a towel around the base of the toilet for spillage.
* Place a smaller towel on the open toilet seat cover, so your loved one does not lean on plastic with bare skin.
* Place your loved one on the toilet seat.
* Fill small plastic measuring cup with warm water .
* Pour over their groan area from front and back.
* Repeat a few times.

**THE GROIN AREA SHOULD BE WASHED EVERY MORNING AND EVENING.
FOR PARTIAL BODY WASH, USE A SMALL PLASTIC MEASURING CUP.**

HAIR AND SCALP

You need to wash your loved one's hair at least once a week. While performing the morning shower, simply add the hair washing part.

Prepare a mild hypoallergenic shampoo and conditioner and soap up the scalp and hair once or twice as needed. Leave the conditioner in hair while you are washing the rest of the body.

Be very careful and avoid getting any soap into their eyes by tightly holding your hand on their forehead, gently covering their eyes with one hand, while rinsing the hair with the other.

Simply rinse hair and body at the same time in the end of the showering.

Always use mild baby hypoallergenic shampoo and conditioner for appropriate hair type. Elderly people tend to have a dry scalp and brittle hair, so chose accordingly.

MAKE SURE THERE IS NO SHAMPOO RESIDUE LEFT ON SCALP THAT COULD IMMEDIATELY CAUSE A DRY, SCALING AND ITCHY SCALP. RINSE VERY WELL.

Use gentle towel dry and finish up blow-drying after they are safely seated in recliner or in bed. Place a protective towel on the shoulders to avoid any wetness.

By all means, avoid all drafts while your loved one has wet hair or they may catch a cold. Do everything you can to prevent that from happening. If you are quick and thorough, everything should go smoothly and your loved one will feel wonderful and refreshed.

If scalp becomes dry at any point, immediately apply some soothing cream. You could use anything from vitamin E, aloe, chamomile to jojoba cream or a mild natural oil. If the problem persist and worsens, get the advice of your family physician or medical professional.

SKIN CARE

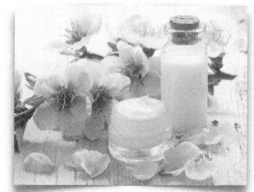

SELECT NATURAL, HYPOALLERGENIC
AND ORGANIC SKINCARE PRODUCTS

Skin is a great indicator of our overall state. When we are dehydrated, it will lose its elasticity and luster. Dehydration is often a challenge with elderly, but when properly addressed, it can be quickly corrected. Of course the first step towards great healthy skin is proper hygiene.

Whenever the body is showered or washed, you need to apply a moisturizer right away while the skin is still moist and absorbency is good. Body lotion needs to be applied at lest once a day, preferably in the morning. If the skin is extra dry in certain regions, you need to keep moisturizing it throughout the day.

Use hypoallergenic, perfume-free, skin sensitive, especially formulated for-dry-skin lotions. Avoid excessively perfumed lotions. For the delicate areas like the behind, you will need special cream that promotes bed sore prevention, redness, dryness or wounds. There are a quite a few on the market, I personally prefer CaRezz. Use it very sparingly, but regularly. It is also great for any other areas that are sensitive, problematic and vulnerable for an open sore. Vitamin E cream from DermaE is also excellent.

Creams for face and neck are also important. Gently wash your loved one's face at least every morning and evening with a facial washcloth. Keep a supply of specific color washcloths only for facial use. A light facial cream should be applied to the face and neck area. If your loved one has super dry hands, feet or heels, address those areas and assure that they are properly moisturized at all times. Find more suggestions for dry skin in Chapter *Holistic Caregiving Remedies.*

THE MOUTH

Another great indicator of overall microbalance in the body, is the oral cavity. Very often the elderly patients sleep with their mouths open. Because they do not tend to swallow regularly, it can create a few problems in the mouth cavity. They may have excess mucus that hardens on the walls of oral cavity during the night.

To clean the mouth with an astringent is a big mistake. You could instantly create a large raw sore and your loved one would suffer greatly. It would drastically affect their ability to eat and may be detrimental to their overall state. Every detail of your loved one's care matters and when you are tedious and alert about any changes, you can balance and immediately help remedy the problem.

It might be suggested to use special rubbing alcohol cotton swabs - Q tips to help keep the oral cavity clean. But in case of morning dry and mucus filled mouth, **I strongly discourage you from using the swabs.** The cotton swabs contain rubbing alcohol and that can be very damaging to the already sensitive skin inside the oral cavity. Instead, you need to balance the mouth flora as soon as possible.

FIRST THING IN THE MORNING UPON AWAKENING, GIVE YOUR LOVED ONE 1 TEA-SPOON OF COCONUT BUTTER.

That will help soothe, oil, cleanse and moisten the oral cavity. Then you can proceed with balancing the ph balance in the mouth.

The one remedy that truly is miraculous is organic kefir drink. Kefir is prepared by inoculating cow, goat, or sheep's milk with kefir grains which are a combination of body friendly bacteria, yeasts, proteins, lipids and sugars. Kefir has many antioxidant properties, and can be used to prevent oxidative damage in the human body. Kefir also aids in lactose digestion.

When you want to avoid milk products, use kefir drinks that are made with milk substitutes such as almond milk, soy milk, rice milk and coconut milk. Kefir can be found in any food store. Have a kefir drink always available for your loved one. A half a cup of kefir drink will almost immediately repair and help maintain a healthy balance in the oral cavity. After the tiny spoon of butter, it should be the very first thing in the morning, that you offer them.

The oral cavity is the source of all sorts of dangerous bacteria. In fact there have been quite a few studies conducted on direct adverse effect of the periodontal disease on healthy brain function.

PERIODONTAL DISEASE IS ONE OF MANY CAUSES OF DEMENTIA.

I cannot stress enough how important it is to keep your loved one's teeth as clean as possible. You can be almost certain that if your loved one has dementia, their teeth and gums are not in good shape and most likely have not been for quite a while. Regular and professional teeth cleaning is very important, although it may not be possible for a dementia patient.

If your loved one wears dentures make sure the hygiene is diligent and regular. If your loved one has no teeth it is better to avoid using dentures, as they will only collect food and become a nightmare to clean and could present a very serious health problem. By keeping removable dentures in the mouth at night you are especially magnifying the possibility of a serious bacterial infection.

It is simple to blend all foods when preparing meals for your loved one and makes it also easier to digest. Keep whatever teeth they still have clean and keep a check on maintaining healthy gums. At this point, it is healthier to avoid dentures and keep everything as clean as possible.

If you decide to have your loved one keep the dentures during the day, then you must remove them before they go to bed and clean them every single night.

DEMENTIA PATIENTS OFTEN REFUSE TO WEAR THEIR DENTURES WHICH IS FINE. THE CLEANER AND BACTERIA FREE MOUTH, THE BETTER FOR THEM.

LIPS

When you spoon-feed you loved one, there is always a chance that it might get a bit messy. Unless your timing is perfect in coordinating your spoon with their opening the mouth, you will have a spill or some dripping.

Out of a habit, you will wipe the lips with a napkin or correct the spillage with the spoon. That adds extra wear on your loved one's lips. You must not wipe them each time, no matter how crazy it drives you.

BY CONSTANTLY WIPING YOUR LOVED ONE'S LIPS WHILE THEY ARE HAVING MISHAPS WHEN EATING, THE DELICATE SKIN ON THEIR LIPS WILL GET IRRITATED. THIS COULD RESULT IN SWELLING, RAW AND CRACKED LIPS.

To avoid this from occurring you need to regularly apply a mixture of soft organic lip balm. The lip balm in stick form is too hard and could damage the lips. I suggest you cut and crush the lip-balm stick into small pieces and mix them into a paste, then add some coconut butter for easier application.

APPLY THE NATURAL LIP SOOTHING BALM THROUGHOUT THE DAY.

Apply lip balm first thing in the morning, every time after each feeding, anytime during the day that you notice the lips getting a bit dry and especially in the evening, before putting them to bed.

By constantly moisturizing the lips you will assure comfortable eating and prevent lips from drying or chapping. Another important detail is to always use a small spoon when feeding. Large spoons can further damage the sensitive and dry lips or mouth corners. Do not dismiss this as less important. Every small detail matters and helps complete a perfect care regimen.

EARS AND NOSE

A good caregiver has to be paying attention to every detail of body care, which includes proper hygiene of ears and nose. After you washed your loved one's hair, it is a good idea to gently clean their ears as well. The outer ear is the part of the ear that can be seen and it includes the earlobe as well as the edges of the opening to the ear canal. It is safe to clean and should be part of regular hygiene routine.

Gently wipe the outer ear and behind the ear. Cotton swabs can be used to clean the folds of the outer ear. It is not recommended that you insert a cotton swab into the ear canal. This can push the wax further into the ear as well as damage the inner ear.

IF THE EARLOBES ARE DRY, APPLY HYPOALLERGENIC LOTION, VITAMIN E CREAM, OR A VERY SMALL AMOUNT OF COCONUT OIL.

When it comes to cleaning the nose, we often forget the simple luxury we have as a healthy person, to blow our nose. The ideal option would be if your loved one could blow their nose with your help. You can ask them to blow through the nose, while you hold the prepared handkerchief on their nose.

However, it is most likely that at this late stage of the illness, your loved one cannot blow their nose by themselves. It is therefore very important that you help them keep the air passageway clear. If the nose is not cleaned, your loved one will constantly breathe thru their mouth, which will among other things create a lot of difficulty when eating and sleeping.

First thing is to maintain nicely moisturized air in your loved one's room and prevent very dry air, which could cause the nose stuffiness to harden and that's really difficult to deal with. In the Chapter *Preparing Your home*, I describe the proper way to keep the air ion the room humid with an air purifier or humidifier. That should help a bit.

The best time to clean the nose is immediately after the shower, when nostrils are still wet.

FOR EASIEST AND MOST HYGIENIC WAY TO CLEAN THE NOSE PASSAGES, YOU WILL NEED A NOSE ASPIRATOR.

Usually you can find it in the baby section at the drugstore. The newest versions of nasal aspirator use disposable reservoir nozzles. The disposable tips have been specially designed to eliminate bacteria build-up inside the mechanism to safeguard users from potentially harmful germs.

With standard nasal bulb syringes, germs get trapped and can remain inside the syringe after use, even after they are rinsed. With the nose aspirator all you need to do is simply replace the disposable, flexible silicone reservoir nozzle tips after use. It is definitely worth getting an aspirator, to avoid all the unpleasantness with this task and make your loved one as comfortable as possible, while ensuring clear nasal passages at all times. Read Chapter *Holistic Home Remedies* for the photo of the nasal aspirator.

If you do not have the nose aspirator, take a small soft paper handkerchief and moisten in with warm water. Gently insert it the slightest bit into the nostril, turn and pull out. Chances are you will manage to remove an unwanted bugger. Repeat if necessary. Always explain to your loved one, what you are doing and how important this is.

It is very sad when nobody bothers to wipe the nose of an elderly person. How torturous is it to live with a permanently stuffy nose? Do everything you can, to help them ease this discomfort.

If your loved one develops a cold, you need to repeat this procedure a few times a day. If you keep wiping their nose with a Kleenex, make sure that they do not develop a raw red rash under the nose. Always apply some gentle coconut oil or vitamin E cream lightly around the nostrils to keep the area moisturized.

HANDS

Pampering your loved one's hands and feet presents a perfect opportunity to help calm them down, enjoy physical attention of touch and help them feel loved. Use daily applications of a hypoallergenic lotion to assure their hands and feet are never dry or have cracked skin. Because your loved one is not using their hands for daily activities, their hands become very soft and beautiful.

NAILS

Your loved one's nails will most likely grow easily. Nails need to be clipped and filed at least once a week, so they are smooth, short and clean. This will help prevent any unnecessary scratching injuries to your loved one, as well as yourself. In their helpless state, they often swing their hands all about, grab onto anything they can, or unintentionally scratch. The best opportunity to trim the nails is after shower, when they are soft and easy to trim or clip. Apply lotion to hands and always keep them clean and well moisturized.

If your loved one suffers from nail fungus on their hands, use the technique and remedies described in Chapter *Holistic Caregiving Remedies*.

FEET

The feet lose calluses and all their require is a regular moisturizer. Make sure the socks your loved one wears are breathable and preferably made of cotton and do not have a tight elastic. If your loved one suffers also from diabetes, it is extra important to keep their feet in absolute top shape, clean and free of any infections, injuries, unkempt broken nails or nail fungus.

Every day, place the feet into a small bucket, add warm water and a 1/2 cup of organic apple cider vinegar. Soak the feet for a couple of minutes. This will help prevent growth of any bacteria and nail fungus. Trim the toe nails at least once a week.

If your loved one suffers from nail fungus on their toenails, which is very common, you can find the detailed description how to help effectively eliminate this condition once and for all with natural remedies. Follow the technique and remedies described in Chapter *Holistic Caregiving Remedies*.

PHYSICAL MOVEMENT

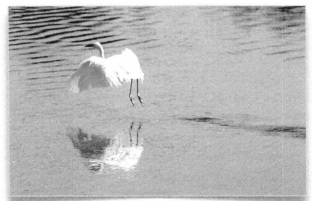

MOTION IS HEALING FOR THE BODY, MIND AND SPIRIT

When my Mother lived in a nursing home for a while, I took her to a beautiful park every day and drove her around in her wheelchair. Sometimes she would get out of her chair and take a very short walk, while I supported her. She seemed to enjoy it.

But in the late stage of her illness when she lived again in our home, she preferred sitting in her recliner and enjoying the tranquility of beautiful nature that surrounded her. She wasn't much interested in the walker neither. She was way too independent for that. The walker frustrated her.

However, I encouraged her daily walk in our garden and she kept it up for quite a long time. She needed assistance of two, one on each side, or one strong person that could offer sufficient support. I walked with her often alone. We would make a big circle around the edge of the rose garden and then return to her room. She could not look at the flowers very much. The walk took much concentration and energy out of her.

Eventually, her daily walks became shorter. We walked to the bathroom and back, but towards the end, she did not want to do that either. She was too tired and weak. I respected her wishes and did not push her. Even when her speech and communication ability was very limited, I always asked her beforehand, if she wanted to walk for a bit or go out into the garden. But she preferred to remain content in her recliner, gazing at the garden roses from afar and eating her favorite food - steamed fish.

I always respected her wishes and preferences, so she still kept some control of her life. It consoled and calmed her.

THE IMPORTANCE OF MOVEMENT

One cannot assume, that just because a person is chair or bed-bound, they do not require any exercise. In fact, regular gentle movement is even more important for maintaining their overall state of health and comfort. Certainly they will not be able to exercise on their own. However with gentle assistance, your loved one could retain basic mobility and flexibility to help them feel as comfortable and pain-free as possible.

Keep in mind that over time, sitting or lying down in a restricted or stagnant position can become very painful. Muscles constrict and cause discomfort even with the smallest movements that are necessary for proper caregiving.

> **REGULAR MUSCLE STRETCHING, LOW INTENSITY STRENGTHENING AND GENTLY ASSISTED RESISTANCE EXERCISES WILL HELP PREVENT MUSCLE LOSS - ATROPHY, MUSCLE CRAMPING AND DIMINISHED FUNCTIONAL CAPACITY.**

Gentle exercise will also contribute to a better functioning digestive system, which is essential for an overall healthy physical state. Always keep a log on any physical activity that you undertake with your loved one, such as a short walk in the garden, inside the home, or simply a few steps in their room. Even standing upright when getting changed, will offer an opportunity for a brief back and posture exercise. Keep track of their physical abilities and decline.

WALKING

While your loved one can still use a walker, assist them in actively using it at least a few times a day. When this ability diminishes with time, encourage them to hold on to the walker while standing, when you change their incontinence pad. It will make your job much easier and will also help them maintain a certain level of physical strength. In late stage dementia, your loved one's ability to walk will decline and eventually diminish. However, even when they are chair or bed-bound and can no longer stand, you can still help them maintain a level of physical comfort by gently moving their arms and legs and incorporating a hands-on gentle massage. The goal is to keep them as pain free as possible and help them retain some level of flexibility, even if they are very limited in movement.

USING A WALKER

No matter what the circumstance, you should definitely have a walker as part of necessary and required equipment. Preferably select the kind that is light weight, folds up and can be easily put away. A walker can be helpful with various changes throughout the day, when you are changing the incontinence pad or while they are on a recliner. It will make it easier if they manage to stand up, hold on to the walker, while you quickly change the pad and clean up. So a walker is very valuable and multifunctional.

If your loved one was more active in the past, you might have gotten them a really high quality walker with rollers and a small seat. As the illness progresses, a basic walker is sufficient for all your needs. If it has rollers on the front two legs, they need to have safety brakes. I recommend a basic walker with no rollers. Keep in mind that your loved one's needs or walking capacity can change daily and you need to keep a close eye on the situation. It could be from one day to the next that suddenly they can no longer safely use the walker.

If they have a desire to walk for a bit around the house or garden, never let them out of your hands! It all seems well, until that unexpected fall occurs and then your loved one will suffer and have to struggle with healing an injury and the care will instantly become much more demanding. So if your loved one would like to take a walk, by all means encourage them. If you are a tall and strong and they are smaller and lightweight, you will manage just fine. But if they are taller and heavier than you, I recommend that you have someone help you.

If they walk just a few steps in their room, you may manage to do it alone, but need to be securely standing in front of them, holding them firmly with both arms and guiding them. You are walking backwards while they walk forward. Use this only for very short distances of a few steps to and from bathroom or when going to bed.

A WALKER CAN BE A VERY HELPFUL TOOL, ESPECIALLY IF YOU ARE THE ONLY CAREGIVER. ALWAYS HAVE IT ON STANDBY TO HELP YOU KEEP THE LOVED ONE STANDING.

Never wander too far from your loved one, in case they get a sudden wave of weakness, lose coordination or suffer from a sudden motor block. I encourage you to keep your loved one mobile as long as possible, but once they do not enjoy it, want it and obviously fight it; you should respect their wish and let them be.

Eventually it will be more and more difficult for them to walk, such is the usual progress of this illness. Always be prepared for a change. When they can no longer walk or use the walker, you will be moving them about the room with a foldable, lightweight and narrow wheelchair that will easily pass through any doorway. When not in use it can be simply folded and put away.

STANDING

If your loved one can remain standing while supporting themselves with a walker, encourage them to do this for a few minutes each day. This simple standing position is excellent for keeping the strength in abdominal and back muscles for better posture and comfortable sitting.

SIT AND STAND EXERCISE

A simple sitting and getting up movement repeated a few times a day is a very useful exercise, for maintaining the muscle strength that is needed for essential activities, such as using the toilet or getting in and out of chair and bed. Keep it a regular part of day movement for as long as possible.

BALANCING EXERCISE

If your loved one is still able to stand, encourage them to stand on one leg while holding on to the walker or you, and then repeating the movement with the other leg. This is a very simple exercise to help maintain a sense of balance. Keep in mind that this illness usually causes a loss of coordination, so they may not be able to do that. Certainly in late stage that will probably not be possible.

MAINTAINING FLEXIBILITY

If you leave your loved one in a sitting position the entire day, where they do not move at all, imagine how painful their joints and muscles will feel, when you have to move them. They could suffer from cramps as well as joint and muscle stiffness.

You can help preserve their flexibility by gently exercising their legs with simple exercises. While they are sitting in their recliner, gently pick up one foot, lift it a few inches and slowly help them stretch and bend the knee. Repeat that gently and slowly between 5-10 times with each leg and pay attention to their level of comfort. If they feel any kind of discomfort, immediately stop.

Next, do a similar exercise with the arms. Take your loved one's hands into your own and lift them up so they are comfortably extended forward at the level of their waist. Now gently bend and stretch the arms 5-10 times and observe their level of comfort. If they are receptive and comfortable, continue. If you see any signs discomfort, immediately stop. Do not rush, stay calm, gentle and always encourage them.

STRETCHING

This is the easiest level of exercise. It can be practiced while your loved one is sitting or lying down. Take your loved one's foot in your hand, gently bend their knee and lift it up towards their chest. Then gently stretch the leg, never forcing, and again bend their knee, and slowly lower it back into original position.

> **ALWAYS BE EXTREMELY CAREFUL WITH ALL MOVEMENTS.**
> **NEVER FORCE, BUT SIMPLY MAINTAIN**
> **THE LEVEL OF FLEXIBILITY THAT IS PRESENT.**

If flexibility is poor, then just do the movement in the space of comfort. Practice this stretching exercise with each leg. Next, move up to the arms. Take their right hand into yours and gently help stretch the arm all the way up and again back down. Then slowly bend and again stretch it. Never force the movement beyond the comfort zone. Repeat on the left side. This daily exercise may take only a few minutes, but will help keep their muscles supple.

BODY MASSAGE

Massage can be practiced at any time, but can be especially useful during the late stage of illness. However, if your loved one suffers from Hypersensitivity to touch, massage can be only administered in a very limited way. Learn more in Chapter *Holistic Caregiving Remedies - Skin*.

If your loved one enjoys massage, you can simply begin by applying some mild lotion and massaging their hands and feet any time during the day. In fact, you can make this a part of your daily or evening routine.

For example:
* You can massage their hands while getting them ready for the day
* After the morning shower routine
* After breakfast so they can relax and take a nap
* When they are resting in their recliner
* While they are in bed before going to sleep for the night
* Anytime you need to help eliminate agitation, anxiety, restlessness, discomfort or any kind of emotional upset

You can extend the massage area to their upper arms, and when sitting, all the way up to their shoulders and neck area. Use elongated, extremely gentle and caressing movement. In addition, you may extend the foot massage further up and gently work through their calf muscles, which have a tendency to cramp. It may be helpful to use some soft background music as a soothing element which will further help them to relax.

CORRECT SITTING POSITION

When your loved one spends most of their day in a recliner or bed, they need to be dressed appropriately and require a few extra comfort aids. Follow these suggestions:

- Cover the chair with a protective washable pad at all times.
- Place a paper disposable pad on top of it and change daily or as needed.
- Make sure your loved one is dressed in loose comfortable clothing, nothing to tight at the waist, ankles or arms.
- They will not be wearing shoes or slippers while on the chair.
- Have a few soft blankets ready for covering them when they are taking a nap or you are airing out the room.
- Even if you have a most comfortable recliner, it is advisable you add a few extra small pillows for their optimal comfort.
- One small neck pillow or very narrow pillow for under their head and neck.
- Two small pillows that you can place under their elbows. You need to avoid too much pressure on any bony parts of the body, so support them with soft cushions.
- You may need another pillow for under their knees.

Sitting in the chair the entire day can become difficult on your loved one's back. If it is comfortable to do so, move them slightly about, side to side and gently massage their back and upper shoulders. Help them stretch the knees for a bit and then return the pillow under the knees.

YOU MAY NEED TO CONTINUOUSLY PULL YOUR LOVED ONE UPWARDS ESPECIALLY IF THEY ARE SLIDING DOWN IN THE CHAIR OR EXTENSIVELY SLOUCHING.

HOW TO CORRECT SLIDING FROM CHAIR

Stand securely behind the recliner and lean over to reach your loved one. Place your hands from behind - under their armpits - and gently pull them upwards so that their hips are properly repositioned at the back of the seat. Be careful, very gentle and use one strong and firm motion to accomplish this.

IMPORTANT TIP

Make sure that with this move, the clothing of your loved on is not in any way crinkled or gathered at their back or under their hips as this could create great discomfort or possible bed sore. Smooth out the material and strengthen everything out so they are comfortable.

If your loved on is slouching, immediately move and readjust the positioning on the recliner. Avoid extreme slouching or their head hanging in one direction and straining their neck muscles or otherwise creating discomfort. The neck support pillows that are often used on the planes are ideal for supporting the head.

Remember, your loved one's situation will be changing daily. Their muscles will weaken and with time it will be difficult for them to hold up their head. You must prevent any painful and cramped position they may slide into. Become in tune with their physical positioning and use common sense when searching for a source of their potential discomfort. No matter how helpless they are and look somewhat comfortable in a slouched position, do not be fooled.

> **BY ALLOWING THE HEAD TO HANG IN ONE DIRECTION,
> THE WEIGHT OF IT WILL STRETCH THE NECK MUSCLES
> ON ONE SIDE AND CRAMP THEM ON THE OTHER.
> THAT CAN CAUSE SEVERE PAIN AND SERIOUSLY RESTRICT MOBILITY.
> THIS CAN OCCUR IN ONE DAY!**

Be diligent and continuously prop them up and rearrange the pillows so that they always sit as straight and as comfortable as possible. Surround them with cushions and small pillows. Remember, even a few hours of wrong sitting position can cause a lot of harm. If you have a caregiver, remind them to watch and correct the posture if needed, especially when you are not present.

TRANSFERING

DAY TO DAY TRANSFERRING

Here are a few extra tips for when you are preparing to move your loved one for an outing, move them about the room or around your house and transferring then from bed to shower chair or wheel chair. What may seem easy to do is not, and you need to be properly prepared.

LUMBAR SACRAL SUPPORT SAFETY BELT

I suggest that you get yourself a wide lumbar-sacral support safety belt that will protect your back. Yes, this is the belt that is usually used by professional movers. You will be dealing with dead weight and your back will be the first thing to go. And you cannot afford that.

PREPARE AHEAD OF TIME

Always take your time and well prepare the area where you are moving your loved one to next. If you are moving them from shower chair to the bed, have the bed completely prepared and ready for them. Under no circumstances is it advisable to transfer them and then start looking around the room for proper bed pads and so on.

KEEP AN EYE IN YOUR LOVED ONE AT ALL TIMES

It may seem like they are sitting safely in their chair and are completely inactive, but the moment you turn away, or God forbid, walk out of the room to get something, they could lean forward and fall headfirst to the ground. I need not say more. Never leave your loved one unattended, unless they are secured in their chair. For example; the shower chair has a safety bar that prevents falling out.

HANDICAP PARKING PERMIT

When transporting your loved one to a doctor visit, you need to have every detail covered. If you are driving them to any appointments yourself, it is essential that you have the handicap-parking permit, so you will have easy access to any entrance of the building and the closest parking option.

SUPPLIES FOR ON THE GO

You need to carry with you an extra set of garments in case of an incontinence mishap. Everything that you might need to change them must be in your shoulder bag. In case they are hungry and get easily agitated when surrounded by too many people, you could have their favorite small snack, which will help calm them down. Bananas are great for that.

GET SOME HELP

I suggest that when you need to take your loved one out of the house, you do not do so all alone. If at all possible, have some help. It is simply easier with an extra pair of hands. Keep in mind, a seemingly simple outing with your loved one in tow, will take your whole day and will most likely require equal amount of energy as if you were sprinting around the block ten times.

TRANSFERRING BETWEEN CHAIR AND BED

These are the steps of easy and safe transfer:
- Wear your back support belt at all times.
- Prepare the areas for transfer.
- Stand firmly on the ground with feet slightly apart.
- The wheelchair and bed should be as close as possible.
- Use the manual wheelchair brake to prevent it from rolling away from you.
- Your body should be facing your loved one.
- You are looking straight ahead between the two transfer areas.
- Avoid turning your body as little as possible while lifting, holding and transferring.
- Lift your loved one up by placing your arms under their armpits. Securely and confidently lift them up with one motion.
- Move them to the designated area and gently set them down.
- Avoid turning your body in the waist area.
- Remain with your torso as one unit and turn your entire body with hips still aligned the same way with the shoulders. You will prevent a back injury, straining, pulling muscles or losing your balance.
- Practice on your own first.

CHAPTER ELEVEN

Incontinence Care

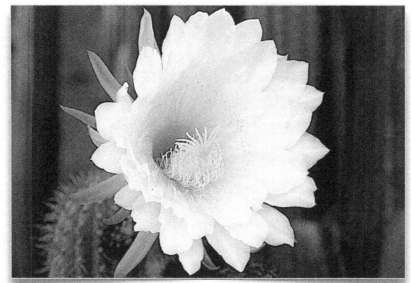

THE LOSS OF CONTROL OF BODILY FUNCTIONS ROBS US
OF INDEPENDENCE, SELF-RELIANCE AND FREEDOM

*W*hen Dad and I prepared for bringing my Mom to live with us at home, I got a simple instruction from the head nurse in the facility where Mom was staying up till then. She said: "At 11pm each night, just change her one last time, as simple as that."

I felt a voice in the back of my mind go off with a lingering feeling, that it will be up to me to do that each night. Brushing the daunting thought away as fast as I could, I consoled myself with the fact that I hired a professional live-in caregiver, who was going to help me with all these chores.

When we finally arrived to our new home in California with Mom in tow, we had endured a long transatlantic flight and were exhausted beyond words. A new caregiver - hired thru a professional highly reputable agency - was waiting for us in the new house. I kindly asked he to change my Mother right away. She hesitated for a moment and then came up with this question: "Can you show me how you do that?"

My heart skipped a beat as I faced the harsh reality. It was going to be my job and I had to learn it the hard way, without instructions. It was not the end of the world, but it was not a piece of cake either. Years later, after I trained numerous caregivers on that specific task, I go it down to a science and was so fast and thorough, that my sweet Mother never suffered from a single bed sore. I am very happy about that. Yes, little things in life can make us happy.

And oh yes, the original caregiver quit the next day. She said it was "Just too much for her." I guess she didn't like my cooking, plus she wanted a bigger bed in her room. Go figure.

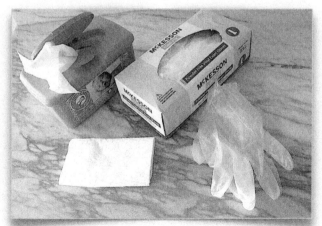

BABY WIPES, PLASTIC GLOVES, TRASH BAG

INCONTINENCE SUPPLIES

Incontinence is without a doubt one of the most challenging and difficult consequences of dementia. When incontinence passes the early phase of just occasional "accidents" you enter a whole new field of at-home care. The best way to describe it is: challenging, energy consuming and a true test of your endurance.

I searched plenty of literature to find some help with this unavoidable daily challenge. More often than not, the advice you will find will say the following:
"When the patient has regular bowel movement – BM – incontinence, it may be a good time to place them into a facility."

That may very well be true, BUT if you do not put them into a facility, then what? This is not a baby we are talking about, the size of a doll, who you can single-handedly pick up and easily change a diaper, in a matter of minutes. You are dealing with a grown up human being, usually extremely upset, humiliated and often angry and frustrated when BM incontinence occurs. This requires some serious attention and expertise.

> **THE KEY MANTRA IS GOING TO BE:**
> **BE PREPARED, REMAIN CALM, ORGANIZED**
> **AND ACCOMPLISH THE NECESSARY TASK**
> **WITH SPEED AND ACCURACY.**

For obvious reasons, you do not want the clean-up to take too long.

WHAT YOU NEED:
- Plastic gloves in your size - better a bit larger than too small. I recommend latex, powder free and clear.
- Small trash bags.
- Baby wipes.
- New fresh, clean undergarment.
- Fresh diaper or pad.
- If needed, protective cream against bed sores.
- Any other fresh change of clothes or bedding that got soiled.

DIAPER OR PAD?

There are a wide variety of incontinence products on the market these days. You can find them in any drugstore. The problem is, when faced with the depressing facts that our loved one suffers from incontinence, we become overwhelmed by all the choices. You can find yourself aimlessly strolling up and down the drugstore aisles or desperately starring at the shelves of a medical supply store. What should you select?

Cost is another fact that is a consideration. Obviously this is a product that you will need continuously and cannot be stingy with. I researched and used many different options. My main concern was functionality and comfort.

I HIGHLY RECOMMEND THE PAD.

This is not a small feminine period-pad that is used with regular underwear. It is a much more absorbent, large-size pad, that is to be used with a light, stretchy mesh undergarment. The undergarment is reusable and provides optimal comfort and air access to the lower body, hip and groin area.

There is nothing more uncomfortable than a huge, hot wrap-around grown-up diaper with no access for air. It is also a fact that a diaper will create moist and hot environment, that is dangerous for potential infections and bedsores.

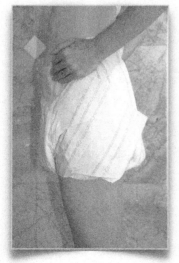 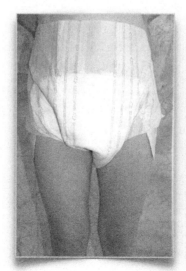 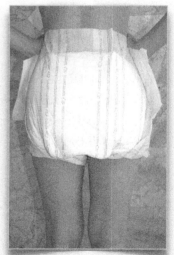

INCONTINENCE DIAPER FROM SIDE, FRONT AND BACK VIEW

In addition, it is much more difficult to change a diaper than a pad. Some diapers need to be removed by completely removing the pants or skirt. Other diapers are removed like disposable underwear, again presenting a fact that you need to completely undress the lower part of the body, to accomplish the clean up and change into a fresh set.

This can be very messy and is not a good option. It will make the whole idea of incontinence change so exhausting to you and such an ordeal to your loved one, that you will be inclined to do fewer changes, which in return will have dangerous consequences.

THE FACT IS THAT BEDSORES ARE COMPLETELY PREVENTABLE, IF YOU PAY ATTENTION AND KNOW HOW TO MANAGE INCONTINENCE CARE.

Research the local medical supplies stores or online selection and find the best pad option for you. I am recommending a pad by TENA, to be used with a mesh undergarment. The loved one will feel more comfortable and the changes will be easier on you both.

The pads come in different sizes. You can choose a lighter one for the day and the heavier, more absorbent one for the night. You may also use the nighttime pad during the day, reducing the changes and still increasing the comfort for your loved one. It will obviously depend on daily food and liquid intake, but you can set up a routine that will work and help you keep your loved one free of bed sores and urinary tract infections.

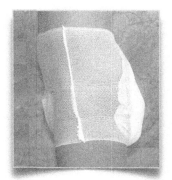 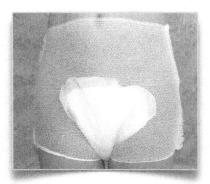 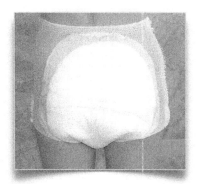

INCONTINENCE PAD FROM SIDE, FRONT AND BACK VIEW
WASHABLE MESH PANTIES HOLD THE PAD IN PLACE

THE INCONTINENCE
HOW-TO CLEAN-UP INSTRUCTIONS

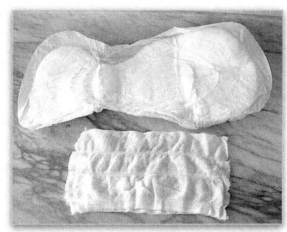

INCONTINENCE PAD AND WASHABLE MESH PANTIES - BRIEFS

HOW TO CHANGE AND CLEAN UP IN THE MORNING

This is most likely the singular and most difficult clean-up time. I recommend you are organized, calm and focused on care. Before you begin the process, prepare everything that you will need.

SUPPLIES YOU WILL NEED
- Plastic gloves
- Baby wipes
- Plastic trash bag
- Shower chair

PREPARATION
- Put on the plastic gloves
- Open the baby wipes box and place on the bed
- Open the plastic trash bag and place in on the bed
- Bring the shower chair to the side of the bed and block its wheels

STEPS

- ❋ Make sure the temperature in the room is appropriately warm
- ❋ Inform the loved one of what you are about to do, every step of the way
- ❋ Uncover the loved one
- ❋ Remove all prop-up pillows and bed railing
- ❋ Completely remove the mesh undergarment - panties. If they are very soiled you can cut them on the side and dispose of. If they are unsoiled, you can slide them off and reuse them after washing.
- ❋ Gently roll the loved one onto their side, away from you and prop their back with a small pillow, so they won't roll back
- ❋ Pull out and remove the soiled pad, always front to back, from behind
- ❋ Immediately place the soiled pad into the trash bag
- ❋ Use the baby wipes to wipe the behind - **ALWAYS FRONT TO BACK**
- ❋ Place the soiled wipes immediately into the trash bag, close it up
- ❋ Roll the loved one back onto their back
- ❋ Gently get hold of their shoulders and neck with one hand and place the other hand under their knees
- ❋ Now slowly pull them towards you and up close to the edge of the bed. Gently lift them into a sitting position.
- ❋ Wait a few moments while they are in the sitting position, so they don't get dizzy
- ❋ Firmly get hold of them under their arms and transfer them from the sitting position of the edge of the bed, onto the shower chair, unblock its wheels
- ❋ Roll the shower chair off into the bathroom
- ❋ Undress the loved one, carefully adjust the water temperature and begin with the shower

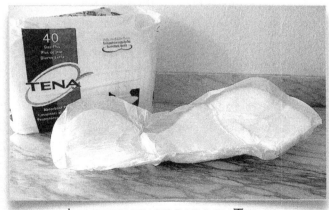

INCONTINENCE PADS BY TENA

HOW TO CHANGE AND CLEAN UP DURING THE DAY

If your loved one is sitting in a reclining chair and needs to be changed, here are the steps:

SUPPLIES YOU WILL NEED
- Plastic gloves
- Baby wipes
- New pad and protective cream against bed sores
- Plastic trash bag
- 2 New protective disposable pads for the chair
- A walker without wheels, or with safety blocks

PREPARATION
- Put on the plastic gloves
- Place the opened box of baby wipes next to the chair
- Prepare a fresh disposable pad
- Open a plastic trash bag and prepare it next to the chair
- Place the disposable chair pad on the floor so it will be directly under their feet
- Place a walker in front of the chair onto the protective disposable pad

STEPS
- Inform the loved one of what you are about to do, every step of the way
- Slowly elevate the chair from the reclining position
- Lift the loved one from the chair into standing position
- Have them hold on to the walker
- Pull down their pants and mesh panties and remove the soiled pad - front to back
- Place the soiled pad immediately into the trash bag
- Clean the loved one with the baby wipes, front to back
- If needed, apply protective cream, then quickly place the new fresh pad in place
- Pull up the sheer undergarment panties to hold the new pad in place
- Pull up the regular pants
- Gently lower them back onto the seat, adjust the recliner to sitting position
- Once they are seated, make sure that the clothing is straightened and smooth under the body or back and no wrinkles or material bulges are pressing on skin

This is the procedure ONLY if the loved one can still stand up and hold onto the walker while you are changing them. Quick, swift action is your biggest advantage.

INCONTINENCE BETWEEN CHANGES

It may happen that your loved one will have a new incontinence accident while you are changing them. Instead of getting upset, clean them anew and get a brand new clean pad to replace the soiled one. To prevent this most frustrating incident from occurring, you need to be incredibly fast when changing the pad. Slow procrastination will leave both of you extremely frustrated and the new mishap will make everything worse. Be prepared, fast, confident but always gentle and kind.

HOW TO CHANGE ON THE RECLINER

If the loved one can no longer stand on their feet and hold on to the walker, you can change them while they remain seated on the recliner.

STEPS
- Inform the loved one of what you are about to do, every step of the way
- Lower the reclining chair into an almost lying position
- You will change the loved one by moving them onto their side
- Roll them over to one side, prop them with a small pillow against the front and back of their body, to prevent them from rolling back onto their backside
- Lower the pants and mesh clear panties
- Pull the soiled pad out, front to back
- Wipe the buttocks with baby wipes, front to back
- If needed, apply protective cream, then place a new pad in place
- Pull up the mesh undergarment and regular pants and return them onto their back
- Once they are again in a sitting position, make sure that the clothing is straightened and smooth under the body, especially on their back and that there are no uncomfortable wrinkles or material bulges pressing on skin anywhere

This change on the recliner is not as safe or comfortable as on the bed. Obviously use your judgment, but once the loved one can't walk anymore at all and exhibits no interest in any activities and mostly sleeps, it might be better to keep them in bed.

HOW TO CHANGE AND CLEAN UP IN THE EVENING

STEps

- ❁ Inform the loved one of what you are about to do, every step of the way
- ❁ Put on the plastic gloves
- ❁ Transfer the loved one from the recliner onto the shower chair
- ❁ Roll the loved one into the bathroom on the shower chair
- ❁ Bring a walker and place it in front of the shower chair
- ❁ Lift the loved one to standing position
- ❁ Lower their regular pants, then mesh panties
- ❁ Remove the pad, always front to back
- ❁ Place the loved one back onto the shower chair
- ❁ Place the soiled pad in trash bag and dispose
- ❁ Remove the walker and proceed with removal of the clothing and the preparation for evening shower routine

NEVER LEAVE THE LOVED ONE UNATTENDED!

I have written this many times before, but here I will get into more detail. The natural decision would be to remove the trash bag with dirty pad and wipes immediately out of the room. This would leave your loved one unattended for a few decisive seconds. This is why you will get into the habit to immediately close off the trash bag that contains the soiled pad and baby wipes. It will remain in the room until you have secured your loved one's safety. This may all sound easy and quick, but believe me, being prepared will get you thru this challenging process.

AIR OUT THE ROOM <u>EACH TIME</u> AFTER A BM INCONTINENCE CHANGE. DO NOT EXPOSE THE LOVED ONE TO DRAFT. ASSURE THE AIR IN THE ROOM IS FRESH AND PLEASANT AT ALL TIMES. IT WILL DO WONDERS FOR YOUR LOVED ONE AND YOURSELF.

If the smell of BM or urine is very difficult for you to tolerate, you may have the disturbing feeling that the unpleasant smell has permanently stayed in your nose. Use natural aroma sprays and have a small aromatherapy oil bottle handy for yourself. Smell the aroma or place a tiny drop on your wrist, and that will immediately cure your situation. Small things like that go a long way.

HOW TO CHANGE A BED - BOUND PATIENT

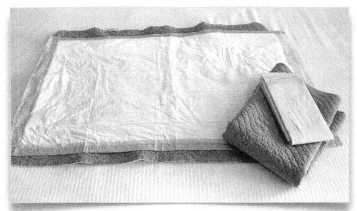

A WASHABLE PROTECTIVE PAD FOR BED
AND DISPOSABLE PROTECTIVE PAPER PAD

If your loved one is bed-bound, you will change them in bed.

SUPPLIES YOU WILL NEED

- Trash bag
- Plastic gloves
- Wipes
- New pad or diaper
- Fresh undergarment-mesh panties that hold the pad in place
- Bed-sore prevention cream
- Disposable flat pad for bed
- Fresh clean nightgown, if needed

STEPS

- Make sure the temperature in room is comfortable for uncovering the loved one
- Put on your plastic gloves
- Gently move the loved one onto their side and prop them with a small pillow against their front and back, to help prevent from rolling either way
- Lower and if necessary remove the undergarment completely
- Pull the soiled pad out, front to back
- Immediately place the dirty pad or diaper in trash bag
- Wipe the buttocks with baby wipes and dispose of them in trash bag

- ❋ Close off the trash bag immediately
- ❋ Put a small amount of bed-sore prevention cream on behind
- ❋ Place a new pad or diaper in place
- ❋ Pull up the sheer undergarment pants and roll the loved one onto their back
- ❋ If nightgown is soiled in any way, change immediately
- ❋ Make sure that the nightgown is straightened and smooth under the body. Even a tiny wrinkle can disturb someone who cannot move on their own to adjust a discomfort.

NIGHT - TIME CHANGES

Basically, the night changes are the same as for the bed bound patient. There are some additional circumstances, which you have to be aware of.

- ❋ If the loved one is awake, always inform them of what you are doing
- ❋ If the loved on is asleep, do everything in silence, with as little light as possible. Avoid making any noise and use slower gestures.
- ❋ If the loved one awakens in the middle of the change, as they often do, immediately calm them down by explaining gently and clearly what you are doing and that you are almost finished
- ❋ Assure them that you will be quick and they will feel much better just as soon as you are done.
- ❋ Often, the loved on will break out in night sweat. If the nightgown is even just a bit damp from perspiration, change them immediately into a fresh one.

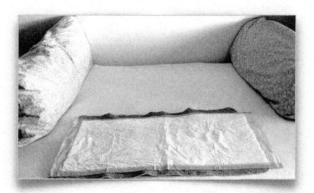

BED SET UP: WASHABLE PROTECTIVE PAD,
DISPOSABLE PROTECTIVE PAPER PAD AND PILLOWS FOR PROTECTION

ESPECIALLY CHALLENGING BM INCONTINENCE CHANGES

What belongs under this category? The super challenging change of them all: diarrhea. That occurrence can send a caregiver into panic or emotional break down. Even when you have everything under control and are organized to the last detail, a severe bout of diarrhea will surprise you, and I mean in a bad way.

I have spoken to numerous caregivers that simply break down at the sight of that kind of a massive clean-up project. Very often this is the breaking and decisive point when family members place their loved one permanently into a facility or hospital. But the consequence does not have to be that extreme. I encourage you to be prepared and know that you are not the first one experiencing this ordeal. I believe you can and will get thru this challenge.

The key is calm, organized and fast action to remedy the situation. You will have to make a few necessary changes to your regular clean up routine. If the occurrence of diarrhea is a surprise, which is most often the case, just stay calm and do not under any circumstances get upset with your loved one. They can't help it.

BM - CHALLENGING CHANGE IN RECLINER

- ✳ Place your loved one fully clothed onto the shower chair
- ✳ Roll them into the bathroom
- ✳ Completely remove all clothing
- ✳ Proceed with a complete shower of the lower body

This is the easier option. If you have previously placed proper padding covers on the reclining chair, you should be in good shape.

SEVERELY SOILED CLOTHING

All clothing that is severely soiled needs to be immediately placed into trash bag and thrown away. Never attempt to pull soiled clothing or dresses over the loved one's head. If need be, cut the severely soiled clothing off with round tip scissors and remove it without causing an even bigger mess. That is one of the reasons you should always dress your loved one into light, breathable cotton clothing with wide neck. Proceed with a complete change, ending with a good airing out of the room.

BM - CHALLENGING CHANGE IN BED

If your loved one is on the bed or is bed-bound while diarrhea occurs, your clean up process is a bit more demanding.

SUPPLIES YOU WILL NEED

Get your clean up and diaper change supplies ready in addition to a new change of clothing and bedding. You will need:

* Trash bag
* Plastic gloves
* Wipes
* New pad or diaper
* Bed-sore prevention cream
* New undergarment-mesh panties that hold the pad in place
* New disposable flat pad for bed
* Fresh clean nightgown
* Clean bedding
* Large round tip scissors

If you have the bed set up with all the security padding as described in the bedding chapter, you will avoid the worst. Nothing should be getting on any part of the bed at all. Everything will be on the padding, where your loved one is lying.

YOUR COMMUNICATION WITH LOVED ONE DURING CHANGES

How you communicate with your loved one while this challenging incontinence change is going on, is extremely important.

Here are a few tips:

* Keep them calm, talk to them kindly and rollup your sleeves.
* While you perform the difficult clean up, assure them that everything will be all right and they will be clean and comfortable in no time.
* Never scold them and show them your frustration, as it will only add to the stressful situation. This experience can be very upsetting for your loved one.
* Remain a picture of calmness, efficiency and fast action.

You will most definitely need to perform a full lower-body shower routine. There is just no way of cleaning someone completely and removing any trace of bad smell without a serious thorough shower.

STEPS

Get a large trash bag and immediately remove and dispose of everything that is severely soiled, there is no chance you will be reusing anything.

- To remove the soiled clothing faster and easier, take the large round tip scissors and cut any undergarment, mesh panties or diaper at the sides on the hip.
- Roll over the loved one to the side and remove the soiled diaper or pad including the cut undergarment and place everything into the large trash bag.
- Assess the scope of soiled clothing and if the nightgown is severely soiled you need to cut away that part of the nightgown and avoid any and all touching of the soiled garment with the rest of the body or bedding.
- Do not attempt to pull the soiled nightgown over your loved one's head.
- If the nightgown is severely soiled you need to dispose of it right away.
- Wipe all the soiled areas of body with the baby wipes and place them into the plastic trash bag.
- Never use regular cotton towels or wash cloths for diarrhea clean up.
- Immediately place all soiled materials into a large plastic bag and remove from the room.
- Prepare for the shower routine.
- Lift the loved one into a sitting position and transfer them onto the shower chair, making sure the removable bucket underneath the shower chair is attached.
- Now roll them into the bathroom and proceed with a complete and thorough shower of at least the lower area of the body.
- After shower is completed, repeat the usual after shower routine with proper creams for skin care and make sure they are clean, nice and dry.
- Change the loved one into fresh clothing,
- Use a large size diaper or pad. You may experience another episode of diarrhea in the near future, until the digestive system calms down.
- Make sure your loved one is secured and sitting in a safe dry chair while they wait for you to clean and prepare a freshly changed bed.

Address the issue of diarrhea with proper diet adjustments and natural remedies. See chapters *Holistic Caregiving Remedies* and *Healthy Diet*.

BED CLEAN UP

Now after you tended to the loved one, you can address the soiled bedding.

- ❋ Throw away any and all severely soiled sheets or pillowcases.
- ❋ Check the under pads on the bed and change any and all bedding. You would be surprised how BM odor can stay present unless you change everything even if it does not look soiled.
- ❋ Keep an eye on your loved one at all times, make sure they are secured in the chair.
- ❋ Tell them that they will be able to return to the comfort of their bed in a moment.
- ❋ Now you are ready to place them back into the fresh clean bed.
- ❋ When they are covered in bed, feeling comfortable, clean, nice and warm, you can thoroughly air out the room.
- ❋ Make sure they are not in a draft where they could catch a cold after the shower.
- ❋ Double-check the room that all soiled materials are gone and use some natural aromatherapy scents to establish a pleasant odor in the room.

This is a very exhausting process and you are a brave and kind human being to have endured it. My respect and sympathies to you! I have been there, I know how it is and I am telling you to just stay strong and know that now, you have become unbeatable! After the ordeal, you are ready to take a shower yourself and have a rest.

ON A LAST NOTE
When your loved one spends the majority of waking hours in a seated position, or is bed bound, you will need to pay extra attention to bed sore prevention.

> **IF YOUR LOVED ONE IS BED BOUND, APPLY THE PROTECTIVE LOTION TO THEIR BUTTOCKS EACH AND EVERY TIME AFTER A CHANGE.**

After you have cleaned them, apply a small amount of lotion to their buttocks in the areas that seem to be getting most pressure when sitting or lying down. You also have the option of placing a small amount of lotion onto the fresh pad where it touches the most vulnerable areas. That may be more comfortable for your loved one. That way you will keep the area constantly protected. Each time you change them, reapply a small portion or the lotion for protection and prevention. Tedious tending to that seemingly meaningless task will prove a true-life saver and will spare your loved one much unneeded pain and suffering.

CHAPTER TWELVE

Healthy Diet

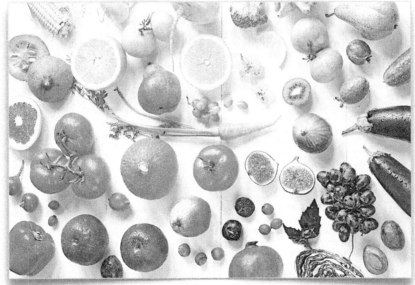

PROPER DIET IS ONE OF THE KEY ELEMENTS
OF EFFECTIVE CAREGIVING

When I prepared meals for my Mother, I used very small glass bowls which measured a cup or half a cup. Each glass cup had a small amount of her favorite food. I enjoyed selecting and preparing the food and looked forward to her tasting every sample. She truly enjoyed her mealtimes and ate throughout the day. As a result, her hydration levels and digestive system were excellent and her weight was ideal.

HEALTHFUL FOOD

Selecting and properly preparing healthy food is becoming increasingly more complex and requires your full attention. Your goal is to establish an optimal balance of your loved one's digestive system, so that it functions properly and there are no additional challenges to their overall state of wellbeing. You also want to make sure that the appetite remains steady and there is sufficient intake of liquids and nutrients absorbed on a daily basis.

Follow these general rules and use only food that is:
* organic, whole and unprocessed
* gluten free
* organic dairy - absolutely no antibiotics
* wild caught fish, no farmed fish
* no junk food such as; salted snack foods, candy, sweet desserts, fried fast food or sugary carbonated beverages
* eliminate all white sugar, replace with natural substitutes such as organic honey, maple syrup, molasses or coconut palm sugar
* use only organic chicken and turkey or meats that receive no antibiotics, are fed organic food that is grown with no pesticides, and live range-free with access to outdoors

USE SEASONAL VEGETABLES AND FRUITS

Obviously, if you live in a climate where there is a big shift in availability of seasonal vegetables and fruits, use what is available and fresh. Adjust the suggested diet accordingly, but keep it healthy, colorful, creative and tasty. Your loved one does not have much excitement during the day, so very pleasant and delicious meals will give them something to look forward to and enjoy.

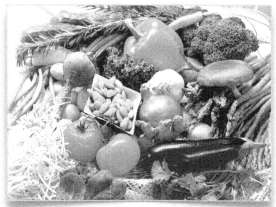

SELECT LOCAL ORGANIC
VEGETABLES IN SEASON

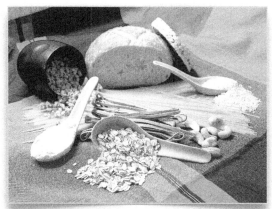

USE ONLY GLUTEN FREE BREADS,
WHEATS AND PASTA

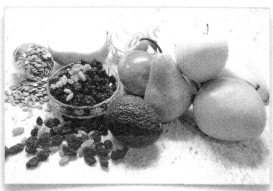

INCLUDE DAILY PORTIONS OF FRESH
BLENDED FRUITS AND NUT BUTTER

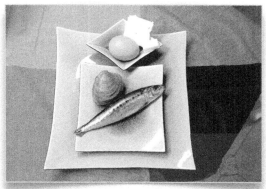

FISH SHOULD BE WILD CAUGHT,
DAIRY MUST BE ORGANIC

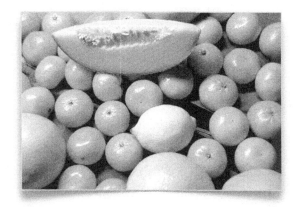

INCLUDE CITRUS RICH IN VITAMIN C

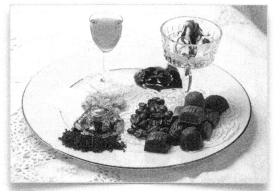

ELIMINATE ALL SUGAR AND CANDY,
REPLACE WITH ORGANIC HONEY,
MAPLE SYRUP

ALKALINE AND ACIDIC FOOD

I recommend a mostly alkaline foods diet, as it helps the body maintain an optimal state of health. Too much acidity in the body creates a thriving environment for illness and imbalance. Keeping the body as alkaline as possible, will help you prevent and manage any challenging situations regarding digestion and overall health.

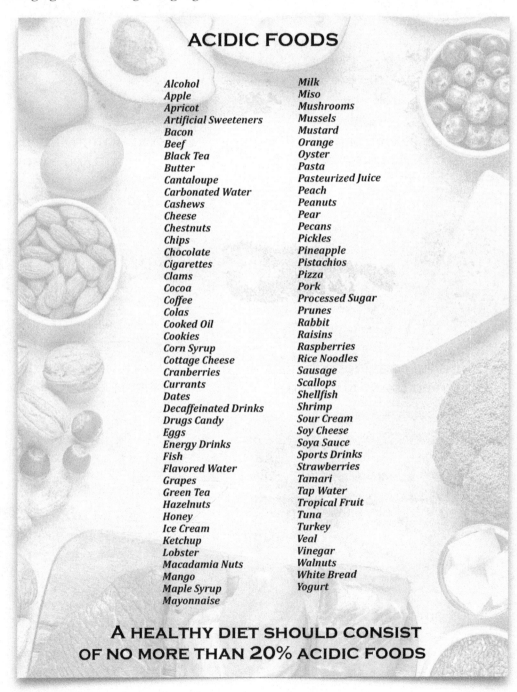

ACIDIC FOODS

Alcohol	Milk
Apple	Miso
Apricot	Mushrooms
Artificial Sweeteners	Mussels
Bacon	Mustard
Beef	Orange
Black Tea	Oyster
Butter	Pasta
Cantaloupe	Pasteurized Juice
Carbonated Water	Peach
Cashews	Peanuts
Cheese	Pear
Chestnuts	Pecans
Chips	Pickles
Chocolate	Pineapple
Cigarettes	Pistachios
Clams	Pizza
Cocoa	Pork
Coffee	Processed Sugar
Colas	Prunes
Cooked Oil	Rabbit
Cookies	Raisins
Corn Syrup	Raspberries
Cottage Cheese	Rice Noodles
Cranberries	Sausage
Currants	Scallops
Dates	Shellfish
Decaffeinated Drinks	Shrimp
Drugs Candy	Sour Cream
Eggs	Soy Cheese
Energy Drinks	Soya Sauce
Fish	Sports Drinks
Flavored Water	Strawberries
Grapes	Tamari
Green Tea	Tap Water
Hazelnuts	Tropical Fruit
Honey	Tuna
Ice Cream	Turkey
Ketchup	Veal
Lobster	Vinegar
Macadamia Nuts	Walnuts
Mango	White Bread
Maple Syrup	Yogurt
Mayonnaise	

A HEALTHY DIET SHOULD CONSIST OF NO MORE THAN 20% ACIDIC FOODS

Remember, fresh clean water with a small squeeze of fresh lemon, creates an instant alkaline drink and is wonderful for flushing out the body's toxins. If your loved one enjoys this simple drink, add it to daily diet.

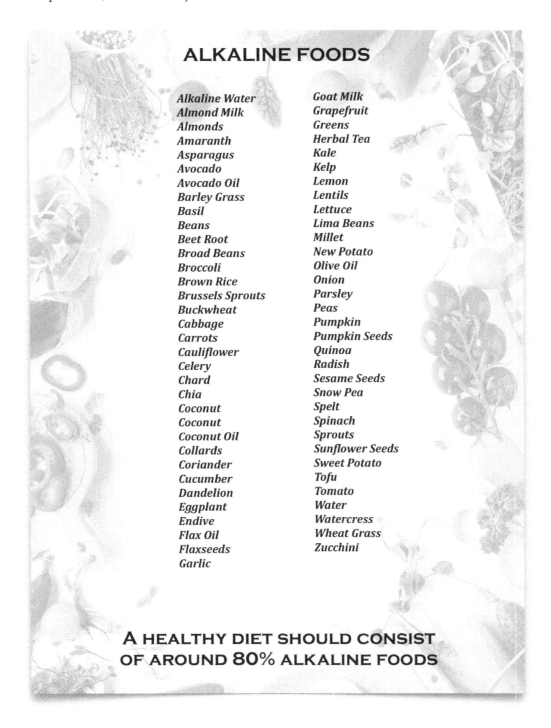

ALKALINE FOODS

Alkaline Water
Almond Milk
Almonds
Amaranth
Asparagus
Avocado
Avocado Oil
Barley Grass
Basil
Beans
Beet Root
Broad Beans
Broccoli
Brown Rice
Brussels Sprouts
Buckwheat
Cabbage
Carrots
Cauliflower
Celery
Chard
Chia
Coconut
Coconut
Coconut Oil
Collards
Coriander
Cucumber
Dandelion
Eggplant
Endive
Flax Oil
Flaxseeds
Garlic

Goat Milk
Grapefruit
Greens
Herbal Tea
Kale
Kelp
Lemon
Lentils
Lettuce
Lima Beans
Millet
New Potato
Olive Oil
Onion
Parsley
Peas
Pumpkin
Pumpkin Seeds
Quinoa
Radish
Sesame Seeds
Snow Pea
Spelt
Spinach
Sprouts
Sunflower Seeds
Sweet Potato
Tofu
Tomato
Water
Watercress
Wheat Grass
Zucchini

A HEALTHY DIET SHOULD CONSIST OF AROUND 80% ALKALINE FOODS

FOOD PREPARATION

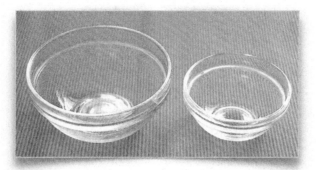

1 CUP AND 1/2 CUP GLASS PREP MIXING BOWLS

You will need a good quality blender since you will be blending all the food. In addition, I suggest you get small glass mixing bowls, which will make keeping track of the quantity of consumed food very easy and helpful. These bowls are dishwasher, microwave and freezer safe. BPA-free glass does not stain or absorb odors and protects the flavor of food. They come in 1 Cup and 1/2 Cup sizes and more. Prepare a small amount of delicious variety of healthy food and place the bowls on a food tray for easy serving.

When cooking for your loved one, follow these principles:
* cook your loved one's favorite foods, while following healthy principles
* select easily digestible foods
* serve a rich variety of foods, so it is never boring
* serve small portions and avoid large portions of the same food
* blend all food, so it is very easy to eat

MEASURING MEAL PORTIONS
Even if it may seem like you have to prepare a lot of food for your loved one, that is not the case. You will be feeding them only small 1/2 cup or 1 cup portions, in order to keep them interested in food and help them enjoy the meals. So you do not have to cook large amounts of food, only a rich selection. It is almost as if you are preparing a tasting tray of various very small portions. This will be very stimulating for your loved one and you will successfully manage proper liquid and food intake.

MEASURING SYSTEM
Tablespoon = Tbsp   Teaspoon = Tsp
1 Cup = 1 glass bowl   1/2 Cup = 1 smaller glass bowl

SAMPLE MENUS

MONDAY

BREAKFAST

PRUNE SMOOTHIE - 1/2 banana, 1 Tbsp flaxseed, 3 prunes, 1/2 cup almond milk

FRUIT YOGURT - 1 cup, mix well

TEA - 1 cup, herbal non-caffeine

APPLE BERRY SAUCE - 1/2 cup

ALMOND MILK - 1 cup, unsweetened

FRESH GRAPEFRUIT & BANANA JUICE - 1 grapefruit, 1/2 banana, blend well

1 SLICE GLUTEN FREE BREAD - cut into small pieces, add eggless tofu spread

OATMEAL WITH CRANBERRIES - 1 cup, add hot water & mix with Tsp of fruit sauce

FRUIT BRAND MUFFIN - mix it well with almond milk

ALOE VERA JUICE - 1 cup

LUNCH and DINER

FRESH CORN SOUP - 1 cup

SMALL DISH OF HUMMUS - 3 Tbsp

AVOCADO - 1/2 cup

WHITE FISH - 1 cup, cook, blend with vegetable broth and a drop of olive oil

KALE - 1 cup , cook, blend with drop of olive oil

SPINACH - 1/2 cup, cook, blend with some olive oil and vegetable broth

SWEET POTATO - 1/2 cup, cook, blend with some olive oil and vegetable broth

CABBAGE - 1/2 cup, cook, blend with cream and vegetable broth

CUCUMBER, YOGURT - 1 cup, blend cucumber, yogurt, cilantro leaf, drop olive oil

ALMOND MILK - 1 cup

FRESH WATERMELON - 1/2 cup, blend

NOTE: This weekly menu includes a smoothie that prevents constipation, as the tendency in elderly is a slow digestive process. In case of a soft stool, simply eliminate the prunes and flaxseed in the smoothie.

TUESDAY

BREAKFAST

PRUNE SMOOTHIE - 1/2 banana, 1 Tbsp flaxseed, 3 prunes, 1/2 cup almond milk

FRUIT YOGURT - 1 cup, mix well

TEA - 1 cup, herbal non-caffeine

APPLE SAUCE - 1/2 cup

ALMOND MILK - 1 cup, unsweetened

FRESH ORANGE & BANANA JUICE - 1 grapefruit, 1/2 banana, blend well

1 SLICE GLUTEN FREE BREAD - cut into small pieces, add organic cream cheese

OATMEAL WITH BLUEBERRIES - 1 cup, add hot water & mix with Tsp of fruit sauce

FRUIT BRAND MUFFIN - mix it well with almond milk

KIWI - 1/2 cup, blend one kiwi

LUNCH AND DINER

GINGER CARROT SOUP - 1 cup

SMALL DISH OF GOAT CHEESE - 3 Tbsp

ALMOND BUTTER - 2 Tbsp

SALMON FISH - 1 cup, cook, blend with vegetable broth and a drop of olive oil

POLENTA - 1/2 cup, cook, blend, add sweet cream and water

BOK CHOY VEGETABLE - 1/2 cup, cook, blend with olive oil and vegetable broth

BRUSSELS SPROUTS - 1/2 cup, cook, blend with 1 Tsp cream and vegetable broth

MUSTARD GREENS - 1/2 cup, cook, blend, with1 Tsp cream and vegetable broth

TOMATO & CILANTRO - 1/2 cup, blend tomato, cilantro leaf, add a bit of olive oil

ALMOND MILK - 1 cup

FRESH GRAPES - 1/2 cup, blend

WEDNESDAY

BREAKFAST

PRUNE SMOOTHIE - 1/2 banana, 1 Tbsp flaxseed, 3 prunes, 1/2 cup almond milk

FRUIT YOGURT - 1 cup, mix well

TEA - 1 cup, herbal non-caffeine

APPLE BERRY SAUCE - 1/2 cup

ALMOND MILK - 1 cup, unsweetened

FRESH GRAPEFRUIT & BANANA JUICE - 1 grapefruit, 1/2 banana, blend well

1 SLICE GLUTEN FREE BREAD - cut into small pieces, add egg salad

OATMEAL WITH CRANBERRIES - 1 cup, add hot water & mix with Tsp of fruit sauce

FRUIT BRAND MUFFIN - mix it well with almond milk

FRESH GRAPES - 1/2 cup, blend

LUNCH AND DINER

SWEET POTATO BISQUE - 1 cup

GOAT YOGURT - 1/2 cup

STEAMED MUSHROOMS - 1/2 cup, steam, blend with cream and vegetable broth

ORGANIC TURKEY - 1 cup, cook, blend w vegetable broth and a drop of olive oil

CELERY - 1/2 cup, cook, blend, add sweet cream and water

GREEN BEANS - 1/2 cup, cook, blend, mix with olive oil and vegetable broth

BUCKWHEAT - 1/2 cup, cook, blend, mix 1 Tsp cream and vegetable broth

MUSTARD GREENS - 1/2 cup, cook, blend, mix 1 Tsp cream and vegetable broth

CUCUMBER & PARSLEY - 1/2 cup, blend, add a bit of olive oil

ALMOND MILK - 1 cup

FRESH STRAWBERRIES - 1/2 cup, blend

THURSDAY

BREAKFAST

PRUNE SMOOTHIE - 1/2 banana, 1 Tbsp flaxseed, 3 prunes, 1/2 cup almond milk

FRUIT YOGURT - 1 cup, mix well

TEA - 1 cup, herbal non-caffeine

APPLE SAUCE - 1/2 cup

ALMOND MILK - 1 cup, unsweetened

FRESH ORANGE & BANANA JUICE - 1 grapefruit, 1/2 banana, blend well

1 SLICE GLUTEN FREE BREAD - cut into small pieces, add eggless tofu spread

OATMEAL WITH BLUEBERRIES - 1 cup, add hot water & mix with Tsp of fruit sauce

FRUIT BRAND MUFFIN - mix it well with almond milk

ALOE VERA JUICE - 1 cup

LUNCH AND DINER

BROCCOLI SOUP - 1 cup

SMALL DISH OF HUMMUS - 3 Tbsp

AVOCADO - 1/2 cup

ORGANIC CHICKEN - 1 cup, cook, blend, w vegetable broth and a drop of olive oil

CELERY - 1/2 cup, raw or cooked, blend, add sweet cream and water

ASPARAGUS - 1/2 cup, cook, blend, mix with olive oil and vegetable broth

BROWN RICE - 1/2 cup, cook, blend, mix 1 Tsp cream and vegetable broth

YELLOW SQUASH - 1/2 cup, cook, blend, mix 1 Tsp cream and vegetable broth

TOMATO & CILANTRO - 1/2 cup, blend tomato, cilantro leaf, add a bit of olive oil

ALMOND MILK - 1 cup

FRESH BLUEBERRIES - 1/2 cup, blend

FRIDAY

BREAKFAST

PRUNE SMOOTHIE - 1/2 banana, 1 Tbsp flaxseed, 3 prunes, 1/2 cup almond milk

FRUIT YOGURT - 1 cup, mix well

TEA - 1 cup, herbal non-caffeine

APPLE BERRY SAUCE - 1/2 cup

ALMOND MILK - 1 cup, unsweetened

FRESH GRAPEFRUIT & BANANA JUICE - 1 grapefruit, 1/2 banana, blend well

1 SLICE GLUTEN FREE BREAD - cut into small pieces, add eggless tofu spread

OATMEAL WITH CRANBERRIES - 1 cup, add hot water & mix with Tsp of fruit sauce

FRUIT BRAND MUFFIN - mix it well with almond milk

FRESH GRAPES - 1/2 cup, blend

LUNCH AND DINER

CARROT SOUP - 1 cup

GOAT YOGURT - 1/2 cup

AVOCADO - 1/2 cup

SALMON - 1 cup, cook, blend, with vegetable broth and a drop of olive oil

BUTTER SQUASH - 1/2 cup, cook, blend, add sweet cream and water

KALE - 1/2 cup, cook, blend, mix with olive oil and vegetable broth

QUINOA - 1/2 cup, cook, mix 1 Tsp cream and vegetable broth

SPINACH - 1/2 cup, cook, blend, mix 1 Tsp cream and vegetable broth

CUCUMBER & PARSLEY - 1/2 cup, blend, add a bit of olive oil

ALMOND MILK - 1 cup

FRESH CANTALOUPE - 1/2 cup, blend

SATURDAY

BREAKFAST

PRUNE SMOOTHIE - 1/2 banana, 1 Tbsp flaxseed, 3 prunes, 1/2 cup almond milk

FRUIT YOGURT - 1 cup, mix well

TEA - 1 cup, herbal non-caffeine

APPLE BERRY SAUCE - 1/2 cup

ALMOND MILK - 1 cup, unsweetened

FRESH ORANGE & BANANA JUICE - 1 grapefruit, 1/2 banana, blend well

1 SLICE GLUTEN FREE BREAD - cut into small pieces, add sour cream

OATMEAL WITH BLUEBERRIES - 1 cup, add hot water & mix with Tsp of fruit sauce

FRUIT BRAND MUFFIN - mix it well with almond milk

FRESH PEAR - 1/2 cup, blend

LUNCH and DINER

MISO SOUP - 1 cup, prepare with water, mix in one spoon of organic miso paste

SMALL DISH OF HUMMUS - 3 Tbsp

AVOCADO - 1/2 cup

WHITE FISH - 1 cup, cook, blend with vegetable broth and a drop of olive oil

BROCCOLI - 1/2 cup, cook, blend, add sweet cream and water

KALE - 1/2 cup, cook, blend, mix with olive oil and vegetable broth

YAMS - 1/2 cup, cook, blend, mix 1 Tsp cream and vegetable broth

CELERY - 1/2 cup, raw or cooked, blend, mix 1 Tsp cream and vegetable broth

TOMATO & CILANTRO - 1/2 cup, blend tomato, cilantro leaf, add a bit of olive oil

ALMOND MILK - 1 cup

FRESH RASPBERRIES - 1/2 cup, blend

SUNDAY

BREAKFAST

**PRUNE SMOOTHIE - ** 1/2 banana, 1 Tbsp flaxseed, 3 prunes, 1/2 cup almond milk

**FRUIT YOGURT - ** 1 cup, mix well

TEA - 1 cup, herbal non-caffeine

APPLE BERRY SAUCE - 1/2 cup

ALMOND MILK - 1 cup, unsweetened

FRESH GRAPEFRUIT & BANANA JUICE - 1 grapefruit, 1/2 banana, blend well

1 SLICE GLUTEN FREE BREAD - cut into small pieces, add cream cheese

OATMEAL WITH CRANBERRIES - 1 cup, add hot water & mix with Tsp of fruit sauce

FRUIT BRAND MUFFIN - mix it well with almond milk

FRESH WATERMELON - 1/2 cup, blend

LUNCH AND DINER

TOMATO SOUP - 1 cup

SMALL DISH OF GOAT CHEESE - 3 Tbsp

EGGPLANT SAUCE - 1/2 cup

SALMON - 1 cup, cook, blend with vegetable broth and a drop of olive oil

TURNIP - 1/2 cup, cook, blend, add sweet cream and water

KALE - 1/2 cup, cook, blend, mix with olive oil and vegetable broth

AMARANTH - 1/2 cup, cook, blend, mix 1 Tsp cream and vegetable broth

RED BEETS - 1/2 cup, cook, blend, mix 1 Tsp cream and vegetable broth

TOMATO & CILANTRO - 1/2 cup, blend tomato, cilantro leaf, add a bit of olive oil

ALMOND MILK - 1 cup

FRESH GRAPES - 1/2 cup, blend

NOTES TO THE MENU

Wherever the menu states Almond milk, you can substitute with any other milk, such as Coconut milk, Oat milk, Rice milk, Cashew milk, Macadamia milk and Hemp milk. Keep in mind, that you will most likely be feeding your loved one a Tsp of peanut or almond butter when giving them medication, if that is their chosen preference. You can substitute any listed vegetable with their favorite vegetable. Adjust the food so that it includes your loved one's favorites.

SPECIAL DIETS

THE BUDWIG DIET

This diet was developed by the German biochemist Dr. Johanna Budwig in the 1950s. The diet consists of multiple daily servings of flaxseed oil and cottage cheese, in addition to vegetables, fruits and juices. The daily serving is 2 ounces - 60 ml of flaxseed oil and 4 ounces - 113 grams of cottage cheese per day. Processed foods, meats, most other dairy products and sugar are prohibited. Cottage cheese is an excellent source of calcium, great for bone health, prevention of osteoporosis, regulating the blood pressure and preventing certain cancers. The diet is prepared with organic cottage cheese finely blended with organic flaxseed oil. It is quite tasty and can be easily included in your loved one's daily diet. Prepare the blend and serve it in 1/2 cup daily portions. It is also an excellent addition to your own diet.

DIET FOR REGULARITY

Regardless of occasional bouts with s constipation or diarrhea, it is wise you keep an established protocol that fits your loved one's unique needs. The usual tendency in elderly is constipation, as a direct result of slowed down digestive movement. As a precautionary measure, you can add daily organic ground flaxseed to any meal. In addition, include a small portion of blended prunes and prune juice. In winter time, when you may not have access to fresh prunes, you can soak dried prunes in filtered water for at least 30 minutes and then blend them into a tasty paste. Use these additions to diet as preventative measure.

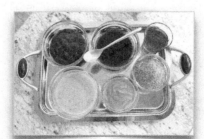

BLENDED PRUNES, GROUND FLAXSEED,
PRUNE JUICE AND BLENDED FRUIT AS DAILY SNACK

SERVING MEALS

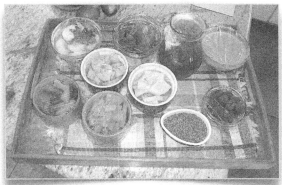

PREPARED FOOD PORTIONS
BEFORE BLENDING

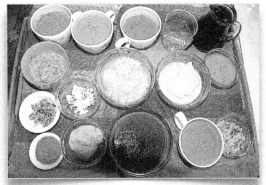

AFTERNOON AND EVENING MEAL

Prepare all the food in the morning, divide it into portions and keep it fresh in covered cups. Before lunchtime, you can blend and mix it with warm vegetable broth, so it can be served at ideal temperature. Keeping all food on a tray will give you easy overview of the amount of food and liquids consumed. It will also make it very easy and fun to serve.

APPETITE

Due to illness, your loved one's appetite may change considerably. It could decline, as the cognitive abilities make it harder to focus on the task of eating, chewing and swallowing. If your loved one has no interest in eating, it is possible they are just tired half way through the meal. They simply become disinterested. There is also the possibility of increased appetite and continuous hunger. This may be caused by antipsychotic and antidepressant medications that are often prescribed for dementia. They can also significantly increase sugar cravings. If that is the case, supplement with healthy substitutes as listed.

MEDICATION CAN AFFECT APPETITE LEVELS.

SUGAR CRAVINGS

Once you implement a healthy diet, that also satisfies your loved one's personal taste and preferences, they will never crave junk food. You just need to be creative. If they desire sweets, add a very small amount of 1/2 of Tsp of honey or maple syrup to blended fruit and that should suffice. Offer a very rich variety and interesting selection of food which will keep them interested, so they will truly look forward to enjoying meal times. It will also help them remember various tastes and will stimulate their senses.

HOW MUCH LIQUID PER DAY?

> ### GENERALLY, YOUR LOVED ONE SHOULD DRINK BETWEEN 9 AND 13 CUPS OF LIQUID A DAY, DEPENDING ON THEIR SIZE AND GENDER.

Let us say the ideal amount for women is 9 cups and for men up to 13 cups daily. The diet you are offering is very liquid and will help you succeed in accomplishing this aim.

WATER

It is very important to keep your loved one very well hydrated. Make all food very liquid. Recommended drinks:

* use only Alkaline or filtered water for all drinks and cooking
* herbal teas from listed selection in Chapter *Holistic Caregiving Remedies*
* use any of the following milk substitutes: Almond milk, Coconut milk, Oat milk, Rice milk, Cashew milk, Macadamia Milk and Hemp milk

FEEDING YOUR LOVED ONE

Feeding an elderly dementia patient requires real skill, tremendous patience and intuition. I cannot express enough how very important it is to feed them properly. If you will give yourself plenty of time and apply this approach, your loved one will receive proper nutrients and liquids, feel well and avoid the usual digestive challenges.

> ### ALL FOOD NEEDS TO BE BLENDED. LIQUIDS ARE MORE DIFFICULT TO SWALLOW, SO YOU NEED TO THICKEN THEM UP BY MIXING WITH SOLID FOODS.

Before a meal, make sure your loved one is clean and comfortable. You cannot expect them to enjoy a pleasant meal, if they have a soiled incontinence pad and need a change. Make sure this is not the case. When they are ready, elevate them up into a comfortable, upright sitting position.

Lift them up sufficiently, so that the head position is straight. Prop them up with pillows, if necessary. If your loved one is bed-bound, elevate the head of the bed sufficiently high, so that their head is as straight as possible and they are able to swallow comfortably.

SWALLOWING

Swallowing is a real challenge with late stage dementia. Pay special attention to assure they swallow properly. Here are a few helpful suggestions:

IF YOUR LOVED ONE IS BED-BOUND OR IN A RECLINER, ALWAYS MAKE SURE THAT THE HEAD IS NOT LEANING BACK WHILE FEEDING THEM, AS THEY COULD EASILY CHOKE. ALWAYS BRING THEM INTO AN UPRIGHT POSITION.

I suggest that you mix liquids with other blended foods, just to create a thicker texture. For example, an orange juice can be mixed with a blended banana. Coconut water can be mixed with blended prunes and so on. Be creative.

It is easier to swallow colder liquids, so if you want to try and feed a liquid-drink, make sure it is at room temperature, not freezing, but also not too warm.

If the loved one starts coughing, it means they are having a problem with swallowing and you need to be especially careful. Feed them very, very slowly, make sure the head is straight and keep a very calm atmosphere. There should be absolutely no rushing. If they start coughing and seem to get frightened, stay very calm and with a soothing voice assure they will be just fine and encourage them to relax. If they continue to cough, pat them gently on the upper back. If you are careful with the feeding process, this will not happen.

ALWAYS FEED BLENDED FOOD, OR CUT BITES INTO VERY, VERY SMALL PIECES THAT DO NOT REQUIRE MUCH CHEWING.

Always test the temperature of the food with a corner of your pinky finger joint. You need to make sure that you will never burn their tongue or feed them freezing food.

STRICT HYGIENE

Keep the utmost hygiene with utensils and dishes. You need to be very organized, because most likely you are dealing with BM and food in the same room. Wear disposable gloves and wash your hands each and every time after dealing with anything regarding incontinence or diaper change. Be extra careful and strict with everyone around your loved one regarding hygiene.

MEAL SCHEDULE

It is ideal to feed a few smaller meals throughout the day. That could mean about FOUR small meals a day, depending on your loved one's appetite and time it takes them to eat.

Your feeding schedule can look like this:
- ❋ First thing in the morning after showering
- ❋ Lunch time
- ❋ A few cups of food a few hours later or throughout the afternoon as they desire
- ❋ A few cups of food an hour before sleep

Be flexible. If your loved one does not eat their portions in the morning, save them until lunch time and so on. I am not suggesting that you save the same cup of food thru the day, but since your menu is custom made for their needs, you can switch back and forth to see what they feel like eating at any particular moment.

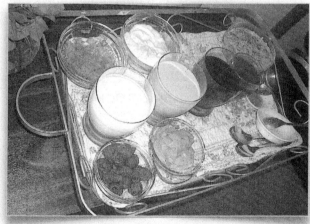

BREAKFAST & MORNING SNACKS

MIX IT UP

Remember, it is not really fun to eat one bowl of food from beginning till the end without mixing it up with other foods. Think about various tastes and flavors and how the eating experience can be more enjoyable. The mixing of foods has to be done really well. If you feed your loved one a cup of kefir drink, mixed with flaxseeds and half a banana, you could add a few spoons of pureed prunes, every few bites. No one can eat an entire cup of blended prunes without some change for the taste buds.

Perhaps you can add a few Tsp of coconut water in between and create an interesting taste that is pleasant and comfortable to eat. It really depends on your observation skills. If your loved one seems to be getting bored with a certain food, immediately switch to a different food and observe their reaction. Perhaps after a few spoons, you can return to the original food and that way ensure that they will eat the necessary foods that their digestive system requires. You will need to really spend some time feeding and observing, especially if you have the challenging issue of trying to manage as case of constipation or diarrhea.

I was always astounded when I noticed perpetually the same menu in nursing facilities, no matter what condition someone's digestive system was in. It is obviously difficult to make specific meals for every resident. That is one of many great advantages of having your loved one at home with you. You will be creating meals for their specific needs. And that will occasionally mean, that you won't decide on their daily diet until determining their regularity in the morning. However, if you have them on a balanced diet, that includes all preventative and remedy measures listed in this book, you will most likely establish a great regularity and will not have these challenges.

The feeding needs to be carefully mixed up, as if you were eating the food. Always put yourself in your loved one's place. Would you feel like eating ten straight spoons of prunes or mix it up with some kefir in between? Pay attention and really patiently take your time. I know sometimes you might feel worn out and just want the long feeding process to be over with. But if you do this correctly, your loved one will be really comfortable, they will feel full and satisfied and will most likely take a nap right afterwards. And there is your break!

It is important that you manage to administer the ideal amount of food and liquid intake that is needed on a daily basis. So it will definitely pay off to do this right.

> **USE SMALL TEA SPOONS, WITH ESPECIALLY SMOOTH EDGES,
> SO THAT YOU ARE NOT HURTING THE CORNERS OF THE MOUTH.
> DO NOT SCRAPE THE EDGES OF THE MOUTH,
> IF SOME FOOD SEEMS TO BE FALLING OFF.**

Since you will be spoon feeding your loved one sometimes for years, you could really create a problem with dry, cracked or bruised lips. Always be very gentle and light with your touch, administer food carefully and slowly. Do not fill the spoon over the edge. Give your loved one plenty of time to chew, even when the food is completely blended. Sometimes they will seem to be chewing blended food, even when there is nothing to chew. Never rush your loved one to eat faster. If they are not interested in food, never force-feed them. Respect their feelings and inclinations and be there, but do not linger impatiently with the spoon in their face. Nobody wants that. The meal should be peaceful and not rushed.

MAKE MEALS A PLEASANT OCCASION

It is a good idea to have a one way conversation when you are feeding you loved one. They most likely won't be looking at you, but will be completely focused on eating. But it will make it more pleasant if you talk to them. Imagine you were being spoon fed by an impatient and quiet person. Your meals would be torture. If you make eating a pleasant experience, your loved one will have a good appetite and will most likely need a rest after feeding. When you notice they are getting tired and don't seem to open the mount anymore, stop feeding them, lightly tap the lips with a soft tissue and apply a layer of natural lip balm.

> **IF AT ANY POINT DURING THE MEAL THEY GET SLEEPY,
> IMMEDIATELY STOP FEEDING THEM.
> ALWAYS MAKE SURE THEIR MOUTH IS EMPTY, BEFORE A NAP.
> IF NEED BE, PUT ON A PLASTIC GLOVE AND GENTLY OPEN THEIR MOUTH
> TO CHECK. ANY FOOD LEFT OVER FOOD COULD CAUSE CHOKING.**

After you are assured their mouth is empty, you may lower the head level to a 30% angle, make them comfortable with a blanket and give them some privacy and peace. Never lower the head into a completely flat position. Keep an eye on them and make sure that they are comfortably resting.

CHAPTER THIRTEEN

The Mind-Communication

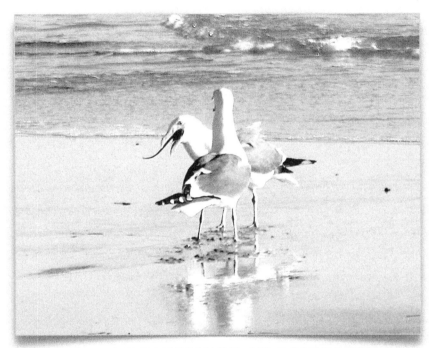

THERE ARE ENDLESS WAYS OF COMMUNICATING

*T*hru the years that I tended to my Mother, I spend long hours at her side trying to understand and communicate with her. There were times where no words were spoken for weeks at a time and then suddenly she would say three clear sentences in a row. That was a very special event and Dad and I were both thrilled to hear her speak.

Later in her illness, her speech diminished almost completely. I figured out a technique to get her to answer to me with a "Yes" and "No," but only sometimes. Other times she just nodded. That was enough for me. If I was not in her room and she let out a discontented frustrated cry that I heard over the ever-present baby monitor, I was immediately at her side. Even when the caregiver watched over her during some hours of the day, so that I could work in my home office, I ran to her side whenever I heard her. I could not bear keeping her in a frustrated state of not being understood.

She was always relieved at the sight of me as I assured her that I will make everything better and that I understood her. I caressed her beautiful hair and smiled at her even though I received no smile in return. Not because she would not want to smile, but because that capacity had been stolen from her. She was frozen in time. But she looked at me with her hazel eyes and we both knew we were communicating.

I did not need to hear the spoken words. I saw her eyes and felt her spirit. It was my honor to be there for her. I am grateful for that opportunity.

One late afternoon when I was at her side, she looked at me in full awareness, lifted he hand and softy caressed my cheek while looking right into my eyes so deeply and with such love and gratitude, that it made my heart burst. I smiled back at her and quickly ran off to another room.

I did not want her to see me cry. But I knew she loved me profoundly and was aware that I was with her… and that's all that mattered to me. Our communication was speechless, but completely connected.

ABOUT COMMUNICATION

The illness with its persistent progress slowly robs your loved one of their basic life functions. Speech is one of them. You can do a lot to preserve speech capacity for as long as possible, but sooner or later it will begin presenting a real challenge.

Assuming that your loved one is in late stage of dementia, their speaking ability will largely depend on how well it has been preserved. In other words, if you have spent a considerable amount of time helping them to continuously retain their speaking abilities, chances are, you will be able to still communicate with them. But if they were left alone, forgotten and no-one engaged with them in conversation, then they will disappear into their own unreachable world.

> **IT IS VERY IMPORTANT THAT YOU DO EVERYTHING YOU CAN,
> TO KEEP GOING WITH AT LEAST THE BASIC CONVERSATION
> FOR AS LONG AS POSSIBLE.
> THAT MEANS AT LEAST A YES AND A NO.
> BUT SOMETIMES YOUR LOVED ONE WILL SURPRISE YOU
> AND IF YOU CATCH THEM JUST AT THE RIGHT MOMENT,
> THEY MAY SAY A WHOLE STRING OF SENTENCES.**

One of the most important facts about keeping the conversation going is that you remain consistent and speak with your loved in the same tone as you used to, before their illness. Never speak to them like they are a little child or a baby, just because they cannot respond properly or quickly.

This illness does not mean that they are turning back into a baby who doesn't speak. They are slowly loosing the capacities they had, but can often still very well understand what is being said. Being silent and not speaking does not mean they do not understand you. They may just be unable to coordinate words and utter a reply.

Imagine you lose you capacity to speak and suddenly everyone starts talking to you like you are two years old. It could very well drive you completely mad. If you see your caregivers addressing your loved one like they are a child, immediately inform them that they need to speak to them respectfully as an adult.

It is also important that you do not speak about your loved one in their presence, as if they were absent. For example, when communicating with other family members or a caregiver in front of your loved one, do not behave as if they are not there. They can very well hear everything. Various negative comments about their dire situation, behavior or overall state could be very upsetting for them. Be conscious and respectful of them.

A person with dementia is still a person with their past, preferences, tendencies, habits, likes and dislikes. They still feel proud, but observe and sense things in an entirely different way. They may seem to have disappeared into a shell, but they are still there.

> **A HIGHLY INTELLIGENT OR PREVIOUSLY CAPABLE PERSON
> WHO IS NOW SUFFERING FROM DEMENTIA,
> COULD GO LIVID WHEN YOU TALK TO THEM AS IF THEY WERE A CHILD,
> OR IGNORE THEM WHILE SPEAKING OF THEM TO OTHERS.**

And that is understandable. You may only notice that they seem agitated, when in fact your ignorant behavior is making it worse for them. Imagine if the situation was reversed, and you were in their distressing circumstance.

Those aspects are not to be dismissed and ignored. A dementia patient is suffering thru a massive humiliation and loss of all control over their life. Do everything you can to help them retain a sense of respect and independence. Even if they are completely incapacitated, when you communicate with them, please treat them as if they are the same person they were. Yes, you can speak in simpler, clearer and easier to understand words, but you must remain respectful and very kind.

> **PROPER COMMUNICATION WITH YOUR LOVED ONE
> IS MOST CRUCIAL WHEN YOU ARE TRYING TO ASSURE THEM,
> COMFORT THEM, UNDERSTAND THEIR NEEDS
> AND GIVE THEM WHAT THEY WANT OR NEED.**

If you fail to make a decent effort in communicating with your loved one, it shows your very own shortcomings such as impatience, frustration or even pent-up anger. If you cannot quickly figure out what your loved one wants, needs or what is disturbing them to such an extent that they are screaming, you need to remain calm and considerate.

You do not have the luxury of loosing your wits. Use your intelligence and insight and imagine how you would feel in precisely their situation. They could be screaming for a million reason, whereas a deficient observer will only notice the screaming and fail to find the source. But the point is to learn and understand what is bothering them or what they are trying so desperately to convey to you. A good caregiver will conquer this challenge and patiently gain the ability to understand the language of someone who is captured in a speechless world.

> **YOU, DEAR CAREGIVER WITH A GOLDEN HEART,**
> **NEED TO BECOME A MASTER AT DECIPHERING**
> **YOUR LOVED ONE'S SIGNALS, SOUNDS AND HIDDEN EXPRESSIONS.**

THIS IS NOT ABOUT YOU

One of the challenges is, to not slip into a typical defensive position and assuming that your loved one's discontent is a personal attack on you. In fact, their discontent probably has nothing to do with you. If you think that they are angry with you, rebelling against you, or intentionally resisting you, rest assured you are wrong.

They are in their own very limited environment, where their ability to communicate has been drastically restricted or stripped away. Their anger or agitated outburst are caused by their frustration at the impossible predicament they find themselves in. You are not the cause, you are only the witness. Taking things personally is a crucial misconception. Your loved one is not being difficult on purpose. They are simply expressing their extreme frustration, anger, or complete dismay about their desperate state. They feel demoralized, incapacitated in the worst of ways. What to do?

> **DO NOT TAKE IT PERSONALLY, GET DEFENSIVE,**
> **REACTIVE AND RESPOND WITH YOUR OWN OUTBURST.**
> **INSTEAD, REMAIN CALM, PEACEFUL, SOOTHING AND CONSISTENT.**

This will help you reestablish harmony and will reassure them that they are cared for, heard, understood, unthreatened, safe and loved. You've managed to turn around the difficult dynamic and have succeeded it making it more bearable, manageable and harmonious.

COGNITIVE DISORDERS

It is important you become familiar with the most common cognitive conditions associated with Alzheimer's Dementia. They can manifest in many different ways, depending on individual's natural vulnerability or sensitivity, therefore the symptoms can vary from person to person. If you recognize one or more of these cognitive conditions in your loved one, it will help you better understand their challenges. It will also help you refrain from your own emotional or reactive response, when problematic situations arise. By being properly informed, you will perceive and comprehend your loved one's reactions, confusions and overall cognitive challenges. They will be more obvious on some days and less on others. You need to know that these conditions are not something your loved one can control. Never take their frustration, anger, disorientation or confusion personally.

ANOSOGNOSIA is a lack of understanding, acceptance or awareness of one's own medical illness. This can be quite obvious and more difficult to manage in early and mid - stage of illness, when your loved one is more combative and firmly convinced that they are not ill. In late stage your loved one will be physically weaker and more passive, but may still not understand that they are ill. They may perceive that they have a short illness and will eventually get better. Since they often exist in somewhat of a time vortex without any real sense of days, months or even years passing by, they can't implement that aspect into their grasp of the situation. By understanding that your loved one suffers from this condition, you will not attribute their persistent denial or confusion to their difficult personality, but will know that they are challenged and cannot understand their own state.

AGNOSIA is a cognitive condition where a person is unable to recognize sensory stimuli, such as visual, auditory or tactile - a sense of touch. An example of visual agnosia is when your loved one does not recognize a familiar location, building or object. A specific form of this condition is called **prosopagnosia**, where the person cannot recognize faces of friends and family. Auditory or verbal agnosia is an inability to understand spoken words, and tactile agnosia is an inability to recognize objects by touch.

APHASIA is a cognitive disorder where person loses their ability to speak or understand speech, as well as reading and writing. This is a very challenging aspect of illness. As caregiver you need to understand this condition, so that you communicate with your loved one by using very simple approach. Do not use a multi-choice question, but ask for a simple Yes and No answer. Anomia a form of aphasia in which the patient is unable to recall the names of everyday objects.

APRAXIA is a cognitive disorder that affects voluntary motor skills and the body's physical ability to function. It is often believed that Alzheimer's dementia simply causes people to be forgetful, when in fact in later stages of illness, the person becomes quite incapable of carrying out desired movements and gestures. It may take a major effort to simply scratch their nose. As a caregiver you need to be aware of this condition, so that you can properly assist your loved one when they really need your help. This will require a very tuned-in disposition, so that you can understand and sense their unspoken words and facial expressions.

ALTERED PERCEPTION is a cognitive disorder that changes how your loved one understands the world and other people. This will cause misperceptions, misidentifications, hallucinations, delusions and actual time-shifting. They will lose the basic concept of time and function in their own version of it.

AMNESIA is a cognitive disorder that causes loss of memories, facts, information and experiences. Retrograde amnesia is memory loss that is limited to the period before your loved one developed Alzheimer's.

APATHY is cognitive disorder that is a symptom of earlier phase of dementia when a person loses interest in what is happening around them. They lack motivation, don't care about what's going on and stop engaging.

ATTENTION DEFICIT is an early sign of cognitive decline and becomes more obvious as dementia progresses. Your loved one's attention span and concentration will decrease, they are easily distracted and have difficulty focusing on task at hand.

UNDERSTANDING YOUR LOVED ONE'S NEEDS AND FEELINGS

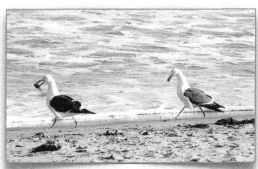

BE PATIENT AND LISTEN

One of the most important elements of successful caregiving is being able to keep communicating with your loved one. You need to understand how they feel and what they need. This will require you learning to think as logically as possible and putting yourself in their shoes.

Your loved one is helpless, dependent, confused, fearful and probably angry about not being in charge of their own body, mind and life in general. Their speech capacity is often completely diminished and the ability to smile has long gone. As their caregiver, you have to learn how to become a fine-tuned instrument with a deep capacity for understanding. Instead of taking their bouts of frustration personally, you need to distance your ego and become an observer and advisor. Of course they are still your loved one, but your previous equal way of communicating is a thing of the past.

FAMILY MEMBER CAREGIVERS OFTEN COMPLAIN
HOW THEIR LOVED ONE IS SEEMINGLY MEAN AND SAYS UPSETTING
THINGS OR ACTS OUT AGGRESSIVELY TOWARDS THEM,
NEVER SMILING OR EXPRESSING ANY GRATITUDE
FOR ALL THE SACRIFICE THEY HAVE ENDURED FOR THEM.

THIS IS NOT THE PLACE OR TIME TO EXPECT PRAISE AND APPLAUSE.
YOU NEED TO RISE ABOVE IT, FOR YOUR FACULTIES ARE NOT IMPACTED.
YOU ARE THEIR GUARDIAN AND PROTECTOR NOW.

When your loved one loses the ability to smile, how do you expect them to smile at you when they see you? When your loved one is stuck with incontinence and depends on others for their basic needs, do you really expect them to stay calm?

By loosing their sense of dignity and pride, don't you think it's understandable for them to lash out or say something upsetting? Think about it. Your loved one may seem like a different person, but somewhere deep inside is still that independently proud individual, who loved life and could be kind and gentle. Now they are trapped in an ailing body and mind and depend on the kindness of others to function, be clean, eat and survive. Their situation is beyond upsetting. It is extremely challenging.

> **THIS IS THE TIME FOR YOU TO BECOME A MASTER OBSERVER,**
> **AN INTUITIVE MENTALIST AND A SPIRITUAL DETECTIVE.**
>
> **YOU MUST LEARN TO UNDERSTAND A MIND PUZZLE,**
> **HEAR A SPEECHLESS WORD**
> **AND READ A MOTIONLESS SIGN.**

A DIFFERENT PERSPECTIVE

How can one imagine a situation that differs from their own?
Only by expanding their mind and envisioning themselves in such a situation. Good actors imagine living in a different body while experiencing a particular life under diverse circumstances. That is how they try to embody another person's existence and help the audience understand their character's actions and behavior.

> **THE HIGHEST SPIRITUAL TEACHINGS**
> **ENCOURAGE US TO NOT JUDGE OTHERS.**
> **TRUE NOBILITY ENTAILS AN OPEN MIND AND HEART**
> **WITH NO JUDGMENT.**

Develop the understanding that various life experiences and events make people see the world differently than you.

- ❋ If you have an allergy to milk, can you understand that someone loves to drink milk?
- ❋ If you enjoy eating meat, can you understand others who physically can't tolerate it?
- ❋ If you like cold showers, can you understand someone who hates standing under cold water?
- ❋ If you live in a city, can you understand a country dweller who is unfamiliar with the subway?
- ❋ If you watch TV five hours a day, can you understand someone who doesn't have a TV?
- ❋ If you live in a free country, can you understand how it is to live in a war zone?
- ❋ If you can easily get food, can you possibly understand how it feels to starve?

Expand your mind and attempt to embrace the diversity of this world and its people. Then you will have an easier time understanding the drastically limited life-circumstances of your loved one. Perhaps you will get less irritated with the situation and see the true value in your service to another human being who is so fragile and utterly vulnerable.

> **EVERY HEALTHY AND FULLY FUNCTIONING PERSON HAS THE ABILITY TO IMAGINE.**
> **OUR MINDS ARE FREE TO EXPLORE AND IMAGINE ANYTHING.**
> **WHAT A LUXURY!**

In order to understand your loved one, put your mindset into a different mode and use your imagination while learning non-judgment and compassion in the deepest sense. If you are facing a challenge when trying to understand your loved one, always imagine you are in their position. It will help you understand a source of possible discomfort or the reason behind their fearful, agitated state.

I invite you to explore this simple exercise that will help you understand how your loved one feels under their extremely challenging circumstances.

EXERCISE FOR A DEEPER UNDERSTANDING

Let's begin with a visualization of the morning events.

Imagine you wake up and find yourself lying in bed, soiled and uncomfortable. You do not recognize the room you are in. It seems familiar, but you don't know where you really are. You are confused, and don't quite understand the source of your discomfort. You feel lost, frightened, embarrassed and frustrated. You try to scratch your nose and can't. Your hand doesn't budge. There is a crumpled sheet under your back, feeling sweaty and uncomfortable. You try to move and cannot. You have a cramped leg that seems to be stuck in the same position for hours. Your body feels stiff and foreign. Nothing listens and obeys your directives.

Imagine you can't find the words to express a simple things like: "I want to get out of bed" or "I think I am wet and want to go to the bathroom." You try to speak, but can't. The words don't seem to want to come out of your mouth. Instead, a loud noise seems to fill the room. You are the one that's making this noise and can't seem to even control yourself. No words, no sense, just a helpless noisy moan.

A person appears at your bedside and you do not recognize them. This is even more confusing and upsetting. You try to convey to them what you need and they don't seem to understand you. They cannot. The more you try, the more frustrated they become and speak loudly back at you. You can't understand what they are saying, it is way too fast and too loud. You are now panicked and frightened.

It seems you are in some strange nightmare. The problem is magnified by the fact that the person does not know what to do and seems upset, less and less patient and finally angry and mean. You try to move your hands but cannot, you try to help them and cannot. Your body doesn't seem yours anymore. It is just a dead weight and you feel exhausted and utterly helpless.

Now they start pulling you out of bed, undressing you, all the while speaking words you can't understand. They seem annoyed with your desperate screams and are incapable of resolving your problem. You don't know what is happening, where they are taking you and why they are undressing you. You are frightened and lost.

Does that seem like a really bad nightmare to you? Well, it is. Except we usually wake up from a nightmare. That will never be the case for your loved one. Their nightmare is continuous and goes on and on. This is the cage your loved one lives in. And it is also an example of a caregiver that is incapable of communication. And yet, that is exactly what is going to happen, unless you get deeply involved and use the keys for better understanding.

Now, let's continue with the last part of our exercise. Imagine the same situation, but the "stranger" behaves nicely. Here is the proper way to communicate in these circumstances:

When you make a sound in your attempt to call for help, a stranger immediately enters your room. They are kind and pleasant. They smile at you, and greet you with a gentle and clear voice. They speak very softly and slowly. The tenderly stroke your head and calm you down. You feel that this is a kind person who will help you. You are comforted and feel assured that all is well. You are not deserted.

They gently explain to you, that they understand you and will make you feel better. And even if you don't understand every word they say, you feel their calm presence, hear their soothing voice, see their nice smile and feel assured you will be all right. When you are calmer you can hear better and sometimes even understand the words they say. You understand when they say: "Everything is fine. I will take care of you, just relax."

Now it doesn't even matter where you are, because you know all will be well. Things are starting to feel familiar to you. The person acts with confidence and you sense that they know what to do. This comforts you and calms you down. They are pleasant and nice to you. They are your friend.

And when you are calmer, you suddenly recognize this is your family member. Thank goodness everything is fine. Now you feel safe.

This is the difference and positive effect on the overall well being of your loved one, who suffers from this devastating illness. You need to know how to relate and behave with them. You must feel confident in your actions, otherwise your best intentions will go unheard and you will end up exhausting yourself and increasing the frustration of your loved one. Apply logic to every circumstance.

IMAGINE HOW YOU WOULD FEEL IF YOU WERE STUCK LIKE THAT. MOST OF US WOULD SCREAM IN FRUSTRATION. THAT'S IS VERY OFTEN THE REASON FOR MORNING SCREAMS.

You need to be aware when the screaming starts and make an effort to be present as soon as possible. With assurance that you understand what is going on and will take care of them, you can calm down your loved one almost immediately.

> **IF A SCREAMING FIT IS LEFT UNATTENDED FOR TOO LONG,
> IT WILL BECOME ALMOST AN AUTOMATIC REFLEX
> AND NOTHING WILL REMEDY IT FOR A LONG TIME.**

The morning routine is beyond stressful and exhausting for the caregiver, so if you can eliminate the desperate screaming of your loved one, you will do everyone involved a huge favor.

SUGGESTED COMMUNICATION FOR THE MORNING

This will most likely feel like a monologue, since you will be talking by yourself. There is a slight chance that your loved one may respond with a tiny answer, since it is morning and their mind is in a different state of deep relaxation. But if you were late in responding to their waking up and they are already upset, you can nor expect any words from them at this point.

No matter how their mood and disposition appear, remain a picture of calm serenity. Never get upset, loud in your communication with them and do not ever scold them. That is completely unacceptable, I don't care how bad your night was or how sleep deprived you are. Muster up your energy and become the helper that your loved one needs at this point.

> **SPEAK SOFTLY, CLEARLY, KINDLY AND SLOWLY.
> HAVE A PLEASANT DISPOSITION,
> NO MATTER HOW TIRED AND OVERWHELMED YOU FEEL.
> IT WILL HELP YOU AS WELL.**

AN EXAMPLE OF YOUR MORNING GREETING:

"Good morning my dear. I hope you slept well. How are you feeling?"
Wait for an answer for a bit, then continue.

"I will be getting you out of bed now. I am always with you.
I heard you and came right away. Just relax."

Regardless of receiving an answer or not, this is the way to start the morning.
If there is some communication always acknowledge that you heard them.

"Did you sleep well?"
Answer: Yes.

"That's great. Would you like to get up?"
Answer: Yes.

"Great, we will do that right away.
Please be patient while I get everything ready.
I want you to be comfortable.
Pause.

"We will get you up, change you and freshen you up.
A great breakfast is waiting for you.
You will like that.
It is delicious."

This way you have done a few things. You have assured your loved one that you understand them and are going to eliminate their discomfort. You have also distracted them with a new and pleasant activity that awaits.

It is important that you do not make a big deal about the fact that your loved one is soiled and can't do anything on their own. Remain kind and pleasant, assuring and comforting at all times. If you cannot manage this, get a caregiver who can. This is what your loved one needs and deserves. No less.

WHAT AGITATES YOUR LOVED ONE - BECOME AN INTUITIVE MENTALIST

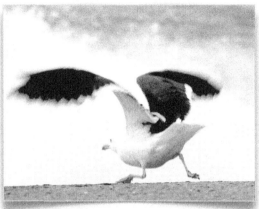

THERE IS MEANING IN EVERY GESTURE

Because your loved one has difficulty in communicating and cannot convey the source of their discomfort or pain, you need to keep a very close eye on them. Pay attention to signs like yelling, moaning, restlessness, grimacing or inability to be still. If you are a keen observer, you will be able to decipher their message and eliminate any unnecessary discomfort or suffering. Remain watchful, every small detail of their behavior matters.

THE PRIORITY IS TO ELIMINATE ANY SOURCE OF AGITATION
AS SOON AS POSSIBLE.
BECAUSE THE ONLY MEANS OF COMMUNICATION
THAT YOUR LOVED HAS LEFT ARE VARIOUS SOUNDS
AND HELPLESS MOANS, YOUR ABILITY TO UNDERSTAND THEM
IS OF GREATEST IMPORTANCE.

Keep in mind; when you attempt to communicate with your loved one and wish to receive a simple Yes or No answer, it is very possible that your loved one will confuse these two options. What will help you decipher the correct answer is the increase in their vocal expression. Their actual Yes answer could be correct, OR the only way they can express an affirmative answer is with a louder vocal moan.

POSSIBLE SOURCES OF DISCOMFORT

Here is the checklist for quick review of possible cause of your loved one's discomfort:

- Incontinence, needs to be changed
- Has to use the bathroom
- Pain
- Leg cramps
- Digestive issues
- Nervousness
- Room temperature
- Awkward sitting or lying position
- Hunger or thirst
- Bright light
- Noise
- Uncomfortable clothing
- Crinkle under back
- Missing neck support pillow
- Needs repositioning of legs or arms
- Sore backside
- Placement of hands uncomfortable
- Other people sitting too close
- Crowded room
- Too much activity in their presence

**FINDING THE SOURCE OF DISCOMFORT
IS OF THE GREATEST IMPORTANCE.
TAKE YOUR TIME, BE PATIENT
AND REMAIN CALM AND KIND.**

STEP BY STEP COMMUNICATION GUIDE

ON HOW TO UNDERSTAND, DECIPHER AND REMEDY UNSPOKEN DISCOMFORT THAT YOUR LOVED ONE IS TRYING TO COMMUNICATE

PROBLEM: Incontinence, wet or soiled incontinence pad

SOLUTION: They need to be changed. Make sure there are no sensitive bedsore start-up areas, as that may considerably increase the discomfort. If you are slow in responding to incontinence needs and do not change them with sufficient frequency, they could very quickly develop bedsores, sometimes in a matter of hours. Another very common consequence could be a reoccurring urinary track infection - UTI, accompanied by unpleasant smell. If left untreated, UTI can quickly spread into kidneys and impair their function. Consequences are very serious.

PROBLEM: Pain

SOLUTION: You need to assess the source of pain. Carefully examine where the pain is coming from. Ask slowly and with a calm and gentle voice:

"Are you in pain?"

If there is no answer, continue assuring them that you will help them. Gently and lightly touch various parts of their body and pay attention, if they vocally indicate increase in pain. If the answer is Yes, inquire further. Slowly touch various areas of the body while asking corresponding question:

" Is it your leg? Is it your tummy? Is it your back? Is it your arm?"

You will soon discover the source. Very often, the answer may be "No!" while they continue with their vocal display of discomfort. This could mean two possibilities: they have confused their answer or they are not in pain. If there is actual pain somewhere, they will confirm it by increasing their vocals when you touch the affected area.

IF YOU TOUCH THE AFFECTED AREA AND THEY YELL OUT LOUDLY "NO" THIS MAY INDICATE THAT YOU HAVE FOUND THE SOURCE OF PAIN.

Now you can address the problem area further. Assure a proper and comfortable position of the body part that seems in pain, then gently massage the area and carefully observe if the pain is relieved. In case of sever persistent pain, immediately notify the doctor. If you choose to ignore the source of possible pain, you could be subjecting them to unnecessary suffering. However, there is a high probability that you will easily find the source of pain and resolve it with a few minor adjustments. If they continue displaying general discomfort, but you did not find a source of pain, and it seems pain is not the cause, explore other possible sources as indicated in this chapter.

PROBLEM: Leg Cramps
SOLUTION: Check for Remedies in Chapter *Holistic Caregiving Remedies*

PROBLEM: Digestive Issues, Constipation, Diarrhea
SOLUTION: Check for Remedies in Chapter *Holistic Caregiving Remedies*

PROBLEM: Nervousness, anxiety
POSSIBLE SOLUTIONS: Check for Remedies in Chapter *Holistic Caregiving Remedies*. Next, carefully examine what the source nervousness. Begin by asking, slowly and softly:
"Are you feeling nervous?"

If the answer is Yes, then assure them that you will resolve the matter. If there is no answer, inquire further. Check all the following possible sources of increased nervousness:

HUNGER OR THIRST

Make sure the loved one is not experiencing hunger or thirst. Gently ask and offer a healthy snack or drink, regardless of your regular feeding schedule. What matters is their continuous comfort. Never forget or ignore their need or desire for food and proper hydration. Quite often a few sips or bites of food will quickly calm down the nervous state.

BRIGHT LIGHT

Make sure the light in their room isn't too bright. Protect them from any direct blinding sunlight with a shade. Never have a strong or glaring neon light directly above their bed or in their room. If brightness was the source of discomfort and you remove it, they will immediately calm down. It may be easier for you to clean their room with a very bright light, but for their optimal comfort and every day use, the light in their room should always be gentle and soft. Check for suggestions on the ideal room set up in Chapter *Preparing your Home.*

NOISE

There should never be too much noise in their room. Request silence from anyone else in the room and create a completely serene environment. There must be absolutely no ongoing conversations or even whispering in loved one's presence for the time being. This will often result in immediate calmness and a more peaceful state. You need to put their comfort before anyone else, since they are helpless and cannot change their circumstance. If you have a caregiver that wishes to watch TV to help pass the time, they need to understand that this creates too much disturbance for your loved one. On the other hand, soft gentle music in the background can do wonders. But if it was noise that got them irritated in the first place, they need absolute silence for a while.

ROOM TEMPERATURE

Check the temperature of the room. Inappropriate temperature – too warm or cold can make them extremely agitated. The temperature needs to be comfortable for them and not you. They are inactive and have different needs. You can adjust your clothing, whereas they depend on you for everything. They should never be sweating or be cold. If their hands or feet are cold, cover and tuck them with a blanket and gently massage them to improve the circulation. Check for suggestions on the ideal room set up in Chapter *Preparing your Home*.

AWKWARD SITTING OR LYING POSITION

Watch out for any uncomfortable physical positioning. Perhaps they slid down in the recliner and feel like they will fall off. Maybe they are propped up, yet feel too slouched and are experiencing stiffness in neck or another body area. Use neck pillow for support. If they are bed-bound, adjust their positioning and readjust any supporting pillows. Maybe they just need to be moved a bit. Gently reposition them and patiently assure comfort. If that was the cause of nervousness, they will respond positively. When you readjust their physical position, make sure that no fabric is gathered at their back causing them discomfort.

UNCOMFORTABLE CLOTHING

Perhaps the cause of discomfort is uncomfortable clothing that feels too warm or too tight in places. Double check for any tight waists or sleeves with tight elastics. Maybe they are simply wearing too much. Keep in mind that certain materials may begin to scratch or irritate the skin, if they are worn the whole day with no physical activity or when perspiring or feeling hot. If they are perspiring, change them immediately into a new set of fresh clothes. Leaving your loved one in sweaty clothing will expose them to danger of painful bedsores.

CRINKLE UNDER BACK

Their discomfort could be caused by a simple thing like a crinkled wrinkle under the back due to a gathered sheet or clothing. It can become very uncomfortable to sit or lie on bunched up material for longer periods of time. If not tended to right away, they could develop a bedsore. Every time you change them or reposition them, carefully and gently smooth all clothing and sheets under their back. Never use any fast or forced movements as you may unintentionally injure their thin and vulnerable skin.

MISSING NECK SUPPORT PILLOW

Perhaps their head is too low and needs to be elevated. Elderly people lose muscle strength especially in the neck, which creates a very uncomfortable circumstance if not tended too. Make sure the neck is well supported and straight at all times. You can use the U shaped travel neck pillow for excellent neck support. If you forget about this problem for even a single day, their head will hang on one side or rest on their shoulder. This will cause severely cramped muscles on that one side and overly stretched muscles on the other side of the neck. Or their head may hang forward as if nodding off without any support. If left unattended, they could completely lose the capacity to keep the head up and their neck will remain seriously curved. All this can cause them severe pain and discomfort. Always watch for this potential problem. Your watchful and ongoing care can completely prevent this issue.

REPOSITIONING LEGS OR ARMS

When sitting in one position without much movement, legs can become especially restless and uncomfortable. Reposition them often and use several different support pillows for under knees, under feet or between knees. Never leave your loved one sitting or lying in the same position for the entire day. If the legs are too low, elevate them slightly by placing a support pillow under the knees. If loved one is left unattended or in the same position, they could develop severe leg cramps, discomfort and pain. Remain diligent and more or less reposition them every hour or two during the day.

SORE BACKSIDE

If your loved one is sitting the entire day, you can only imagine how sore their tailbone, backside and lower back area can become. This can be even worse, if they suffer from hemorrhoids. If that is so, always rearrange their sitting position by moving them more to one side and place them on the softest cushions. In addition, pull them up on the chair every few hours to carefully redistribute their weigh. If they slide down and have all the weight on their lower back, the pain may become unnerving and they could also develop bed sores.

To pull them up on the chair, tell them what you are about to do. Next, step behind the chair and place your hands under their armpits from behind. Then pull them up gently but firmly with one confident move. Examine the clothing to make sure there is no gathered and rolled up pressing material anywhere. Smooth out the clothing under their back to assure complete comfort.

Always use a lumbar support belt to prevent straining your back. Slowly lean them onto one side to get access to their back. Gently massage their back and hip area. Lean them to the other side and repeat.

HEMORRHOIDS

If your loved one seems uncomfortable while sitting and is more agitated during incontinence changes and seems calmer afterwards, this may be caused by a flared up Hemorrhoid. Examine them carefully during the incontinence change and check to see if this is the source of discomfort. Check for Remedies in Chapter *Holistic Caregiving Remedies*.

PLACEMENT OF HANDS

Make sure they are comfortable with the placement of their arms and hands. Unless you are airing out the room and it is cold, do not tuck their arms under a blanket. Leave the hands out and place them with fingers gently stretched on small curved pillows, so that the hands do not get closed, clenched or cramped. If you do not pay attention to hands, in short time they could develop completely closed and clenched fists that can't be undone.

PEOPLE TOO CLOSE

Anyone stuck in a passive position all day can become irritated by constant presence of another human being to close to their face. It can become an overwhelming feeling of claustrophobia and lack of privacy. Make sure that you or a caregiver does not lean into the personal space of your loved one too closely.

Very often a frustrated person will vocally express their discomfort about that, yet since nobody understands what the problem is, the well wishing caregiver will only increase the "too close for comfort" position and magnify it by loud questioning. By wanting to help, they will be doing exactly the opposite. After a failed effort they will feel that the person is just nervous for no reason. Wrong. If you are not aware of this, just the sight of the caregiver could agitate the loved one.

CROWDED ROOM

This can happen during visitations. Your loved one is in need of peace and quiet at all times. Of course, when a doctor is present there will be some activity. But doctors will know to keep things calm, and unless you raise your voice in loud attempts of explanation, the atmosphere in the room will remain peaceful.

However, when there are visitations from relatives or friends you must be aware that people usually do not understand that your loved is now a very different person. Repeated loud random questioning could irritate anyone, especially when their condition prevents them from answering and interacting as they used to. The main occupation for your loved one is to feel comfortable. That is really all that they are capable of concentrating on. Their body and mind are in such a slow operating state that they cannot engage with others, no matter how much they wish to. Everything else is simply too much and overbearing for them. Long visitations will interfere with their usual pace and could have negative consequences. If the loved one suddenly becomes nervous or agitated when visitors are present, they should immediately leave the room without a major ordeal or long goodbye's. Minimize any interactions or visitations that could in any way aggravate your loved one.

TOO MUCH ACTIVITY IN THEIR PRESENCE

No matter what is going on, you can never expose your loved one to stressful circumstances. A loud discussion with the caregiver, furious vacuuming and dusting, or other noisy clean-up activity in their presence, can seriously disturb them. Limit cleaning and vacuuming the room to a necessary minimum, or do it when your loved on is not there. Perhaps you can take them outside while their room is being cleaned. If you are alone with them, and have to clean the room yourself, clean it in small sections and in short segments. Keep most conversation with caregivers outside of your loved one's room. If you are the caregiver, keep other family members properly informed about the need for peace and quiet. All daily clean-up activities can be done quietly, without slamming doors, creating drafts and nervous fury. Be like a shadow of a presence and do everything to keep things peaceful.

These are some of the possible causes for their nervous state. Of course the possibilities are quite endless, but if you cover this basic checklist, you will be closer to figuring out where lies the problem.

IF YOU HAVE TRIED ALL THE ABOVE AND NERVOUSNESS PERSISTS, THEN TRY A DIFFERENT APPROACH - DISTRACTION.

The following suggestions can often resolve irritable nervousness:

- ❋ Offer them a light snack
- ❋ Put on some soft soothing music
- ❋ Air out the room
- ❋ Change their incontinence pad, just to make sure that is not causing the problem
- ❋ Engage them with a light conversation
- ❋ Turn on the TV with their favorite program
- ❋ Go outdoors and change the scenery by spending time in nature. Maybe they just feel restless in their restricted situation.

Any kind of change will help redirect their attention away from their stagnant position. Distraction will also help interrupt automatic repetitive moaning, that may be their way of self-soothing.

If all the above approaches fail, do your best to consider other possible causes for their frustration and discontent. Quite often it will resolve itself with a change of pace, a meal, going outdoors or getting ready for bed.

If the agitation continues for the whole day and does not in any way change or diminish after you feed and wash them and put them to sleep, you need to use the medication on as-needed basis that has been provided by your doctor, for this purpose. However, keep in mind, if you remain patient and persistent, you will most likely succeed in resolving the cause of agitation.

TO CLARIFY, WE ARE TALKING ABOUT A GENERAL MOODY, AGITATED, NERVOUS STATE AND NOT AN ACUTE, AGONIZING, PAINFUL SCREAMING STATE. IF THE LATER IS THE CASE, ALWAYS IMMEDIATELY CALL THE DOCTOR.

If you continuously call on the physician with the same minor complaint, without beforehand exploring all options for possible solution yourself, they will simply prescribe proper medication - a sedative - for this condition. You cannot expect the doctor to spend hours at your house exploring all the possible causes of nervousness. If the doctor comes for a home visit even as fast as the next day, there is always the possibility that by then, your loved one may be perfectly fine. That is challenging, but very often the case.

This is why it is important that you become well versed at understanding your loved one. Paying attention to any considerable changes with your loved one is your responsibility as a caregiver. Always notate them in the specific log, so you are properly prepared for the doctor's visit. If you have checked and carefully paid attention to all possible causes of your loved one's discomfort and have successfully remedied them, you have done your job.

If the doctor feels a small dose of medication is needed, just to help keep the patient less nervous, that makes perfect sense. Ideally, the doctor can give you anxiety reducing medicine that you can give your loved one on an as-needed basis. This way you are prepared for the next agitation episode. As said, this is of course only after you have not been able to remedy the situation with a simple comfort adjustment.

It is a tragic fact that people usually don't take the time to figure out an often simple cause of discomfort of their loved one. They simply announce that the person is nervous for no apparent reason, and insist on medicating them. That way, they can leave them soiled, heavily sedated and hanging off the recliner, hungry, dehydrated or otherwise uncomfortable. They simply quiet them down with often unnecessary and overprescribed medication.

However, a mild sedative for occasional use, on an only as-needed basis, can be very useful and helpful, if they are in a particularly agitated state. Use it sparingly and it will be more effective. When used continuously, the doses will have to be increased in order to have an effect.

I FIND THE APPROACH TO RANDOMLY OVERMEDICATE THE ELDERLY, IN ORDER TO KEEP THEM QUIET AND NOT PAY ANY ATTENTION TO THEM, INEXCUSABLE, UNACCEPTABLE, AND TRULY TRAGIC.

Don't misunderstand me, I believe proper medication can and is a real lifesaver. But only after you have explored all other logical options and have not resolved the source of the discomfort.

OBSERVATIONS

One of the key skills in observation is to sharply concentrate and focus on the ongoing condition of your loved one, without getting too emotional. May I kindly remind you, that the descriptions here are specific for the advanced stage of Alzheimer's dementia.

When you see your loved one every day, from morning till evening, it is often more difficult to notice any ongoing changes. They occur gradually and you simply get used to them. However, your ability to discern the progress of illness, carefully focus and observe the visual appearance and behavior of your loved one, is essential.

Pay especial attention to the following aspects:

- Is there a different expression in the eyes, a more distant gaze?
- Are they still answering your questions?
- Do they visually look different?
- Are their hands more cramped?
- Are they less mobile?
- Are they less interested in walking?
- Has their appetite decreased?
- Do they still recognize you?
- Are you still able to communicate with them in any capacity?

All those indicators of the ever evolving and changing situation are especially important for the purpose of your fine-tuned understanding of how they feel. Your logging booklet is going to prove more valuable than ever. Notate any and all changes, so you can properly track your loved one's condition and are able to keep the doctor well informed.

> NO MATTER WHAT THE PROGRESS OF ILLNESS IS,
> ONE THING YOU CAN ASSURE YOUR LOVED ONE
> IS OPTIMAL COMFORT AT ALL TIMES.
> AND THAT IS INVALUABLE.

UNDERSTANDING SOUNDS

When your loved one is not feeling comfortable, there will be a few ways they will try to alarm you of their troubling situation or discomfort. Here is a list of usual efforts when they are trying to communicate with you, and a list of possible causes and remedies.

CALLING YOU, BUT NOT ABLE TO FOLLOW-UP OR EXPLAIN

Come to their rescue and assure them that you heard them and are always here for them.
MOST LIKELY REASON: fear, isolation, confusion, discomfort, needs assurance

RANDOM CALLS OF DISTRESS

Assure them that all is well and you are watching over them and they are never alone.
MOST LIKELY REASON: distress, discomfort, thirst, fear, and confusion

YELPING

Calmly soothe them and remind them that they were heard and all will be taken care of.
MOST LIKELY REASON: feeling helpless, abandoned, sad, fearful

YELLING

Immediately assure safety and comfort. A lukewarm washcloth pressed to the forehead may help in calming them down, changing their focus, and getting out of that state.
MOST LIKELY REASON: bad dream, fear, pain, left unattended, confused

MOANING AND WHINING

Gently inquire what is the problem. Check everything again and calmly state that everything is fine and there is no reason for worry.
MOST LIKELY REASON: very often the person will slide into an almost self induced self-soothing chant-like moaning rhythm, that seems to keep them occupied and releases tension or frustrated pent-up energy of not being able to form words and properly speak.

HELPLESS LIFTING AND REACHING WITH ARMS

It is heartbreaking and frustrating to watch this and not know what to do. Hold on to their hand and let them know that you are paying attention to them and will remove their discomfort shortly. Go thru the checklist while informing them of what you are doing. Assure them that you will take care of everything and make them comfortable.
MOST LIKELY REASON: Often they just need you to be present and hold their hand. It gives them a feeling of comfort and reduces their fear of helpless abandonment.

READING FACIAL EXPRESSIONS

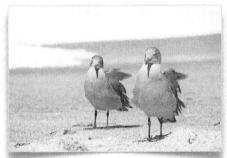

OBSERVE AND LEARN

FROWNING AND GRIMACING WITH NO WORDS

You can get a lot of information, by cautiously observing your loved one's facial expression. If they seem troubled or uncomfortable, they will frown and grimace. To make sure it is not just a frown out of habit, stroke their forehead gently and see if they relax. Frowning can indicate pain, discomfort, depression, unease, fear and frustration among others.

I suggest that you go thru the check list and assure that nothing is missing. You may not always experience a crying call when something is amiss. So be diligent and check on everything. Gently assure them that you are checking everything for their comfort. Most likely you will find the source and their face will relax.

LOOKING AT THE FLOOR

Possibly sad, tired or completely disinterested. They need proper rest, but also pleasant distractions to see if their mood improves. When they look down, they feel down.

GAZING INTO THE DISTANCE

They could be reminiscing and are far away with their thoughts. Let them be and enjoy their daydreaming. As long as they are peaceful, they are most likely comfortable.

FROWNING

There is a discomfort somewhere and you need to figure it out. Check the list of possible discomforts and all the while soothe them with your voice that everything is fine and you are helping them be more comfortable.

STRUGGLING EXPRESSION

Make sure there is no problem with incontinence or constipation.

OPENING THEIR MOUTH, NO SOUND

Most likely they are hungry and need feeding. A spoonful of food will calm them down.

EYE CONTACT

Make sure you project assurance, comfort and kindness when making eye contact. Your loved one is always yearning to feel supported, protected, safe and loved.

ANGER OR SUSPICION

It is possible that your loved one is momentarily confused about who you are. They may feel threatened and mistrusting. Stay pleasant, calm, relax your eye contact, smile, be very gentle, so they can relax and feel safe. Step away for a few moments and then calmly return.

Try gently saying: "It is me, your daughter, son, partner ..." and repeat your name. Remind them that everything is fine and you are there with them. Assure them, you are taking care of everything and all is well. You can help relieve their mistrust by gently stroking their hand or their hair while speaking with soft and kind vice. They will eventually relax. Do not make a big deal about their confusion and it will diminish faster.

CREATING A COMFORT ZONE

The environment is most certainly the key element in creating the optimal comfort zone. But without you - the loving and confident caregiver - everything is meaningless. Human connection is as important as ever. Every one of us needs human touch, gentle words, loving heart and kind care.

> **DO NOT ASSUME THAT BECAUSE LOVED ONE CANNOT SPEAK OR MOVE, THEY DO NOT REGISTER IF YOU ARE THERE. THEY MOST CERTAINLY CAN. THEY CAN FEEL A LOVING PRESENCE OR IF THEY ARE CONSIDERED A NUISANCE.**

Be as loving as you can, for any human that is stuck in such a helpless a situation deserves the kindest and most compassionate care. They will feel it, sense it and if it's meant to be, you will see their appreciation in their eyes. Their soul is present and knows everything. Make no mistake. This is not only a test of their endurance. It is also a rigorous test of your character and capacity for unconditional love.

YOUR VOICE

When used properly, your voice is an incredibly powerful healing tool. Even if the loved one is incapable of understanding the words you try to convey, they will sense the tone and emotion behind them. Speak slowly and clearly, never repeating the same thing too many times. Not all elderly are hard of hearing and often people repeatedly, impatiently and continuously yell loud questions into their ears. That is ignorant and disturbing.

ALWAYS USE A GENTLY SOOTHING VOICE, REASSURING THEM THAT YOU ARE UNAFRAID AND RELIABLE. NEVER DISPLAY YOUR HURT FEELINGS, DESPAIR OR SADNESS.

It could further confuse and upset them. There is no good purpose in letting them see you sorrowful, even thou you may feel like that. Yes, this is the time to put on a brave face. Even when things are very challenging and difficult, you must remain the calm in the storm. If you manage to do that, you will be pleasantly surprised when an unknown source of energy will come from within you, and help you remain calm and gentle, even when everything seems to be falling apart.

No matter what chaos may be happening around you, remain the picture of strength and love. Using a calming voice will help in calming you down as well, so you can create and maintain an ever peaceful, secure and loving environment.

HEALING TOUCH

A few things are as comforting as the soothing, healing touch of your hands. Use a gentle light stroke to caress your loved one's head and their hands. Gently massage away any tension from their face and induce a general state of relaxation. Every morning and evening when you apply their facial cream, use the same slow, light and gentle touch and it will become a soothing part of daily routine, that could instantly calm and relax them.

If they enjoy this interaction, you can implement a daily light massage of their hands, arms, legs, and feet. Understanding this from a subtle energy perspective, your hands have an amazing ability to disperse comforting energy through your intentional healing touch. This positive energy exchange can become an intricate part of your daily care as a powerful soothing tool of your healing-touch routine.

TIPS FOR CALMING DOWN

When your loved one is voicing their discomfort, calmly approach them from front and check thru the basic check-list to assure their well-being. To help immediately calm them down, I suggest that you softly and calmly inform them that you heard their calls, with following assurances:

OPTION ONE

" I am here and I will help you. Everything is all right. I will take care of everything."

OPTION TWO

"You are not alone. I am always here for you."

OPTION THREE

"Let's see why you are uncomfortable. Everything is fine I will just change you and freshen you up. We will be very quick and done in no time. Don't worry, everything is all right."

Keep the communication to a few clear words that you convey calmly and slowly. While you are speaking to them, do a quick review of their situation with the basic check-list. Move and adjust the various support pillows to address the possible discomfort. Sometimes that is all it will take to remedy the situation.

Usually you will quickly find the source of the problem. Keep in mind they might not stop crying or yelling right away, so it is up to you to determine, if something obvious is creating discomfort, such as a soiled incontinence pad or undergarments. After you eliminate the problem, assure them that it is taken care of and they are all right. Hopefully they will calm down shortly. Gentle soothing music in the background may be helpful.

If you need to change the pad, always inform them of what you are about to do. It will help eliminate confusion about what is going on. Remember, they cannot understand their momentary state and need to be reminded, even if you did this particular task a million times before.

When you are eliminating a problem, here is the most effective formula:
The quicker you find the source of discomfort, the faster they will clam down. That is the priority in this particular challenge. Even if the source of discomfort is such, that you cannot resolve it instantly, your kind voice, a gentle caress of their head or hand, will substantially calm them down fairly quickly.

NEW RULES FOR CONVERSATION

When you interact with your loved one, remember that they are not able to be your communication partner as they used to be in the past. The dynamics have shifted in most profound ways. The opportunity for conversations where you complained and shared your heartaches are long gone. This is also not the time to criticize your relatives or others, while feeling sorry for yourself. Do not complain about how lonely you feel, how exhausted you are, and how your life stopped in it's tracks, and you are a mess.

> **ANY EXPECTATIONS YOU HAVE OF YOUR LOVED ONE FOR THEIR SYMPATHY OR FEELING SORRY FOR YOUR CIRCUMSTANCE AS A CAREGIVER IS UTTERLY UNREALISTIC.**
> **THEY ARE STRUGGLING TO BARELY FUNCTION, AND YOUR SITUATION IS NOT SOMETHING THEY CAN POSSIBLY GRASP OR UNDERSTAND.**

Even if they wanted to comfort to you, they cannot. Don't be self-absorbed in your heartache, it won't be helpful. Instead, make an effort to find someone else you can talk to, perhaps a friend, a caregiver support group or a therapist. That can be a very beneficial and positive experience.

But with your loved one, the days of them helping you solve your problems are gone. That can be especially challenging, if you were very close. Now you are here for their comfort and safety and that is a non-negotiable fact. All that remains is a very limited, kindhearted exchange of a few words, if you are lucky.

You may tell them that you are tired and will go to bed, or that you need to rest, but keep it light and not in any way upsetting. This is your time to stand mature, solid, unwavering, uncomplaining and unconditionally loving. It is a true test of your endurance and strength of character.

Find more suggestions for caregiver emotional wellness in the following three Chapters: *Spiritual Wellness*, *Your Life* and *Self Care for Caregivers*.

HAPPY STORIES

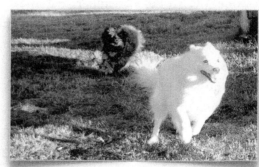

My DOGS HAPPY AND DIDI ARE A STORY OF HAPPINESS

There is still a glimmer of joy you can experience when interacting with your loved one. Speaking to them can become a different kind of wonderful experience, even if they can't respond or say a word. You can reminisce about old, happier times, when you were laughing or living through fun adventures together.

Tell them the stories slowly and in a relaxed way. They will hear you and listen to you and if you are a good storyteller, you may even get them to smile or laugh. It will mentally and emotionally stimulate them and perhaps they will even utter an unexpected sentence. You will be surprised. Select happy stories that go far back in time, so there is a better chance that your loved one can remember. Long - term memory can sometimes last amazingly well, so keep that in mind.

> **A DAILY HAPPY STORY**
> **WILL HELP KEEP THEM SOMEWHAT MENTALLY ACTIVE**
> **AND WILL DEFINITELY CHEER THEM UP.**

You need to be able to almost imagine their answers or questions and lead a conversation that way. If you were very close, you know how they would usually react or what kind of question they would pose. As you go along with your recollections, you will notice their eyes widen with attention, or perhaps look at you with interest. When you conclude your story, they may gaze into the distance with a slight smile. It is good to remind them of happy times and you should strive to keep those memories alive and well.

YES, YOUR LOVED ONE HEARS YOU

Despite appearing as if the loved one cannot hear or understand you, do not assume it is so. They can hear you and possibly also understand you, but are unable to respond. Which means, that if you are talking about them as if they are not there and describing their inabilities, mishaps, accidents, difficult behavior, or even complaining about your caregiving hardship, it is very possible that they hear everything. That can become extremely upsetting for them.

Therefore, I strongly suggest you do not talk about sad, unfortunate events or facts. They need to be moved far into a back drawer of your mind and need not be opened. Not right now and not with your loved one listening in. Even if the sense of hearing diminishes with age, it remains active. So, be selective and pay attention to what you say in your loved one's presence.

NEVER SPEAK ABOUT NEGATIVE PROGNOSIS OF THEIR ILLNESS.
REMAIN LIGHT AND CHEERFUL
AND IF YOU NEED TO DISCUSS ANYTHING DIFFICULT,
STEP AWAY AND MAKE SURE THEY CANNOT HEAR YOU.

It is not in your loved one's best interest to be exposed to some sad, lamenting and depressing descriptions of their difficult circumstance. Protect them and sustain a peaceful, pleasant and calming environment in all possible ways. I am not saying that you should look them in the eye and lie that they will get better and have a happy life. I do not find that correct. But I also do not see the purpose of exposing them to a negative way of thinking and telling them something disturbing or sad. Their situation is difficult enough, no need to repeatedly speak about it. It could trigger a nervous agitated reaction and truly disturb their hopefully serene state.

Keep a pleasant and cheerful disposition at all times. The long journey through this illness will go on and there is no need to remind them of it. Believe me, on another level of consciousness, they know. Do everything you can to uplift them and yourself.

LEARN TO TRULY LIVE IN THE MOMENT.
AND MAKE THAT MOMENT A HAPPY ONE.

THE HEALING POWER OF MUSIC AND PICTURES

Music is one of those magical mysteries that can help us travel through time. Just hearing a song from our past will instantly transport us back to that time and place. The magnitude of the sensory healing power of music is immense.

Music therapy is a fantastic tool to get your loved one to utter a few words or maybe even sing along. The long-term memory sometimes stays amazingly intact and your loved one could suddenly remember the words to a song from the era when they were young, happy and singing. Maybe it was just a song that played on the radio at a particular time in their life, but will have very therapeutic effects and do wonders for memory.

> YOUR LOVED ONE WILL LIVEN UP AND POSSIBLY REMEMBER
> SOMETHING HAPPY AND FUN FROM THEIR PAST.
> IT COULD HAVE A VERY PEACEFUL AND CHEERING EFFECT ON THEM.

Another way to use the healing and soothing power of sound is to play a nice musical selection in their room. Gentle, sleepy but comforting music to play in the evening before bedtime will automatically help them fall asleep. You can also use healing music when they are agitated or restless.

Repeating the same music CD again and again can establish a sense of familiarity and remind them of various activities that occur while listening to certain music. Stick with a good music selection that helps them fall asleep and do not change it. They will associate that particular sound or song with sleep-time. You could use different music for various times during the day. You should only play your loved one's favorite music in their room.

Do not play music that you or a caregiver prefers, because your loved one probably can't relate to it. Their room is their domain and everything there should be for their optimal comfort and peace and not to entertain others.

Same goes for TV or films. Play their favorite old favorite movies, but not all the time or every day. Do everything in moderation and closely observe their reaction. If it seems to agitate them, turn it off. If it gets their attention and they seem to enjoy it, you have cheered them up and that is always a good thing.

Talk to your loved one while watching TV and help them understand the narrative. Remind them of familiar actors in that particular film. What will usually stimulate them is a film from the era when they were younger. For example, if they liked Katharine Hepburn, then seeing her in a movie might trigger a positive reaction. You could say: "Look, it's Katharine Hepburn, she looks lovely, remember her? "

Your loved one may suddenly react with a word or two. Or they may stay silent, but their facial expression will reveal they are enjoying themselves. That is a success and you are doing great. Anything that helps them recall joyful occasions is positive.

> **THEIR LONG TERM MEMORY WILL RESURFACE, ACTIVATE THEIR LIFETIME LIBRARY OF HAPPIER TIMES AND RECREATE A WONDERFUL "TIME CAPSULE" MOMENT FOR BOTH OF YOU.**

Revisiting old photographs may bring up mixed emotions and could be more difficult for them to process, depending on the family dynamics or members who are no longer with you. Anything that could potentially upset your loved one should be avoided at all cost. They need to be shielded from any emotional distress, sorrows or sad reminders. Focus on this very moment, the peaceful tranquility and loving care that you are offering them. Do everything in your power to keep them content, comfortable and undisturbed.

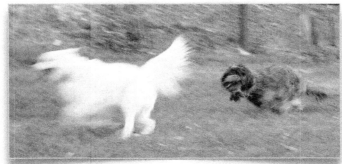

EVERY CAPTURED MOMENT IS A TREASURE CHEST.
OPEN IT UP AND REVISIT.

CHAPTER FOURTEEN

Spiritual Wellness

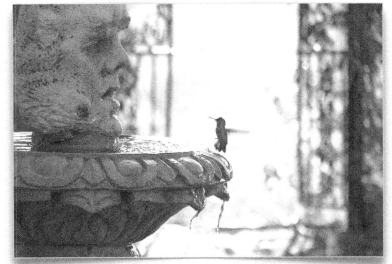

DRINK FROM THE UNIVERSAL WELL OF LOVE

I am a seeker. I like to search for a deeper meaning and true purpose of everything that is happening around me and I am experiencing. I have to decipher it and understand its true purpose. I love to observe people and discern why they act in a certain way. It fascinates and inspires me.

The desire to constantly strive and help others exists in every fiber of my being. If I know I have information that may be helpful, I simply have to spread the message. Then, it is up to an individual if they use it.

When I faced my Mother's merciless illness, all my previous beliefs were put to a severe test. Nothing made sense to me, and I was beyond devastated. My Mother was my unwavering anchor and my very closest, dearest friend and confidante. When she fell ill, I fought tooth and nail for her. Everything else fell by the side, because it was less important than her.

When the final chapter approached, I felt like an exhausted lonesome bird that endured wind, storm, cold and hunger. But I held on and was not going to crash and fail her. I was going to stand by her side forever. But what helped me profoundly, is when I started to have an ongoing heart to heart conversation with God. It saved me from complete and total despair.

In the morning I would say: "I am still here, I wake up at any and all hours of day or night to be here for her. I am doing everything and anything I can to ease her suffering. The rest is up to You. I just show up every day, that's all I can do." And then, an interesting shift happened. I sensed a sudden big relief. Somewhere, someone was listening to me and heard me. I could feel it.

My conversations with God deepened as time of my Mother's departure neared. I would ask Him to give me strength and keep me from crying, whenever I gave her a sponge bath or changed her. A wave of serene peace and amazing fortitude would come over me. I did everything I had to do with full concentration and awareness. Within me was a deep, calm, peaceful feeling and I truly felt that I was not alone.

One has to overcome many storms to realize the unbeatable Spirit that sustains us. But more often than not, we can only realize its power once the tests are long gone, and we can safely observe the reflection of the past that we endured. That is a part of ever evolving self-realization process.

Have faith about your enduring strength, for it is He who sustains you and guides you now and always.

YOUR SPIRITUALITY

At one point or another during this journey, your belief system and spirituality is going to endure some seriously challenging moments. You will have questions, doubts and anger. Overwhelming feelings of isolation, devastation and utter hopelessness could linger on.

That is to be expected. When the test of endurance pushes us to the brim, the burden seems intolerable. You may feel that you can't take your daily grind a moment longer. Your responsibilities and duties will bring you to a breaking point. At that particular moment your spirituality will be greatly tested. Again and again.

> **HE WILL NOT GIVE YOU MORE THAN YOU CAN CARRY.**
> **HE WILL STAY AT YOUR SIDE. HE WILL NOT DESERT YOU.**

Those are the encouraging words you may hear from your friends, but the reality seems to stay the same: you are exhausted. What is going to get you thru this difficult time is your unwavering spiritual discipline.

> **REGULAR INNER REFLECTION, PRAYER, MEDITATION**
> **AND COMMUNICATION WITH YOUR HIGHER SELF**
> **IS THE ONLY WAY TO KEEP YOUR MIND AND SPIRIT ABOVE WATER.**

Whatever your spiritual practice is, this is the time to use it more than ever. If you have no spiritual base and have utterly ignored that aspect of your life, the caregiving duties will push you to finally confront and identify your beliefs.

You will ask what is the point of all this suffering, who cursed your loved one, your parent, your partner, your family and you? You will question where is God in all of this? Does he exist? If so, where is he now? You will ponder the meaning of life, and the purpose or reasoning for the tremendous loss that your loved one is enduring.

> **THIS INNER QUEST WILL BEGIN A JOURNEY**
> **INTO THE DEEPEST CORE OF YOUR EXISTENCE.**

The Universal power, God, Divine energy, whatever or whoever is your belief system anchor, that is all you have left, to help you hold on and keep it all together.

**IT WILL BE JUST YOU AND HIM, HER, IT OR THEM -
HOWEVER YOU RELATE TO THE DIVINE POWER.
IT WILL BE A SHOWDOWN BETWEEN YOU AND YOUR GOD.**

You will be forced to search deep inside your soul to find that power and strength, to sense and hear an answer, to know how to go on each and every day. How can you find peace in all of this? How can you endure this journey? How can you overcome the urge to run away from it all? How can you wake up from this nightmare?

This will be a very profound and deeply transformative spiritual journey. There are no coincidences in life, no strange chances and weird senseless happenings. Everything has a certain purpose and even though it may seem cruel beyond words, there is a hidden meaning, a higher learning you are experiencing. This is the process of a true spiritual awakening.

How can you reason and justify within your heart the purpose of this illness, the long years of suffering and the heartbreaking process of seeing your loved one disappear in a most painful and harrowing decline? What is the meaning of all this? Again and again, you will ask yourself these questions. You will wave your fists and yell at the sky, and in the end, you will cry to God. With every cell of your body you will feel the agony, sadness, despair and magnitude of this illness. Your battle with anguish, hopelessness and pain will open up your heart and soul.

In that most tender sacred space, you will cross an inner invisible threshold. A mysterious gate will open and you will enter a new realm. You will begin to experience your life in a new, altered way and will eventually emerge forever changed. How?

**YOU WILL UNDERSTAND THAT WITHIN LIFE'S TOUGHEST BATTLES
LIE MOST PRECIOUS HIDDEN GIFTS.
AND THE PROFOUND WISDOM GAINED ON THIS JOURNEY
IS THE GREATEST TREASURE YOU CAN FIND.**

You will fathom how very blessed you are, for you have received an invaluable gift of a deep spiritual awakening. While going through this process of ascension, you will need to understand and overcome a few decisive obstacles. Take your time and pay attention to every and each one of them, so you can swiftly move ahead and master this assignment. Here are the stepping stones of your journey.

FAITH

Faith is your anchor to help you thru the days and nights while taking care of your loved one. Faith, that you will survive this ordeal and there will be something left of you at the end of this hard journey.

And even though there will be countless times where faith will feel but a far forgotten shadow, each time you will call its name, it will return and gently take your hand. You will swallow your tears and keep persevering, with faith in your brave heart and resilient mind.

Faith will keep you going with hopes and prayers that your loved one won't suffer too much and that you will stay strong and valiant while holding everything up. Faith will help you stay optimistic. Faith will help you remember that our actions, deeds and sacrifice, are rewarded with countless blessings in disguise.

YOUR HEARTFELT CONCERN AND LOVING CARE ARE NOTED, FOR NOTHING ESCAPES THE ETERNAL EYE OF THE UNIVERSE.

You are truly an angel with a beautiful heart and selfless spirit.
You are sacrificing so much for your loved one.
You are giving up your time, sometimes months and even years.
You are offering your vital energy.
You are sacrificing a level of your health, which is undoubtedly challenged.
You are giving up your personal freedom, which is extremely limited.
You are willing to let go of your relationships that may not survive this ordeal.
You are pausing your career or livelihood, that is compromised.
You are canceling your carefree evenings and vacations, and giving up your life as it was.
You are abdicating a great deal of yourself on this journey, for this odyssey cannot go on without your unconditional and selfless service.

It is the ultimate test of your endurance, strength, discipline and … Faith. But I promise you, by keeping faith, you shall live to see a brighter day.

KEEP THE FAITH IN EVERY BREATH YOU TAKE AND REST EASY IN KNOWING, YOU ARE DIVINELY PROTECTED.

THE HIDDEN GIFT OF KARMA

It is amazing to me when someone says as a matter-of-factly, as if they were counting apples: "Well, it is obviously your karma to do this." Needless to say, that is a very ignorant remark.

First of all, nobody can have such tremendous all-knowing insight to make this kind of a generalized statement. It is merely an indicator of how they categorize life's challenges, but that does not mean it is true. What I especially dislike about this kind of oblivious remark, is that it makes it sound as if you deserve to be going thru this difficult time. In their simple-mindedness, you must have obviously done something pretty terrible in a previous life to have this punishment descend upon you now.

Karma is undoubtedly involved in every aspect of our lives - *what you sow, so you shall reap*. However, let us look at principles of karma with a little more depth. As humans, we have a tendency to fear what we don't know or understand. And while people usually use the easy way out and blame karma for every terrible thing that occurs, they are missing a crucial point. Karma can in fact bring you amazing gifts as well. Karma certainly does not necessarily mean punishment. It is something entirely different.

> **KEEP IN MIND, EVERY LUCKY MOMENT OR BLESSING IN YOUR LIFE IS A DIRECT KARMIC GIFT.**

And if the purpose of our life is to learn how to overcome adversities, while inspiring and uplifting others, how can one best prepare for that mission? Perhaps you have to live through a challenge in order to truly understand it. In such a case, karma has given you a gift, wrapped up in a tremendously demanding assignment. Perhaps the bigger the obstacle, burden or responsibility, the bigger the blessing, hidden in its core. Let's reflect about that for a few moments. Perhaps on some deeper spiritual level, this caregiving journey is a karmic gift.

> **REMAIN OPEN TO THE POSSIBILITY, THAT A THREAD OF LIGHT IS CAREFULLY WOVEN THROUGH EVERY HARDSHIP WE ENDURE. SOMETIMES THE GREATEST BLESSINGS COME IN THE DARKEST OF DISGUISES.**

YOUR FREE WILL AND CHOICE

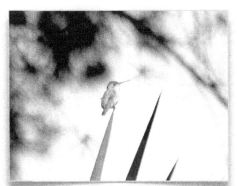

THE HUMMINGBIRD IS A HEALER HELPING SPIRITS IN NEED

I believe that all of my Mother's suffering and my sacrifices have not gone in vain, because you are reading this book at this precise moment… and I know you will gain some useful advice. This will help you and hopefully minimize your hardship. This way, my Mother and I have created something very positive and helpful for you.

That has been my choice of belief and I am at peace with it. I was given the opportunity to help others. As indescribably difficult as it was, I remain grateful and determined to accomplish this mission.

No matter how the circumstances of your loved one's illness developed and what was going on before you landed in the position of a caregiver, there was a moment when you had to make a decision. The choice was yours to take and yours only.

Of course it may have seemed that you had no choice. Maybe you were the only one left to take care of your loved one. Still, there is always a choice. After all, you could have put them in a nursing home, never visited them or disappeared, and that would have been your choice as well. Instead, your choice has been to stay very involved, and even if they are in a facility, you are present in their life as much as you can. You are the primary caregiver.

And if you have kept your loved one at home and are their primary caregiver for their final years, that was also a choice that presented itself and you bravely went ahead and took it. Even if it appeared you had no other choice, it was still your choice. Maybe it seemed unfathomable to do anything else. But considering your character, your kind heart and your belief system, you made the best choice that you could. And that is what free will is all about.

Nothing is carved in stone, for there is always room for choices. Even if there are only two choices with minor variables, the choice is still there. So make no mistake, karma might have been the one to present this situation to you, but it has been your choice to proceed as you have. You used your free will. That is what making choices and decisions is all about.

TAKING RESPONSIBILITY FOR ALL OUR DECISIONS IS SELF-EMPOWERING AND SPIRITUALLY MATURE.

So let's not make any mistakes about it, I do not believe that bad karma has put you into this predicament. You were presented with certain difficult options and you made a free-will choice. And even if it seemed that you had no other options, you made the right choice by not abandoning your loved one or running way, which could have also been a choice, but a poor one.

YOU CAN BE PROUD OF YOUR DECISION AND WILL FULFILL IT WITH LOVE. MUCH GOOD WILL RESULT FROM YOUR CHOICE.

We could look at this from another perspective. Perhaps we make certain choices even before we are born. Maybe we choose our life's challenges and assignments, long before we embark on our life's journey. It is possible we even made previous arrangements with our loved ones, as future parents or life partners and knew we would become their caregiver.

Why would someone chose such a difficult assignment? The possibilities are endless, but they definitely entail learning, selfless service, unconditional love and gained wisdom. If the knowledge gained would make it possible for us to help others who are going thru a similar ordeal, we will truly make a positive difference.

Think about how your choice will have positive consequences and how your free will has guided you through this journey. Trust your intuition and the choices it lead you to make. Remember, every choice you make has direct consequences. Making no choice is also a choice, usually a considerably less favorable one.

LIFE DEMANDS CHOICES. BE BRAVE AND FACE THEM.

YOUR INTENTION

What is the most important aspect in karmic sense? Your actions are certainly decisive, however, think about what precedes them? The answer is - your intention.

IN YOUR SOUL'S EVOLUTIONARY PATH, YOUR INTENTIONS CARRY THE MOST SIGNIFICANT WEIGHT.

If your true intention is to help someone, but there is an unpredictable mishap and your help is not effective, in the karmic sense - you did nothing wrong. Your intention was clear and well meant.

On the other hand, if one has a bad intention and as a result of their actions another person suffers, that is very negative in karmic sense. So while we certainly cannot always control the outcome, we can control and master our intentions. Your intention as a caregiver is crystal clear - you want to alleviate your loved one's suffering and are offering them the best care possible. That is your intention, even if you don't always succeed.

AS A CAREGIVER, YOUR BIG-HEARTED INTENTION CARRIES THE HIGHEST FREQUENCY OF LOVE. IN KARMIC AND SPIRITUAL SENSE, YOU ARE ON AN ELEVATED AND NOBLE EVOLUTIONARY PATH.

Reflect on this principle and how you intentions apply to your life circumstances, situations and various relationships. To have loving, kind and good intentions is key to attracting positive events and loving people into your own life.

Think and project love and kindness and you shall receive love kindness. Like attracts like. Reflect on your intentions every morning and evening. It will help you keep a clear perspective on the "bigger picture" while staying on track with your mission.

YOUR LOVING INTENTIONS HOLD THE KEY TO YOUR AUSPICIOUS FUTURE.

YOUR MISSION AND PURPOSE

When embarking on a mission to fulfill your purpose, you have to know the rules. You cannot waver, falter or give up before you succeed.

So the question I ask of you is this:

* ❋ Have you reflected on your life purpose?
* ❋ What is your mission as a caregiver?
* ❋ Is it to help your loved one feel loved, comfortable and cared for?
* ❋ Is it a desire to protect them, watch over them?
* ❋ To ease their journey?
* ❋ To teach or help others from your hard-gained knowledge?
* ❋ Is your mission and purpose to help alleviate all suffering?

> **EVERY MISSION REQUIRES SACRIFICE.**
> **YES, I WILL REPEAT THAT,**
> **EVERY MISSION REQUIRES SACRIFICE.**

So you see, these two things go together. You cannot have one without the other. Keep that in mind. If you are able to make the required sacrifice, you will accomplish the main objective of your mission. It may not be everything you wanted, but the most important aspect will be achieved. If you always complain about the sacrifices you endured, you will forget the mission you accomplished, as a direct result of those sacrifices.

> **REMIND YOURSELF OF YOUR GREAT ACCOMPLISHMENTS,**
> **AND DON'T DWELL ON THE LOSSES.**

GREAT EXPECTATIONS

Another challenging dynamic to master is your expectations concerning every part of your life. This includes your health, the ability to function physically, emotionally, mentally, spiritually and certainly financially. You may also face concerns about how the caregiving duties are affecting your general sense of success and the reality of placing your dreams and ambitions on an indefinite hold.

You may wonder about how much time will remain of your life, to accomplish what you once desired. You will also ponder, how long before your life can return back to any sense of normalcy. You are reflecting on this, because this is a part of your daily reality.

Well, my dear caregiver, the truth is, your life will never be the same. It will never truly go back to the "same old normal" that you knew before. The caregiving experience will expand your understanding and observation skills as a human being to such a degree, that you will begin to see life very differently.

You will gain inner wisdom, an open and perceptive heart and profoundly deep insight about the complexities of life.

YOU ARE IN THE PROCESS OF MASTERING A MOST CHERISHED ABILITY FOR COMPASSION AND SERVING WITH UNCONDITIONAL LOVE. THIS WILL GREATLY ENRICH YOUR SOUL.

AS A CONSEQUENCE, YOUR OWN EXPECTATIONS ARE EXPERIENCING A PROFOUND TRANSFORMATION.

To help you let go, consciously reflect on your deeper feelings, inner thoughts, old fears and previous priorities. You are learning to discern which old beliefs can be tossed aside and abandoned. Once that occurs, you will feel liberated.

You may have encountered a challenge from people in your immediate environment, your partner, other family members, your old friends or acquaintances. Maybe they preferred, liked and loved the old version of you, where you were able to give them a generous amount of attention, time and energy.

They may continue to have these expectations of you and suddenly your transformation will not fit their needs. You are becoming someone else and that may be very confusing, inconvenient, or even unacceptable to them. At such juncture it becomes important that you stay true to yourself and allow the caregiving experience to change, mature and ripen you as a human being. As a result, the old expectations may become impossible to fulfill and you will experience a significant change in your relationships and friendships. It is to be expected.

If a partner or friend can remain a loyal companion and a supportive presence thru your caregiving journey, your relationship will deepen, while entering an exalted level of unconditional love and friendship. So you see, you will gain great insight into the true nature of partnerships and friendships in your life.

ONLY THE AUTHENTIC PARTNERS, FRIENDS AND LOVERS WILL REMAIN AT YOUR SIDE.

It is certainly possible that a partner loves you, but cannot manage to stay with you while you are a caregiver. Yes, they love you, but not enough. They are simply not capable of that kind of sacrifice and unconditional love. Or they may not want to share you and want you all to themselves. Their love therefore is not authentic or spiritually compatible with the evolutionary process of your own soul. Their love is restricted and in fact, conditional.

When you successfully release the burden of self-imposed expectations, you allow a new, more mature and secure person to emerge. That is the new you, accepting the uniqueness of your life journey. Even if it seems that you are at a standstill and nothing is happening, except the all-encompassing caregiving duties, be gentle with the expectations of your future. Allow time and space to open new doors, new ways of thinking and new wisdom.

And the last piece of advice is this: do not impatiently wait about how long this experience will last and when will it come to an end. It will last as long as it is supposed to, and the sooner you truly understand, accept and stop anticipating and fearing the end, the better for everyone involved.

WHEN YOU RELEASE YOUR EXPECTATIONS, THE UNIVERSE WILL BLESS YOU WITH UNIMAGINABLE AND SURPRISING NEW OPPORTUNITIES.

PATIENCE

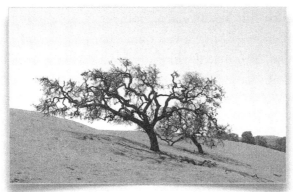

THE IMMEASURABLE PATIENCE OF A TREE

Your patience will be profoundly and continuously tested. If you were an impatient person before, then this is going to be one of your major challenges.

You will feel tested every moment of your caregiving experience. If you hire caregivers, dealing with them will be an incredible test of your patience. When you explain to someone what needs to be done and then see the reoccurring mistake, you will need to be kind, diplomatic and yes, extremely patient.

Dealing with your partners, friends, relatives who will at times offer well-meaning, but ignorant and utterly unrealistic advice, will also require loads of patience. And finally, you will certainly need tremendous patience when dealing with your ailing loved one, who may at times chew one spoon of blended food one-hundred times, while you wait with the next spoonful to feed them. How can you do that without enduring patience? You cannot. Embrace the fact that patience is now your very best, loyal, diligent and predictable friend.

ONCE YOU MASTER PATIENCE,
YOU WILL CONQUER THE ILLUSION OF TIME,
EITHER GOING TOO FAST - WHEN MISSING YOUR FUN TIMES
OR PASSING TOO SLOW - WHEN PERFORMING YOUR DUTIES.

AFTER ALL, TIME IS ONLY AN ILLUSION OF THIS EARTHLY EXISTENCE.

ELIMINATING FEAR

There are many things to fear at any given moment in time. Foremost, you may fear the inevitable pending departure of your loved one. That fear will take a permanent presence in the back of your mind. You may dread the moment when it happens. To help ease your way, I write about all the complexities of final transitioning and how you can better navigate through that process, in the final chapters of this book.

You may also fear that you will not last thru the caregiving, that you will lose your strength, your friends and everyone that's close to you. You may fear that you will end up all alone, unable to financially survive and that your health will decline.

**AND FINALLY, YOU MAY FEAR THE GREATEST FEAR OF THEM ALL,
THAT YOU TOO MAY ONE DAY SUCCUMB
TO THE SAME ILLNESS AS YOUR LOVED ONE,
BUT WITH NO ONE TO TAKE CARE OF YOU.**

These fears can drive you out of your mind. You may feel helpless in that there is nothing really you can do to erase them. All your fears seem well founded and real. You are not just being paranoid and imagining things. It could happen.

What you can do, is face these fears and address them one by one. They will diminish in their persistence. Plan your financial future, communicate in your personal relationships with partners and friends and become a warrior against obstacles.

**REMAIN A PIONEER IN TAKING GREAT CARE OF YOUR HEALTH,
SO THAT YOU STAY HEALTHY FOR A LONG, LONG TIME.
BE SUPREMELY DISCIPLINED IN PROPER SELF-CARE.**

In addition, I highly recommend that you do not obsessively dwell on these fears, as they will drain you of energy and hope, and leave you in a depleted state. Mind is a very powerful tool and whatever thoughts we allow to drift within our mindset, they have a good chance of becoming our reality.

VISUALIZE ONLY GOOD AND POSITIVITY.

Like an athlete who in their mind practices a perfect ending to their race, that is how you need to practice a positive mindset and control your thinking patterns. Negative thoughts, or imagining something bad, sad, desperate and tragic, will only vibrationally attract or create such circumstances.

There is nothing positive about feeling fearful and agonizing over what could happen. The caregiving is demanding enough without you dwelling on what could go wrong. Instead, concentrate on the positive, strong, winning, conquering and victorious thoughts and outcomes.

BE THE WARRIOR OF COURAGE, OPTIMISM AND HEALTHY LIVING.

To help gain the ability and conquer your fears, ask yourself: what is your biggest fear? Identify and look right at it. And then remember, that all fears come from the ultimate fear of death. Since eventually we all die, there is certainly no point in dwelling on it.

Face the fear you carry and release its hold and power over you. It will help you discover, that fear itself is nothing to fear. You have a choice to obsess over it, or just let it be.

I prefer to ignore fear and leave it alone, because I am not interested in investing my precious energy in a negative direction. Fear will try to stop you from doing things that your heart desires. And as a consequence, you will find yourself drowning in regret. If you allow fear to hold you back, you will not be able to fully live your life.

LIVE FEARLESSLY IN THIS VERY MOMENT,
BECAUSE ALL THAT TRULY MATTERS IS RIGHT NOW.

PACE YOURSELF

In difficult times, every moment seems like an eternity. When someone says to you: "Take it one day at a time," it is because we can handle stress easier in smaller increments. If your day begins with overwhelming challenges, you need to pace yourself. That is why thinking about one day at a time truly helps.

> **YOU JUST NEED TO THINK ABOUT THE NEXT TWELVE HOURS. IF THAT STILL SEEMS TOO MUCH, WHY NOT TAKE EVEN SMALLER STEPS. JUST TAKE ONE MINUTE AT A TIME.**

Simply stop whatever you are doing, be still and ask yourself this question:
"What should I do right now, at this very moment? Not tonight or tomorrow, or this week, but just now, this very instant, what should I do?"

The momentary answer will come to you and the sense of overwhelm will gradually diminish. Take a deep breath of relief in knowing that you have overcome the crisis. From this moment on, you can move to the next with greater ease. You can successfully manage a highly stressful state with this simple technique, of just getting by one moment at a time. In the bigger picture, your pace plays an equally important role. Assess ahead of time if your plan of chores and duties is realistic. Prioritize and address only the essential important obligations.

> **CONSERVE YOUR ENERGY WHENEVER YOU CAN.**

Avoid getting into a pattern of perpetual activity, because you energy level will quickly diminish and you will exhaust and deplete yourself. Non-stop activity can cause adrenal burn out. Imagine you are running a marathon. Obviously, you don't want to run at the highest speed right from the start. Establish a realistic easy going pace and develop endurance. This principle will help you sustain a healthy level of energy for a long period of time.

> **WHEN YOU MASTER YOUR OWN PACE, YOU WILL DEVELOP STAMINA, STRENGTH AND STAYING POWER.**

YOUR INNER VOICE OF GUIDANCE

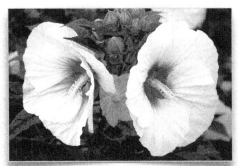

FIND YOUR DIVINE WHISPER WITHIN

When things are challenging, we all need guidance. Counsel is welcome even when things are good, but that is not the time we seek it. Perhaps one of the reasons for facing challenges is, that it offers us an ideal opportunity to learn. We are presented with difficult situations and suddenly forced to evolve, grow, learn, seek new information and guidance. Learning to rely on your own inner guidance is very liberating and empowering. When you find yourself in despair, search for your intuitive inner voice, that holds the answer to your crisis.

CONSCIOUSLY CONNECT WITH THE DIVINE WHISPER, THAT IS GIVEN TO EACH AND EVERY ONE OF US.

The key is to be able to hear it, especially when you're in urgent need. That inner voice can be heard only when you are completely calm, perfectly still and breathing with a calm, deep and slow breath. When you reach that state of inner calm, you can ask a clear question. And the answer may be very simple, such as: "Do nothing, just wait and be still. This will resolve itself."

Use all the tools we've mentioned in this chapter: your faith, patience, wise pace and a clear sense of your mission and purpose. And then take a deep breath and listen.

WHEN YOU LEARN TO HEAR YOUR INNER VOICE, ALL ANSWERS ARE RIGHT AT YOUR FINGERTIPS.

SURRENDER

We have now arrived one of the most demanding aspects of your spiritual growth and empowerment. No matter how much you pray, mediate, sit in stillness and listen to your inner voice, there is one more quality you need to learn. This can be a challenge for those of us who like to be in charge. You need to learn what is means to surrender.

SURRENDER IS A DEEPLY PEACEFUL AND ATTUNED STATE OF MIND WHERE YOU REALIZE AND ACCEPT THAT YOU CANNOT POSSIBLY CONTROL EVERYTHING AND EVERY SITUATION.

In the particular case of caregiving, your learning process to surrender can be exceptionally harsh. You can do everything that is in your power to help your loved one, but then you have to consciously surrender to the fact, that they will not recover from this illness.

While you are a caregiver, your need for surrender is also required in numerous other areas of your life. You can do everything possible to keep your normal sense of life alive, but the fact is, you are a caregiver and have to surrender to that duty. That is your primary obligation. It is a non-negotiable fact.

You may feel that life is passing you by, and it may seem that way, but it really is not. You could be as free as a bird, with no caregiving duties and life would still seem to be passing you by. It is all about our momentary state of mind and timing. When good and happy times are supposed to come your way, they will find you, no matter where you hide. Surrender to the fact that you cannot control everything.

**THERE IS A HIGHER POWER THAT IS IN CHARGE.
SO ONCE YOU'VE GIVEN IT YOUR BEST EFFORT,
GIVE-UP THE EXPECTATIONS, GOALS AND OUTCOMES.
SURRENDER IT ALL.
THE UNIVERSE WILL DECIDE.**

And if you belong to the ones who avoid being in charge and permanently wait for someone else to make the decisions for them, this lesson will be different. You will have to surrender to the fact, that not everything can be decided for you.

You have to take responsibility for your passive avoidance, get out of your comfy chair and make an honest effort. Surrender to the fact that you participate in creating your scenario, your choices or lack of them, and need take full responsibility for it. So you see, the lesson of surrender applies to every one of us differently.

Since you are the primary caregiver, chances are, you are most likely a goal-oriented person who knows how to take charge and go to battle. You will stand up for your loved one, fight to win over their brutal illness and do everything for their comfort. Your fight has the purest of intentions, fighting for survival and comfort of your loved one. That is your mission.

But no matter how much you hate it, you have to surrender to the fact that this journey is going to take as long as it has to. You cannot control everything, even if you jump out of your skin. So after you have done the impossible, take a step back, exhale and surrender to the higher power.

THIS IS A DIFFICULT TOPIC AND MUST NOT BE MISUNDERSTOOD. IT DOES NOT MEAN THAT YOU GIVE UP, LET SOMEONE SUFFER OR DON'T HELP THEM IN EVERY WAY. IT JUST MEANS THAT YOU CANNOT CONTROL EVERYTHING AND MUST LEARN TO LET GO OF THE OUTCOME.

You need to spiritually surrender in awareness, that your loved one will never recover. So your goal is to assure their optimal comfort and quality of life, while they are here. There is an enormous difference between living with Alzheimer's dementia in excellent care, or in neglect and suffering from additional physical pain. It is incomparable. So your mission to assure optimal comfort and care is clear.

However, surrendering to the fact that the pending departure is near, will help you live in peace and not in emotional pain. After you have done the impossible with your exceptional care and self-sacrifice, close your eyes, say a prayer and surrender. Please. Everybody will be relieved. As will you.

MASTERING THIS QUALITY WILL HELP YOU OPEN UP THE HIGHEST LEVEL OF CONSCIOUSNESS.

YOUR INNER PEACE

Once you sort out in your mind, heart and soul, why you are in this situation, and take responsibility for choosing this assignment, you should have a much easier time achieving the very important next step that will help you sail thru this storm.

You are now in pursuit of inner peace. The key element is to find this quality within you, so you are completely at peace about everything. This is partially what this entire journey is about.

YOU CAN ONLY TRULY EXPERIENCE INNER PEACE, WHEN AND IF YOU HAVE MADE PEACE WITH YOUR OUTER WORLD.

Your inner peace will be a tremendous ally thru your time of caregiving. Imagine yourself peaceful, strong, calm and collected in any and all situations that you face. Would that be helpful? Of course it would. So you should strive towards that. When dealing with your loved one, taking care of them, cleaning them, feeding them, helping them thru difficult days and nights, your inner calmness will help them feel more secure, protected and safe.

Your loved one is very sensitive to your subtle energy state and demeanor and if you are nervous, impatient, angry or depressed, it will affect them in a negative way. You must strive to gain this peace and calmness every day and night. When you are awakened at 3 am and need to change your loved one while they are screaming in your sleepy and tired ear, the only friend you will have is your inner peace.

By staying calm and peaceful, you will take care of the problem, console your loved one with a calm voice and afterwards go back to bed without being beside yourself with agony, nervousness, anger, impatience and despair. Everything is easier when you have inner peace. You become untouchable, unbendable and victorious in this battle. And that is what you want for yourself and what your loved one needs.

ACHIEVING INNER PEACE WILL MAKE YOU INVINCIBLE.

YOUR SPIRITUAL PRACTICE

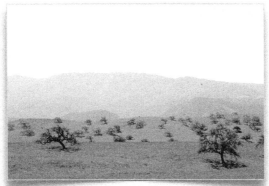

THE DISCIPLINE OF TRANQUILITY

Everything we learned about the various aspects of your spirituality that is tested and challenged, cannot work without your dedicated spiritual practice.

EACH AND EVERY DAY, YOU SHOULD DEDICATE SOME TIME TO SIT IN COMPLETE STILLNESS, ENGAGE IN INNER CONVERSATION, SELF-REFLECTION, CONTEMPLATION AND SPIRITUAL REPLENISHING. THIS IS YOUR SACRED AND NECESSARY TIME TO RECALIBRATE YOUR SPIRIT.

I know very well how challenging your caregiving schedule is. There simply does not seem a possible time for this spiritual routine. You may be awakened in the middle of the night, will try to steal a few extra minutes of sleep in the morning and have a demanding day ahead of you. If you have caregivers, privacy is rare, and if you are doing everything alone, you're managing a million tasks. In the evening, you collapse into a sleepy exhausted daze in front of TV, before you need to prepare once again for the midnight change. After that is accomplished, you finally crash into bed. There are not enough hours in day to get everything done.

When could you possibly find a moment to sit still and meditate or pray? As important as everything else is, so is your daily spiritual practice. You simply must find a few minutes to remember who you are, find your inner peace, stay calm, and hear your inner guiding voice.

The best time is in the morning when you wake up. It will help you begin your entire day on a good note. Take at least ten minutes to sit still and close your eyes, breathe and become serene, calm and peaceful. Breathe through the nose, concentrate on the solar plexus area, deeply inhaling and exhaling all the stress, anxiety and exhaustion you might carry in your body. Practice for a few minutes and remain in complete stillness for a few minutes afterwards. Feel your body relax and release all negativity. With each breath, recharge and fill-up with power, inner peace and strength that can endure anything. Begin with your inner dialogue and contemplation.

IF YOU HAVE A PRESSING QUESTION, ASK AND WAIT FOR A RESPONSE. IF YOU HAVE A WISH, ASK AND RELEASE IT INTO THE UNIVERSE. IF YOU NEED EXTRA STRENGTH, ASK AND THANK FOR IT.

Remember to express gratitude for all the blessings that you have received. Even if things are beyond challenging, there is surely something to be grateful for. Remember simple blessings, like a comfortable bed to sleep in, a roof over your head, food on the table, the ability to care for your loved one. Express gratitude for everything that is given to you. This will establish a positive mindset and fill you with a sense of contentment.

Carry that peace within you the entire day and if it becomes challenged, disappear into a room by yourself for a few minutes and repeat the exercise. At night before retiring, repeat the spiritual practice for at least five minutes. Find your stillness and peace and exhale all the burdens of the day. You will feel lighter and ready to return to your safe cocoon of inner peace and contentment.

YOUR MOST POWERFUL TOOLS ARE MEDITATION AND PRAYER.

This are your anchors that will help you remain healthy and resilient while you endure all the challenges that are placed upon you during this journey. Any kind of light exercise, such as a few yoga stretches a day, or walking in nature are very beneficial. You daily spiritual practice will keep you healthy and sane. Be as disciplined about your meditation and prayer time, as you are about giving the best of care to your loved one.

A CAREGIVER CAN BE MOST EFFECTIVE ONLY IF THEY PRACTICE GOOD SELF-CARE.

FINDING JOY IN SERVICE

This is the final principle to conquer. Learn to feel inner joy in every act of care. Instead of feeling overwhelmed and upset when dealing with mundane tasks like cleaning, feeding, and patiently taking care of your loved one, it is not enough to feel peaceful, calm and kind. What is going to help you endure this long assignment, is the ability to do each and every task with a sense of joy.

You might say that is simply impossible. How can one feel joyful while going thru such a draining, inexplicably sad experience? How can you feel joy when all your days entail endless duties and painfully limited communication with your loved one? Where is joy in watching your loved one diminish and suffer in a speechless, helpless stupor?

There is joy in service. There is joy in loving your dear one, offering them the highest level of care and comfort, being there for them, providing them with good healthy food, warm kind hands and gentle peaceful conversation, even if there is no response.

FEELING JOY IN SERVICE IS THE FINAL STATE OF SELFLESS GIVING.

When you are joyful and present while caring for them and easing their journey, you will feel an even deeper sense of joy.

You will feel grateful and blessed that you are lucky enough to be there for them.
You will feel joy in the opportunity to be protective, kind and caring.
You will feel the grace and kindness of the heavens that allowed you to take care of them and reduce their suffering.
There is joy in that.

CHERISH THIS OPPORTUNITY, THE BLESSING OF YOUR STRENGTH AND ABILITY.

Now you have successfully mastered the final task of this demanding assignment. Your spirit is maturing, becoming brighter and aware of life's true purpose. It is all about Universal love.

When you tenderly care for your loved one, the joy in your heart will magnify and expand. You will become who you are supposed to be. An enduring messenger of tireless selfless service, everlasting kindness and unconditional pure love.

YOUR LOVED ONE IS SO APPRECIATIVE
OF HOW WELL YOU ARE MANAGING EVERYTHING
WITH THE UNWAVERING INNER PEACE YOU CARRY WITHIN.

FROM SOME OTHER, HIDDEN PLANE OF EXISTENCE
THEY SEE AND KNOW EVERYTHING
AND ARE SO VERY GRATEFUL AND PROUD OF YOU.

CHAPTER FIFTEEN

Your Life

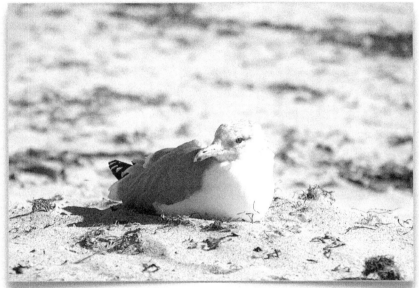

WHAT ABOUT YOU, MY DEAREST CAREGIVER?

*B*efore my Mother started showing the first signs of this brutal illness, my life was pretty carefree. I was happy, lived on the bluffs in Malibu with a lovely fiancée and wrote best selling self-help books. I was planning to start a family, was full of great ideas, projects and fantastic plans. But of course, they all evaporated into thin air, after she got ill. Suddenly it felt like someone pulled the plug off a sound system that played beautiful violin music. There was no music now. There was just a huge void, full of deafening silence and a dark, heavy cloud hovering over my head.

Keep in mind, my life was not always easy. I earned everything on my own with hard work, perseverance and tenacious discipline. There were many sacrifices, big and small. However, it seemed that I finally arrived at a great place I worked so hard to reach, and all was going to be lovely from now on. Of course that is not how life works.

Since this illness takes such a long, sneaky and secretive way of creeping into a person's life, there is a good chance you may miss it, or even misunderstand the first tell-tale signs. But my circumstances were a bit different. I lived in Malibu, far away from my parents in Europe, and when I saw them on my regular visits at least twice a year, the decline in my Mother's appearance always startled me. A tight grip of worry squeezed my heart each time I got off the plane and noticed her increasingly fragile state. She was an incredibly capable and beautiful woman in her mid sixties and appeared perfectly healthy, but obviously tired and burned out. Her nerves seemed frazzled, she was irritable and something was amiss.

When her state of health took a dramatic turn, I was devastated and my heart was heavy. I made the agonizing decision to leave my dear fiancée and beautiful life in Malibu and move to Europe. My plan was to stay there for a year, and somehow manage life on both continents. But that quickly proved impossible and my stay in Europe turned into six long years. The ever increasing challenging situation at home made matters worse for my Mother's condition and I needed to step in.

My life changed completely. The bottomless abyss of the devastating illness spread its destructive tentacles, reaching deeper and deeper into the family. The situation became all encompassing and mercilessly demanded every second of my time and every ounce of my energy. I had to deal with one crisis after another and time for myself simply evaporated.

The me and the life I knew was gone. I was spinning in the eye of a violent tornado and had no idea how, when or where it was going to release me. I felt that by the time it might be over, there would be nothing left of me.

WHERE IS YOUR LIFE?

The moment your loved one gets diagnosed with this illness, your life is changed forever. Nothing is the same. The time between early detection and the slow process of the illness could take years and when late stage of Alzheimer's dementia sets in, your life in general will be entirely different.

This illness is cruel, harsh and merciless. Its slow and persistent progression will be present with you every day. As a child, partner or immediate family member of an Alzheimer's patient, your own personal relationship with them will irreversibly alter, your career choices will have to adjust and most of all, you as a person will undergo a profound transformation. Your loved one will be fading slowly and persistently into a different unreachable world, while you watch, feeling helpless and fearful. These are the undeniable facts.

In the last stage of illness, your role as a caregiver becomes increasingly more demanding. There are times when you feel that your life has simply vanished and is non-existent. Those are tough moments, but every caregiver lives thru them. The caregiving assignment is simply so demanding, that you are constantly challenged to battle for a few stolen moments of much needed peace and rest.

This situation affects everything, your mornings, days, evenings, nights and more of the same. For weeks, months and possibly years. The uncertainty of the duration of this devastating illness adds additional aspect of difficulty. If one knows how long a marathon will last, one can prepare and endure it. But, if the marathon lasts seemingly forever with no clear idea of an end in sight, that reality adds additional sense of hopelessness that can feel debilitating. Yes, someday the agony will end, but when? Most likely years from now. There seems to be no break, no breathing room for you.

I say this because that is the reality of situation. While you go thru this period of your life, you will experience some real lows and depressing periods. It comes with the territory. But even with a seemingly hopeless and devastating situation like this one, believe it or not, you still have a choice. A big choice.

YOU CAN BECOME A BITTER PERSON OR A BETTER PERSON.

What does that mean? It means that you simply make peace with the situation life has dealt you and make the very best of it. You can perceive these tests of endurance, patience, optimism and strength, as character and spirit building opportunities. You can conquer it all, and in the end remain standing tall, older but indescribably wiser.

In the spiritual wellness chapters we talk about staying peaceful and holding on to your faith. All techniques that work for you in order to remain calm and resilient are now put to the test. You will often wonder where your life has disappeared, or what has happened to your seemingly trouble free existence from years ago.

Well, it has changed. You are in a different period of your life and are going thru a journey that is very important. And it just so happens, that most valuable experiences are often most difficult.

> **REMEMBER THAT NOTHING LASTS FOREVER AND EVENTUALLY THE TIME WILL COME WHEN YOU WILL BE RELEASED OF THE CAREGIVING DUTIES. MAKE SURE THERE WILL BE NO REGRETS. FULFILLING YOUR CAREGIVING OBLIGATIONS OFFERS YOU THE PERFECT OPPORTUNITY TO ASSURE THAT.**

You will always have the consolation, that you have done everything possible to maintain your loved one's ultimate comfort, kept them in physically pristine condition and helped alleviate their suffering.

> **IN FACT THIS PERIOD RIGHT NOW, IF HANDLED PROPERLY, COULD PROMISE YOU YEARS OF INNER PEACE AND SETTLED CLOSURE. THAT IS INVALUABLE.**

It could also provide you with an opportunity to spend ample time with your loved one. Even if the quality of your interaction is limited and you cannot have a normal conversation or even speak with them, an entirely different kind of loving communication is taking place. Your loved one feels, hears and knows that you are with them and that they are loved and supported. When they need you the most, you are not deserting them or letting them down. That is a huge accomplishment.

You are loyal and protective of them. That can offer you great consolation and will help diminish any regrets, feelings of guilt or sorrowful anguish, that you did not do everything possible to ease their suffering or spend enough time with them. You are there for them now and the present moment is what matters most.

> **SO WHEN YOU ASK YOURSELF,**
> **"WHERE IS MY LIFE? WHAT HAS HAPPENED?"**
> **THE ANSWER IS CLEAR:**
> **YOUR LIFE IS EXACTLY WHERE IT NEEDS TO BE RIGHT NOW.**

You are providing your loved one with essential and most important personal care and learning valuable insight while at it.

When everything else seems to be falling apart, keep unwavering faith that at this very moment, you are dealing with one of the most important assignments of your life. Nothing else matters as much. Commit wholeheartedly, do your very best and you will notice how frustration, anxiety and anger will diminish.

> **EVERYONE'S LIFE AND TIMING IS UNIQUELY DESIGNED FOR THEM.**
> **YOUR LIFE AND YOUR PARTICULAR TIMING**
> **CANNOT AND SHOULD NOT BE COMPARED**
> **TO ANYONE ELSE'S.**

By accepting the situation and making the best of it, you will ease the challenging aspects and find the true purpose of your experience.

THE BATTLE FOR YOUR TIME

Once you understand that there is a higher purpose behind your circumstance and make a conscious effort to enjoy your caregiving assignment, you will experience an instant shift.

TIME WILL BECOME YOUR FRIEND AND NOT THE MUCH-DREADED ENEMY.

You will overcome feeling like a desperate victim and will regain a certain level of control. The true challenge at this particular time, will be juggling all your responsibilities while also finding valuable time for yourself. Those moments will be rare and few between, but keep in mind, your daily spiritual routine will set your pace and disposition for the entire day that lies ahead. Early morning is the ideal time to establish your daily meditation and prayer time.

Whenever you have an opportunity during the day, find a few moments to take a short breather and recharge. Maybe you can escape to a movie, enjoy tea time with a friend or go into nature. It is important to get away for a bit and still remember how it feels to walk amongst regular people, where no one expects or needs anything from you. You can just be yourself and enjoy some carefree time.

If you cannot get away, and have no caregivers to help you out, then the only recharging opportunity you can enjoy is quiet time at home. Depending on the schedule with your loved one, there must be an occasion during the day, when they take an extensive nap and don't need you. Usually that is when caregivers frantically try to accomplish a long list of errands and overdue chores.

But you cannot possibly cram everything into an hour of spare time. What to do?

**PRIORITIZE BY MAKING A TO-DO LIST IN ORDER OF IMPORTANCE.
INCLUDE SOME PRIVATE RELAXATION TIME FOR YOURSELF
WHEN YOU CAN REST AND BE STILL.**

Certain chores require less time and attention that others. Maybe you can take care of your monthly bills when your loved one is awake and you are keeping an eye on them, but are still able to do your work. Maybe the laundry can be done while your loved one is awake. It could actually help calm them down to watch you do a mundane task such as folding the laundry.

Be inventive with tasks that can be done in your loved one's room, without disturbing them, so you easily watch over them. It is also a nice distraction for them to see a regular daily activity in their room, as long as it is peaceful and just with you.

The ideal time for your recharge is when your loved one is actually sleeping. That can be your golden opportunity to just let go and relax. I know this may be difficult, because you are geared to keep on working and taking care of chores, especially when you feel like you can finally catch up. Your impulse is to accomplish as much as possible. But believe me, you will be able to achieve much more, if you take a well deserved break.

> **WHEN YOUR LOVED ONE TAKES A NAP DURING THE DAY,**
> **DON'T RUSH TO CATCH UP WITH THINGS TO DO.**
> **INSTEAD, RELAX, READ A BOOK, MEDITATE,**
> **JUST BE STILL AND ENJOY THE PEACE.**

It will help you rejuvenate and be more alert and full of energy when you are needed. When your loved one wakes up, you can switch back to your multitasking. But not now, when they are asleep and you can escape, even if just in your mind. So it is truly up to you how you navigate your schedule. Give yourself the well deserved necessary breaks, set aside time for yourself and make sure you can properly recharge. Stay quiet and relaxed with no demands and no one to please. Create and cultivate this private time by always including it in your list of chores.

YOUR PERSONAL LIFE:
YOUR PARTNER, RELATIONSHIPS, FAMILY AND LOVE

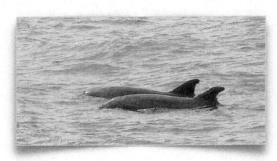

EVERYONE NEEDS LOVE AND COMPANIONSHIP

This is a very challenging aspect of your new life as a caregiver. If your spouse or relationship partner is the one suffering from this illness and you are their primary caregiver, your situation has its own uniquely difficult dynamics. Your relationship has been going through a long term change for some time and it is important to recognize the difference between personality changes that are a direct consequence of the illness and your partner's true nature.

Their love for you may be stronger than ever, despite the fact they are experiencing an increasing sense of helplessness and social isolation. You need to understand that their mood changes, mishaps and unreasonable behavior have nothing to do with their love for you. It is a clear indicator of the illness.

In the late stage of illness, the dynamics may change once again. Your role as a caregiver requires an enormous adjustment in relationship, often in the very opposite direction from what it usually was. The biggest help in adapting is your access to information, so you can clearly understand what is going on and prepare the best you can. Read more about this particular dynamics in Chapter *Your Loved One and Your Past.*

But if you are the caregiver to your parent or another close relative, your other intimate relationships and partnerships will suffer in a different way. I can't just wrap this into a colorful paper and say everything will be rosy. It simply won't be. Your partnerships, marriages, relationships and love life in general will undergo a crucial change. This illness demands an excessive amount of your time and attention, which will cause suffering in your personal friendships and especially love relationship.

When you are caring for your ill and helpless parent who depends on you for every single function and basic survival, there is really no negotiation about what is more important. When your parent needs to be changed, it needs to happen right away. When they need to be fed, you need to have patience and time to feed them properly and keep everything running smoothly. When they feel uncomfortable and you need to spend an hour or the entire morning figuring out what is creating their discomfort, that is your priority. There is no doubt about order of importance. You cannot abandon your loved one in need. By the time you are done with your caregiving responsibilities, there is very little left of you.

EVEN THE MOST WONDERFULLY AMAZING PARTNER THAT LOVES YOU TO PIECES, MAY FLEE THIS PREDICAMENT. THEY SIMPLY WILL NOT BE ABLE TO HANDLE BEING WITH YOU, BUT NOT REALLY BEING WITH YOU AT ALL.

They would have to live with your parent's illness and watch you prioritize them right out of your partnership. It does not mean that they don't love you and your parent, or understand what needs to be done. But they have their level of tolerance, as well as their own needs. They may simply not be able to endure this kind of a shift.

Their love has limitations and conditions. And suddenly they feel they are not getting anything in return. Many partners will not be able to watch how hard you work through your caregiving assignment, it will be too heavy, sad and depressing. That is the price this illness may claim - your most precious relationship. Your big love, your husband or wife, boyfriend or girlfriend - you will most likely lose them as well.

This is when the situation truly becomes overwhelming. Not only are you stuck in a very difficult and sad circumstance, challenged about keeping yourself afloat, tending to your own wellbeing, or making basic ends meet. You are sleep deprived, tired, sad, hopeless about this depressing and merciless illness stealing your parent, and now you might lose the big anchor of your life as well. This point in the crossroad becomes a test of gigantic proportions. I have lived thru it myself and have seen it countless times. Yes, there are the golden rare exceptions, but let's be honest, they are truly rare.

IF YOUR PARTNER REMAINS LOYALLY AT YOUR SIDE WHILE YOU ENDURE THIS GRUELING CAREGIVING DUTY, THEN HOLD ON TO THEM TIGHT, FOR THEY ARE EXCEPTIONAL, INDEED.

If the worst case scenario comes through and you in fact lose your partner, there is really no need to further worry about your love life, for there will be none. How can you live like that? Well, for the time being, you just do.

At that time in my life, I lost the love and emotional support of my partner. His love had limitations, conditions and considerable needs. I felt like an avalanche of heartbreaking events wanted to bury me underneath a heavy weight of reality. My survival skills kicked in high gear and I just concentrated on getting thru this ordeal, one step at a time. I was so occupied, it was simply impossible to even imagine another person expecting or needing my attention. I feel it is much harder to have a partner in your life that you cannot spend any quality time with, or a frustrated discontent partner, than having no partner at all. A supportive partner is a true godsend, but a demanding partner is impossible to maintain in this situation. Keep in mind, a great partner remains with you through sickness and in health. After all, life also has plenty of dark days and not every day is soaked in perpetual sunshine. Caregiving tests all your relationships, especially love alliances.

And I must say, when you are going thru this kind of experience, there is very little left of you, and not much to offer a partner anyway. If you manage to hang on to your partner, it will require a conscious effort to help keep everything really clear and not endure an increasingly resentful situation, because they feel neglected. If you speak openly about the amount of energy left for your relationship and they are secure, strong and dedicated enough, they will remain at your side and simply direct their focus into a different area of their life, such as their work, business or personal growth.

Such time-out periods might prove decisively beneficial and will salvage your relationship. At the end of the ordeal, you will still have each other. But do keep in mind that everything will take a period of adjustment. If they will be used to having you near, but in a very distant unavailable way, that could completely diminish the passion. You are physically there, but then again, you are not really available at all.

IF YOU ARE IN A RELATIONSHIP WHEN YOUR PARENT'S ILLNESS STRIKES, HAVE AN HONEST CONVERSATION AND PRESENT YOUR PARTNER WITH ALL THE FACTS.

They must hear that you still love them, but this situation will simply demand an enormous commitment of unpredictable length and you really need to be there for your ailing parent.

Very often, even if a partner wants to make it work and remain at your side, they simply won't be able to. In that case, it is a good idea to speak openly about true reasons why the relationship won't last thru this and accept it as peacefully as possible.

THE EX- PARTNER COULD STILL REMAIN YOUR CLOSE FRIEND AND PART OF YOUR MUCH - NEEDED SUPPORT SYSTEM.

I highly recommend that. Do everything you can to keep them somewhat present, even from a distance. It may help you a great deal.

If you lose the relationship and the communication is bad, full of anger, resentment and hard feelings, then it is best to take compete time off and reduce the interaction to a minimum or eliminate it all-together. If they decide to move on with a new partner, it may be too painful for you to keep them as a friend.

ALWAYS ASSESS WHAT IS THE BEST OPTION THAT WILL CAUSE YOU LEAST UPHEAVAL, TURMOIL OR SUFFERING. YOU NEED TO SAVE YOUR HEALTH, AND A RELATIONSHIP TUG OF WAR CAN BE SERIOUSLY DRAINING.

If you decide to prioritize and save your love relationship and therefore place your parent into a facility, then I urge you to make peace with that decision in the deepest chambers of your heart. Resentful and angry feelings, because you deserted your parent for partner's sake, could eventually ruin the relationship anyway. In that case you will end up a complete loser, firstly by feeling guilty for deserting your parent, and secondly by resenting your partner who could not support your wish to take care of your parent at home.

I believe it is always better to face the facts, embrace the true feelings, admit the honest desires and give it a go. Whichever man stands tall in the end, will do so with a clear mind, open heart and peace in their soul. Choices will be extremely difficult, but if you follow your heart, you will make the best decision.

IN THE END, YOU ARE THE ONE THAT HAS TO LIVE WITH YOUR CHOICES AND CONSCIENCE, NO ONE ELSE.

CAREGIVING AND YOUR CHILDREN - THE SANDWICH

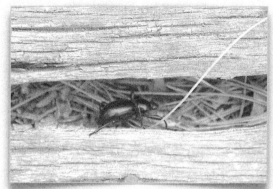

EVEN A TIGHT SPACE HAS BREATHING ROOM

If you find yourself in a squished sandwich generation of having a family and children of your own in addition to caring for your parents, my heart really goes out to you. If one of your parents suffers from Alzheimer's, your primary caregiving duties can become overwhelming. You are required to perform an amazing juggling act.

I think caregiving is very difficult to undertake when you have small children. You will definitely require outside help and can hopefully have that. If your children are pre-teens, your schedule can be saturated with school homework and driving them to various afternoon activities that require a lot of time and great planning. Once your children are in your teens, your parenting skills need to include good oversight and strong guidance, which adds a different kind of pressure.

THE ONLY REALISTIC AND WISE SOLUTION IS THAT YOU INVOLVE YOUR CHILDREN IN PERFORMING A FEW LIGHT CAREGIVING DUTIES RIGHT ALONG WITH YOU.

Obviously they will not be able to do the most demanding tasks, but perhaps checking on your parent, sitting with them for an hour or so, helping you in the kitchen and with other small tasks may prove extremely helpful. You will have less time for your teens so they will learn to be more self reliant, efficient, independent and certainly less spoiled. It will also educate them by example, that grandparents need respect, care and love and that this are your family's principles, duties and choices.

No matter how you look at it, your situation will be draining and exceptionally demanding. Yes, your plate is full, but I will remind you of the positive side. Keep in mind one very fortunate aspect: by having had your own children before your parent got ill, you have fulfilled your personal family desires.

YOU ARE NOT IN A CHILDLESS AND HOPELESS SITUATION. RECOGNIZE AND APPRECIATE THIS VERY FORTUNATE FACT.

There are many caregivers who lose their opportunity to have a family or their own children, very often precisely because of caregiving duties. When you are taking care of your parent as a primary at-home caregiver, there is no way you can even begin to think about bringing a child into this world. That is simply unrealistic and basically physically, emotionally and mentally impossible.

Those caregivers have to make peace with the fact that unless they are still young enough to have children later in life, they will not have a biological child of their own. It would be a rare case, where a caregiver was still young enough to have their own children after caregiving duties for their loved one are concluded.

This of course is especially the case for women, since they are most often in the primary caregiver role. A male caregiver has a considerably longer and practically limitless opportunity to have their own children and reinvent a brand new life for themselves, whenever their caregiving duties are over.

BY BRINGING YOUR CHILDREN UP IN A SITUATION WHERE THEY CAN LEARN FIRST - HAND HOW IMPORTANT IT IS TO CARE FOR AND RESPECT THE ELDERLY, YOU ARE SETTING A WONDERFUL EXAMPLE FOR THE FUTURE GENERATION.

Recognize also the positive side that your wonderful children help bring a permanent youthful presence into your home. It is a continuous reminder that life can still be happy, exciting and full of new joyful events. You are surrounded by a fresh optimistic energy and that alone will sustain you thru the caregiving experience. You can in fact look forward to an exciting future of your continuous family life.

That is not the case for a caregiver who is all alone, childless, without a partner and therefore facing a very different dynamic. They are on their own while going through the entire ordeal with the ill parent, often in addition to supporting the other remaining parent.

That creates a very sad feeling that can be very difficult to endure and overcome. They have no children that bring some young energy or something to look forward to in the future. All they have is a sad scenario with an obvious and unavoidable ending, once both parents perish. They are facing their parent's end of life dying process, death and eventual total aloneness and isolation.

> **SEE YOUR GOOD FORTUNE**
> **THAT YOU HAVE YOUR CHILDREN WHO REMIND YOU**
> **OF HAPPIER TIMES AHEAD AND**
> **FUTURE OPPORTUNITIES TO CELEBRATE LIFE.**

While your predicament of feeling squished between two needy generations is certainly not easy, just remember the positive aspects of your own circumstances. That is always wise and considerably more productive.

> **ALWAYS RECOGNIZE YOUR BLESSINGS AND AS A RESULT,**
> **THEY WILL MIRACULOUSLY MULTIPLY.**

WOMEN~CAREGIVERS AND THE TICKING CLOCK

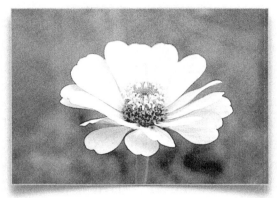

YOUR FUTURE IS OPEN

Considering that two-thirds of dementia caregivers are women and about one-third of them are daughters, I want to give some attention to the unique and irreversible challenges these wonderful women face. Most often, the main caregiver for the parent becomes the daughter. It is very possible that this daughter is in a relationship, but does not have a family of her own yet. Just when time seems right and all things are aligned properly to have her child, the parent gets ill. Consequently the daughter looses the partner, because the entire situation becomes too challenging. Now the daughter has lost the partner and her chance of creating her own family.

> **AS THIS ILLNESS PROGRESSES THROUGH THE FINAL YEARS, A SINGLE DAUGHTER CAN ENTER A DEEP PERSONAL CRISIS.**

She is loosing precious time of her own personal and professional life, thus the scenario leaves her with no partner, a severely challenged career and livelihood and an increasingly diminishing chance at ever having a family and children of her own. This can be deeply saddening and difficult to deal with.

The woman is watching her life go by, while certain aspects of her future are irreplaceably lost. This adds another very difficult aspect to the day-to-day care giving assignment. She may feel as if her life is ruined. She is alone, childless and presented with a daily list of sad, discouraging tasks that leave her empty and completely deprived of any possible future happiness. She is also facing a high probability that she will remain alone and childless in her old age. How can one accept and make peace with such a devastating and cruel consequence, for doing something as unselfish and kind as caregiving?

Well, the fact is that everything has a reason, and there are no guarantees in life. Even if she was free to enjoy a relationship, it does not mean it would be a happy and fulfilling one. And even if she were to have five children of her own, that does not guarantee she wouldn't end up alone in her old age. There are endless versions of how her life could have or would have turned out, had it not been stopped in its tracks. So I am suggesting that you look at the bigger picture, when trying to understand the reasons why something happened to you.

EVERYTHING IN LIFE HAS A HIGHER PURPOSE AND SACRIFICES OFTEN TURN OUT INTO THE BIGGEST BLESSINGS. REMAIN AN OPTIMIST, BE OPEN TO BEAUTIFUL SURPRISES. HAVE FAITH!

It is impossible to see the big picture now, while you are amidst this caregiving journey. Learn to trust that there is a divine masterplan and someday everything will make perfect sense to you. Be open to marvelous new beginnings that await, once you conclude this assignment. There will be new partnerships, friendships and experiences coming your way.

"When?" I can hear you asking impatiently, with a lingering tear in your eye.

"At the perfect time," is the answer. There must be a reason why your life was turned upside down and your journey was disturbed.

Without trying to analyze it right now, allow life to surprise you in pleasant and unexpected ways. Remember, this experience is supposed to make you better and not bitter. Erase the sad, worried and hopeless expression from your face and know that you are not the only one going thru this difficult time. There are actually millions of people experiencing very similar situations, while facing decisions and feeling sadness. When time is right, maybe you will be able to help someone else in need, since you will understand them better than anyone. Allow your experience to empower and enrich you so greatly, that you will become an even better person than you already are.

AND ALWAYS REMEMBER, IT IS EVER TOO LATE TO FALL IN LOVE , ADOPT OR FOSTER A CHILD. YOUR FUTURE HOLDS ENDLESS POSSIBILITIES.

WHEN YOU FEEL LIKE GIVING UP

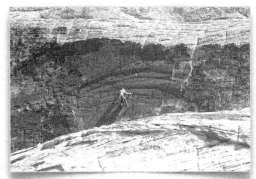

YOU CAN CONQUER THE SEEMINGLY IMPOSSIBLE

No matter how strong of a warrior you are, there will be those days or mid-night ruthless and exhausting moments, when you will feel like quitting and just leaving everything behind. You may feel like you are at the end of your rope and can't go on like this for another second longer. When this happens, you have two choices. First, immediately schedule a much needed break for yourself. A respite where you can leave for a few days would be very welcome.

How can you accomplish this? Keep in mind that at this stage of illness you cannot move your loved one into a short term facility, because it would disrupt the stability you worked so hard to establish and present an insurmountable amount of additional work for you. If you wish to take at least a few days off, you will need to hire a full time caregiver. This will require you to train them, show them where everything is, and implement them into your established-caregiving schedule. That process will require your additional effort and energy.

If that seems too much work and defeats the purpose, your second option may be better.

IMMEDIATELY ESTABLISH A NEW SCHEDULE WHERE YOU CAN TAKE A FEW HOURS IN THE AFTERNOON COMPLETELY OFF.

You will need to hire a caregiver only for those specific hours and days. Maybe you chose three afternoons a week for a helpful respite. The set up for that will require minimal training, it won't be overly demanding, and the cost will be manageable. Schedule your time away during the periods when your loved one usually takes a nap and requires very little assistance, thus very little training of the hired caregiver will be necessary.

Once you gain this window of freedom, do not stay at home, but take this opportunity to leave the house, change your environment, go into nature, get a massage, a manicure, an acupuncture treatment, take a yoga class, attend a guided meditation, or anything you can think of, to pamper yourself and change your mindset. Escape to the movies, to a café, to a bookstore, meet a friend if you are in the mood. If you wish to be by yourself, take a drive, explore the neighborhood, go to the botanical gardens, read a book and stare at the clouds or a body of water. Listen to the birds and just breathe.

YOU WILL BE AMAZED HOW QUICKLY YOU WILL REPLENISH WHEN YOU SPEND A FEW HOURS AWAY, OUT OF THE HOUSE AND PEACEFULLY ON YOUR OWN.

If this break doesn't suffice, and you still feel burned out, then it is time to find a regular caregiver, and engage them for a full day, a few days a week. If you already have a professional caregiver, increase the hours of care and take as much time off as possible. Assist them considerably less and assign a bigger workload to them. Perhaps you can adjust the schedule accordingly for one month, drastically reduce your own duties and just try to recover and regain your sanity.

If you cannot afford a caregiver, inquire with local Caregiver organizations about their support services and volunteer caregivers they may have.

If you have explored all options and still feel you are at a breaking point and just can't manage, then it is time to find a facility for your loved one. If you do not know how to go about it, find a local geriatric care manager, who can inform you about the best options and availability in your area and highest comfort for your loved one.

IF YOU CANNOT MANAGE FINANCIALLY, EXPLORE VARIOUS GOVERNMENT PROGRAMS INCLUDING MEDICARE AND HOSPICE FACILITIES THAT SHOULD BE ABLE TO HELP YOU.

Late stage of Alzheimer's often qualifies for hospice care and perhaps it is time you set that wheel in motion. Accept the fact that you did everything in your power, gave it your best, and simply have to save yourself.

May I forewarn you that there will certainly be a great sense of relief when you do that, but there might be just as big or even bigger sense of worry, guilt and failure that you did not keep your loved one at home.

Therefore I would advise you to really have a thorough conversation with your family members and most importantly with yourself, to make peace with your plan of action. If at this point, you cannot accept within your heart to place your loved one into a facility, and feel that the worry, sense of failure and guilt will weigh you down more than the caregiving itself, then you know the answer.

Maybe this realization will give you a renewed sense of strength and determination, so that you will see this journey till the end and in your home. You have to weigh your options carefully. On one side there is relief about regaining your night sleep, your days and life in general, on the other side there is worry, grief and guilt about failing to see this journey thru. These are your two choices and only you can decide which one you can live with.

REASSESS THE OPTIONS WELL, BECAUSE YOUR DECISION WILL BE FINAL.

Once your loved one at this late stage of illness enters a facility, you will not ever be transferring them again back home. It would be too exhausting and dangerous considering their frail state. If you decide to place them into facility, accept it and make peace with it. You have to know how to pick your battles. Give it some deep, and honest thought. Reflect on the details and various options. Make a list of pro's and con's. How can you best eliminate your loved one's suffering as well as your own perpetual worry and stress about their state? When they live in your home, you can see with your own eyes, that they are comfortable and well taken care of. That can be a considerable stress reducer.

Every time the situation wears you down, remember your decision and the reasons behind it. You see, you had the option to make a choice, and you did. Acknowledge that and release any feelings of powerless despair. You have chosen this assignment and I believe you are strong enough to get thru it and successfully complete it. If not, you are still a kind, good-hearted and very special person. Why? Because you gave it your best with the very best of intentions. And that my friend, is what matters most.

MORAL DILEMMAS
AND OTHER PEOPLE'S IGNORANCE

You may think this is not a problem for you. You have wholeheartedly decided to be the caregiver for your loved one and have no doubts about it. However, with time and thru various situations when you speak to friends, relatives or anyone else, you will eventually hear their opinions. Even if they respect your dedication to caregiving, their judgments will make you think or even self-doubt. Maybe you will reflect on their words and begin to wonder.

SOMEONE'S RANDOM JUDGMENT CARELESSLY THROWN AT YOU, COULD CAUSE YOU A LOT OF EMOTIONAL TURMOIL AND AGONY.

Therefore I have decided to address this ever-important topic. Your circumstances may slightly vary, but no matter how you look at it, you are a caregiver. I assume that if you are reading his book, you are attempting to do the best job possible. You're struggling to get thru the setbacks and are searching for better solutions to ease and alleviate any kind of discomfort or suffering of your loved one. No doubt there will be things you wish you could have done better, but don't be too hard on yourself. Do the best you can, each and every day. Here is the usual comment you may hear, that you need to be prepared for:

"Because you are taking such good care of your loved one, you are prolonging their life and also their agony."

The insinuation here is, that you are extending their suffering. These words are very difficult to hear. You are sacrificing your energy, time and life in order to provide care, and don't need to hear this kind of an ignorant comment. Yet you will, even from people who wish you well. They are obviously clueless when it comes to the reality of your situation. Such people should refrain from talking about a subject they know nothing about. Even if they watch you every single day, they are still not the ones actually doing it.

LET'S KEEP IN MIND, THAT THINGS LOOK MUCH EASIER TO DO, WHEN SOMEONE ELSE IS DOING THEM.

If you can change your loved one quickly without a screaming ordeal, then you have mastered it. But someone watching you might naively think that it's easy. Yet, if they had to do it themselves, they would probably quit, break down and cry in the midst of it all.

The absolute fact is that if you can alleviate someone's suffering, it is your duty as a fellow human being to do so. The belief, that if you don't take optimal care of someone, they will die earlier and therefore suffer less, is gravely mistaken. By allowing a circumstance that produces discomfort to go on, you are actually causing and enabling their suffering. It does not mean that the person will expire earlier. But it certainly means and assures that they will suffer. Let's make no mistake what I am talking about.

EXAMPLE CONSIDERING A HEALTHY DIET

Let's say you always prepare the best foods for your loved one. This way you do everything possible to assure healthy digestion, proper hydration, no constipation or diarrhea, no dangerous impactions and certainly no hunger. If someone is of the opinion, that your loved one would stop eating earlier, had you not prepared such good and tasty food, I consider that comment absurd. If your loved one is hungry you feed them, if they decline food, you respect that as well. You are not in charge when they should stop eating. If you spend no time figuring out the proper diet for your loved one, you will consequently cause them difficulty in that area. You may have to deal with applying enemas, which are very uncomfortable for everyone involved. Again, your poor care will create suffering. By not implementing enough liquids you are creating all sorts of havoc in the body.

> ## GOOD DIET IN YOUR LOVED ONE'S LIFE IS IMPROVING THE QUALITY OF THEIR LIFE AND PREVENTING SUFFERING.

EXAMPLE CONSIDERING VITAMINS AND SUPPLEMENTS

If you provide a healthy amount of vitamin supplements for your loved one, you will help alleviate any discomforts that are caused by vitamin deficiencies. A common and very painful ailment like leg cramps, can be remedied with a higher magnesium intake. You are not prolonging their life, but are assuring the best circumstances to alleviate pain.

EXAMPLE CONSIDERING SKINCARE

Yes, bathing and skincare are crucially important. By maintaining your loved one's skin in a healthy condition, you are assuring better resistance against bedsores. Is that going to prolong life? Absolutely not, but it will prevent a tremendous amount of suffering.

EXAMPLE CONSIDERING DILIGENT INCONTINENCE CARE

Someone may suggest, you should allow more time between incontinence changes, so you can sleep better at night. They are wrong. One missed incontinence pad change, and your loved one could have an instant bed sore. This will cause tremendous suffering.

EXAMPLE CONSIDERING NAIL FUNGUS CARE

You will hear that nail fungus cannot be alleviated and what's the point anyway? Here's the point; ignoring this condition could result in a major foot infection. With diligent discipline and natural remedies you can successfully eliminate nail fungus. Are you prolonging life? Hardly. Are you preventing loved one's suffering? Definitely.

I am certainly not talking about serious life and death situations like tube feeding or resuscitation. That kind of dilemma is your doctors's and family's decision and hopefully your loved one left a clear directive, so you don't have to face that difficult choice on your own. In the caregiving situations I listed, we are talking about your dedicated commitment to superior care.

> **THERE ARE NO EXCUSES FOR POOR CAREGIVING.**
> **IN FACT, THERE IS NO HALF WAY THRU HIS JOURNEY.**
> **EITHER YOU DO IT FULL SPEED, OR YOU DON'T DO IT AT ALL.**

So don't let these commentaries from uninformed standbys get in your way. Clearly they have absolutely no knowledge or awareness what kind of commitment it takes, and how important everyday care and maintenance really is. Most importantly, they have to learn that it is morally wrong for anyone else to decide how long someone else should live, just because they are elderly and ill. Still, people's ignorance can be extremely difficult to tolerate.

The final transition is meant to be experienced by each and every one of us in our own way and time. You have no right to rob someone of that experience or rush them, because you are in a hurry to be free of the responsibility. You need to guard them with all your might, so that they do not suffer unnecessarily.

> **KEEPING A LOVED ONE WELL CARED FOR, CLEAN, NURTURED**
> **AND NEVER ALONE, IS A REAL AND TANGIBLE GIFT TO THEM.**

As humans we have to accept that we do not control everything. We think we do, but in reality, we are merely making decisions about a few choices that are given to us. Our judgments, actions and intentions definitely matter. But the final decision? No, my friend. That one is out of your hands. And thank God for that.

*P*ersonally, at that late stage of my Mother's illness, I could never make peace with placing her into a facility and never seeing her again in my home. No matter how worn out I was through certain days, evenings or nights, just the thought of that made me beyond upset, so I never considered it an option.

But I am really speaking from having experienced both choices. As I wrote in the early chapters, during the mid-stage of her illness, due to complex dynamics, my Mother had to be placed into a facility. So I experienced how it felt to have her away from home.

My loyal daily visits to her, including morning and evening calls to the facility, only provided partial relief. I was overwhelmed with the constant worry and my anxiety was extreme. Daily visits only partially dissipated my concern and I sensed how the facility staff dreaded my daily inspections.

I immediately saw and notified them of their oversights, errors, neglect, failures, sloppiness, and disregard for overmedicated residents. My presence did not make their life easier, for my goal was to assure my Mom's wellbeing. The caregiving facility was well respected and supposed to be of the highest quality, the fees were sky-high and I made them earn every penny. Still, there were considerable failures and negligence.

So when my Mother's illness shifted and there was a possibility to bring her back home, I made a brave decision. I took her out of the facility and brought her home. It was an incredibly overwhelming undertaking, but it proved manageable and better for her at that stage of illness.

It felt also considerably better for me, as I was calmer now that I could personally assure she didn't feel abandoned and had the best care possible, every single minute of day and night. I did not allow the need for nighttime changes and my continuously interrupted sleep to discourage or regret my decision.

I was now living the nighttime changes with her, so we both still suffered, but I worried less. And she was content and considerably more comfortable. So out of the two choices, this was definitely the better one.

UNDERSTAND YOUR MISSION

You will wonder about this quite often.
The big question: "What is this about? Why my loved one, why me?

Well, here you are, time is ticking, years have gone by and still you are in this impossible predicament or caregiving for your loved one in your home.

> **I AM NOT ADVISING YOU TO CHOOSE THIS ASSIGNMENT,**
> **FOR IT IS AN INDIVIDUAL CHOICE.**
> **BUT IF YOU HAVE CHOSEN THIS MISSION,**
> **THEN I AM STANDING BY YOUR SIDE TILL THE VERY END**
> **AND SHARING WITH YOU ALL MY HARD - EARNED KNOWLEDGE**
> **I'VE LEARNED THROUGH MY OWN CAREGIVING JOURNEY.**

I am making sure that the time it took me to figure something out, is the time that I saved you. The frustration I experienced, is the one you are spared off. The fear and agony that I felt, has hopefully to some degree eluded you. In the end, this is about eliminating human suffering.

I pray and hope that the way my Mother, our family and I suffered thru this ordeal made way for you, dear reader, to suffer less. Does that make sense? It does to me. Actually this thought is what got me thru a lot of agonizing, sleepless nights and moments filled with utter despair and grave sadness. But you see, what I am talking about is the fact that you are on a mission. I figured out my mission.

What is my mission, you ask? What you are holding it in your hands is a big part of it. A book that can aid someone in the most difficult hour of need. A book that can endure thru years and still help you navigate thru a testy time. A book that will let you know someone else has been on this journey before you. And I am not afraid to write about it, I am not embarrassed to talk about bowel movement and how to clean an incontinent loved one. Why?

Because nobody want's to talk about the ugliest, most difficult parts of getting weak, old, ill and needy. It seems the world is pretending that nobody ages or goes to the bathroom, when in fact the entire world does. Every day and all the time!

As human beings we still have so much to learn. Our ability to perceive needs a great awakening. We desperately need to mature and evolve. If we cannot talk about the inevitable aging process, respecting our elders, what happens when basic bodily functions fail, what does it mean being incontinent, and how to gracefully face the final transition of life thru the gates of death, then we are completely out of touch with the meaning and purpose of life.

**THE FACT IS THAT NONE OF US ARE GETTING OUT OF THIS WORLD ALIVE.
WE SHALL ALL AGE AND EVENTUALLY DEPART.
WHY KEEP PRETENDING IT ISN'T SO?**

No matter how untouchable you feel, death is nearing each and every second. We are not doing ourselves any favors by treating our elderly like they need to be thrown out, dismissed, getting rid off and just forgotten.

Obviously I am not talking about you, my dear caregiver. I am pointing the finger at the ones who are hiding and running away. I am directing the beam of glaring truth at those who abuse and neglect our elder community. Those fragile old souls who find themselves at the mercy of the greedy, ignorant and heartless.

You my friend, are here facing and dealing with it head on, because you have courage, heart and strength. That is you mission. Wear it proudly, teach it to others and set an example.

**THE WORLD DESPERATELY NEEDS A HERO, A SHINNING EXAMPLE.
THE WORLD NEEDS MORE WONDERFUL PEOPLE LIKE YOU.**

LIVE LIFE TO THE FULLEST, EACH AND EVERY DAY!

CHAPTER SIXTEEN

Self-Care for Caregivers

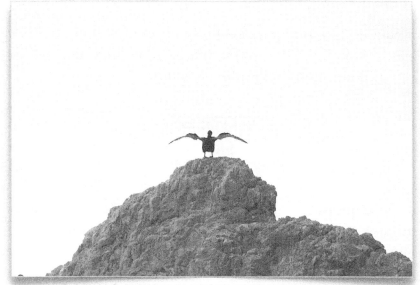

CARING FOR YOURSELF IS PARAMOUNT

SELF CARE

One of the positive aspects about caring for your loved one under *Holistic Caregiving* principles, is the fact that they can be easily applied to you as well. The principle of healthy diet is the perfect example. While preparing the best food for your loved one, you have a perfect opportunity to implement a healthy diet for yourself. If you go by the rules of avoiding all sugar, and consume a strictly gluten free, organic foods diet, you will greatly eliminate the damaging effects of stress and build a stronger resilience.

Our primary purpose is to keep your loved one comfortable and in a loving, optimally healing and peaceful environment. However, you my dear caregiver, are the one that makes everything happen. Without your health, there is nothing.

STRESS

The number one enemy and threat to your health is stress. Your individual endurance and stress response to physically, mentally and emotionally demanding situations affects your overall health. Some people can manage high levels of stress, others less. If you lead a highly stressful life and then suddenly come to a breaking point, your stress tolerance has reached its limit. While occasional stress is a regular part of life, ongoing long term chronic stress can cause serious repercussions to your health.

YOU ARE THE GATEKEEPER OF YOUR LOVED ONE'S SANCTUARY. AS SUCH, YOU MUST PRESERVE AND PROTECT YOUR HEALTH.

As a primary caregiver, you are exposed to the highest level of long term, chronic stress. Your endurance, resilience and strength are severely tested. How can you protect yourself from excessive levels of stress?

Here are a few suggestions:
* Get informed - look for signs of excessive stress in your life
* Assess the level of your stress - mild, medium, high
* Understand the potential negative effects - physical, mental, emotional health issues
* Recognize your existing health challenges and ailments resulting from stress
* Make a decision and dedicate yourself to follow a stress management plan

Stress can sneak up on you and quickly become a normal part of your daily life. Your state of health will undergo various significant and indicative changes, but you may ignore them, assuming they are a normal part of the aging process. They are not.

> **THE LONGER YOU NEGLECT YOUR OVERSTRESSED STATE, THERE MORE EFFORT IT WILL REQUIRE TO REPAIR, RECOVER AND REGAIN YOUR HEALTH.**

You may be quite resilient to stress and have a great natural capacity to withstand taxing situations and ongoing pressure. If you are physically and mentally fit and have a determined resilient character, your endurance may last for quite a while. For example, if you have engaged is sport activities throughout your life, you will have a stronger physical stamina than someone who never exercised. However, no matter how fit you are, a long term stressful lifestyle will eventually burn you out. As a primary caregiver you need to pay great attention to your own state of physical well being.

> **THE FIRST AND MOST OBVIOUS SIGNS OF CAREGIVER BURNOUT ARE EXHAUSTION, FATIGUE, IRRITABILITY, WEIGHT GAIN OR LOSS AND DEPRESSION. THESE ARE ALL PROMINENT SIGNS OF SERIOUS ADRENAL BURNOUT.**

It is crucial that you pay very close attention to your level of energy, sleeping pattern, weight and mental fortitude. In addition, observe the state of your emotional resilience and examine:

- ❋ Are you easily overly excited, irritated, depressed or angry?
- ❋ Has that always been your natural disposition?
- ❋ Are you considerably less patient?
- ❋ Do you suffer from a persistent pain and dismiss it as your "new normal?"
- ❋ Are you losing or gaining weight while stress eating?

If you feel unwell or exhausted, your physical body is sending a clear signal, that you need to pay attention. If you ignore the consequences of stress, the ailments will grow stronger, multiply and establish a long term presence in your system.

Each one of us carries some kind of physical vulnerability within our constitution. When under duress, your weakest link will break first. For example: if you have a sensitive digestive system, you could develop IBS, while someone with hypersensitive skin could begin suffering from a rash or psoriasis.

> **IT IS IMPORTANT THAT YOU KNOW AND UNDERSTAND YOUR INDIVIDUAL PHYSICAL VULNERABILITIES THAT ARE MOST PRONE TO GIVE IN, UNDER CHRONIC STRESS. WHAT IS YOUR WEAK LINK?**

This is why caregiving can become a detrimental factor in caregiver's overall state of health. Despite the fact that you may be naturally a very strong person, with great physical endurance, you are not indestructible. We all are susceptible to damaging effects of stress therefore it is urgent that you pay close attention.

Take look at the list of various damaging effects of stress on your physical health. Ask yourself truthfully if you suffer from any of these symptoms.

PHYSICAL EFFECTS OF STRESS

DO ANY OF THESE AILMENTS APPLY TO YOU?

- Adrenal burnout
- Asthma
- Autoimmune Problems
- Backache
- Chest pain, rapid heartbeat
- Chronic Fatigue
- Diabetes
- Diarrhea or constipation
- Dizziness
- Elevated cholesterol
- Frequent colds
- Heart problems

- High blood pressure
- Infertility
- Insomnia
- Irritable Bowel Syndrome
- Low resistance
- Migraine or tension headache
- Nausea
- Skin Problems
- Thyroid problems
- Ulcer
- Weight gain or weight loss

PSYCHOLOGICAL AND EMOTIONAL SIGNS OF STRESS

ARE YOU EXPERIENCING ANY OF THESE SYMPTOMS?

- Addictions
- Anxiety disorders
- Changed eating habits
- Changed sleeping habits
- Chronic worry
- Depression
- Emotional overwhelm
- Difficulty with decision making
- Grinding teeth in your sleep
- Inability to relax - restlessness
- Irritation

- Isolating yourself from others
- Lack of concentration
- Loss of objectivity
- Loss of sex drive
- Moodiness
- Negative mindset
- Neglecting responsibilities
- Neglecting self-care
- Nervousness
- Panic attacks
- Procrastination

If any if these symptoms apply, you are suffering from stress. When you are a primary caregiver, it is practically next to impossible to stay unaffected and stress free. The daily and nightly grind and sleep deprivation are difficult to sustain for a long term. This is your perfect opportunity to take decisive steps to help regain your health, reverse any damage and protect yourself from future deterioration.

IF YOU SUFFER SERIOUS HEALTH AILMENTS, YOU NEED TO SEEK MEDICAL ATTENTION AS SOON AS POSSIBLE. DISCUSS WITH YOUR PERSONAL PHYSICIAN ALL THE CHOICES AND RECOMMENDATIONS TO HELP YOU REMEDY BURN-OUT AND REGAIN YOUR HEALTH AS QUICKLY AS POSSIBLE.

If you simply feel tired and stressed, but do not have any other serious health challenges, you can reverse the damage and regain your optimal state of wellness by implementing a clean and healthy lifestyle regimen. There is a lot you can do to prevent and regain your best possible health. Practice disciplined self-care, set the rules and boundaries and do not push yourself beyond healthy limits. Dedicate time for yourself and preserve your life force as much as possible.

THE SEVEN PILLARS OF SELF-CARE

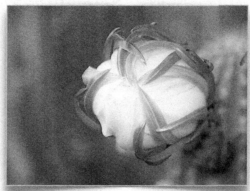

YOUR BODY IS NATURALLY RESILIENT

By living like a guard on duty, a midnight nurse on call, and constant primary caregiver you can wear out faster than a candle burning on both ends. You urgently need to create a routine of self-care. Nothing else will work if you burn out, fall apart and crash.

**IT HAS BEEN OFTEN SAID
THAT THE CAREGIVER DECLINES FASTER
THAN THE PERSON THAT ACTUALLY HAS ALZHEIMER'S.
THAT MAY VERY WELL BE TRUE.
BUT YOU MUST NOT ALLOW THAT TO HAPPEN.**

What is expected and needed of you is definitely exhausting beyond words. Here you are, working tirelessly around the clock. But if you know how to keep a healthy attitude and reserve some time for your own health support and maintenance, you will be able to get thru this period of your life, without suffering lifelong health consequences.

Here are your seven main principles of self-care, that will help maintain your health thru the caregiving challenge.

1. SLEEP

The most important rule in beating stress is sufficient sleep. You require a minimum of eight hours of sleep in order to function normally, especially when under any kind of stress. Sleep whenever you can, steal a nap in the afternoon if possible and remember that watching late TV or surfing the web is not worth cutting your primary sleep hours.

You should be getting at least eight good healthy hours of sleep every night. If you have a challenging night with your loved one, you need to make up for all the lost sleep as soon as possible. If you lose and hour, you need to catch up ASAP with a short nap or two during the day.

**IF YOU LOVED ONE KEEPS AWAKE AT NIGHT,
THEY WILL NEED PROPER MEDICATION,
BECAUSE YOU WILL NOT BE ABLE TO SUSTAIN
THAT KIND OF SLEEP DEPRIVATION FOR ANY LENGTH OF TIME.**

In order to preserve your health and function like a normal person, you need your sleep.

Of course your loved one can catch up on their missed sleep on the following day anytime they so desire. While you run around a million errands, sleep deprived, sluggish and exhausted from the previous night, they will take a wonderful nap.

If the sleepless nights continue without you managing to catch up on lost hours, I can guarantee that you will burn out very fast. Even one week of sleep deprivation could have disastrous consequences on your health. No one can function on no sleep and you are no exception.

A twenty-minute quick nap will leave you feeling refreshed and recharged. You owe it to yourself and your loved one to stay well, healthy and rested. If you don't replace your sleep, you will quickly suffer from adrenal burn out. Consciously resist your tendency to keep going. Slow down, rest and be as kind to yourself as you would be to your best friend that you love and respect.

2. HEALTHY DIET

The next important self-care rule is proper diet. If you find yourself each evening crashing on the couch, hungry and exhausted and reaching for pizza, cookies and ice cream, that will quickly become your undoing. While under your loving care, your loved one may look like they are on a permanent vacation, while you will appear like you carry the burden of the world on your shoulders and feel a thousand years old. To prevent this from happening, please check the Chapter *Healthy Diet*. You will find valuable information about how create your meals, when to eat and the best nutritional plan for you.

3. SUPPLEMENTS

In order to stay healthy and continue navigating through the caregiving journey, you need to be informed about your physical vulnerabilities and areas of weakness. Proper supplements will help you fortify and strengthen your over all system. Find a health care professional to help you create a healthy regimen with proper supplements. You can find all about natural remedies and supplements in Chapter *Holistic Caregiving Remedies*.

4. EXERCISE

Another key in proper self-care is regular, easy exercise. Whatever kind of movement suits your body best, find time to include it in your maintenance plan. This could consist of gentle yoga, meditation, breathing, easy walking, hiking, swimming, easy stretch, jogging, tai chi, and so on. You should engage your body in physical activity at least a few days a week. The more you oxygenate your body, the better you will preserve your health.

5. CAREGIVER BREAKS

Respite breaks are an absolute must. Organize a caregiving schedule that includes some free time for you. Whether that requires a helpful relative, friend, volunteer caregiver or a hired caregiver that relieves you a few hours each day, one day a week, or at least an afternoon a week. If you can manage to get away for the weekend, that is excellent. I know that is very difficult to do. But you would be amazed what a difference it makes to leave the house at least a few hours every few days. Keep a realistic schedule that includes accommodating your own needs for some down time, so you can maintain a good healthy mindset.

6. PRIVATE TIME FOR YOUR SPIRIT

Another necessity for optimal self-care is regular, peaceful and private time for contemplation, inner reflection, meditation or prayer.

FULFILLING YOUR SPIRITUAL NEEDS IS ESSENTIAL FOR MANAGING THIS LONG AND DEMANDING JOURNEY.

You need to remember who you are, what are your abilities, talents, dreams, interests and possible future endeavors. What is this experience bringing to your life that could be beneficial and positive? Reflect on that and make the best of this given situation. You could be guided into the next area of work, a different circle of friends, a special interest group, or a greater cause. Allow time for prayer, meditation and complete stillness. Give yourself the opportunity to unwind, cultivate inner conversation and contemplation. Write a journal to help balance your emotions and find answers. Read an inspiring book and follow a guided spiritual path that helps sustain you through this journey. Establish your source of inner strength and spiritual resilience.

7. YOUR SUPPORT SYSTEM

A decisive factor in your overall stress management is your support system. That means your loved one's doctors, your team of caregivers - if you have them, your neighbors, relatives, friends and various caregiver support organizations. They will stand by your side thru this, talk to you, offer respite, emotional support and a good ear for listening.

By all means do not allow yourself to get completely isolated in this illness and caregiving journey. Keep connected and communicate with others, for you would be amazed how many people find themselves in a similar predicament. A great support system will help you through every step of the way. When you loved one enters the very final stage of the journey, you should call on hospice and lean on them for support. You need all the help you can get, but remember, only you are the one who can allow the help to come to you. Open your arms and ask for help and you will find it. My dear, you are not alone.

PROMISE YOURSELF YOU WILL ENGAGE IN SELF-CARE. YOUR HEALTH IS YOUR NUMBER ONE PRIORITY. IF YOU DON'T CARE FOR YOURSELF, YOU CANNOT CARE FOR OTHERS.

PROTECTING YOUR SUBTLE ENERGY FIELD

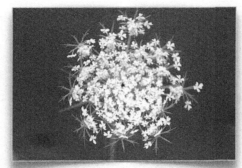

EVERYTHING CONSISTS OF ENERGY AND VIBRATION

There is a complex subtle energy aspect to caregiving that is important to understand. It may seem a bit esoteric, but it should not be taken lightly or dismissed. I will share with you the main principles, so you can get the idea and understand this fascinating and important information.

WHY IS THIS KNOWLEDGE VALUABLE?

Because it will help you understand how your energy level is affected, due to the invisible subtle energy exchange with your loved one. Each and every one of us has an invisible energy field within and around our physical body. This energy body-aura is highly sensitive to various sensory stimulants, such as your environment and people in it.

WHAT RECHARGES YOUR ENERGY FIELD?

Healthy lifestyle, spending time in nature, organic fresh and healthy food, meditation, exercise, self-care activities such as massage and acupuncture or listening to soothing music. Spending time with positive and uplifting people will help recharge and magnify your subtle energy field. Emotions such as happiness, joy, laughter, delight and love will boost your aura.

WHAT DEPLETES YOUR ENERGY FIELD?

Unhealthy lifestyle, addictive substances such as drugs, alcohol, smoking, poor diet, physical exhaustion, illness, stress, depression and disruptive sensory stimulants, such as loud noise and electronic devices. In addition, negative and needy people can be a considerable energy drain on your energy field. Emotions such as fear, hate, anger, jealousy, and sadness will weaken your aura.

When you meet someone, you instantly intuitively sense a certain energy or vibration about them. This is your intuitive awareness. If it feels pleasant, you like them and are attracted to them. You feel good in their company and enjoy spending time with them, because it energizes, uplifts, inspires and motivates you. Their personal frequency is compatible and harmonious with yours, and there is an equal energy exchange.

But if you meet someone and their presence makes you feel uneasy or uncomfortable, and you intuitively dislike them, they are not compatible with you. The feeling of aversion clearly indicates that their personal frequency is not harmonious with yours, and the energy exchange will disrupt or deplete your own energy field.

WE ARE ENERGETICALLY MOST COMPATIBLE WITH PEOPLE THAT WE ENJOY A HARMONIOUS RELATIONSHIP WITH; SUCH AS PARTNERS, LOVERS, CHILDREN, FRIENDS AND OUR PARENTS.

In fact, the invisible and powerful subtle energy bond with your parents is one of the anchors of your energy field. Your Mother's energy field will imprint yours before birth, and both your parents continue to have a strong energy effect on you, that remains with you thru your entire lifetime.

In early childhood, the energy bond with your parents strengthens and sets up definite relationships dynamics. If this bond is good, positive and healthy, you develop into a thriving, independent and confident individual. Your own personality traits also play a decisive role, but the energy frequency that surrounds you cannot be undermined, for it does influence you.

Later in life, when you form relationships and partnerships of your own, you may find yourself in similar pattern as your parents, and simply repeat the familiar energy dynamic. Established energy patterns often follow us throughout our life.

WHEN YOU ARE IN AN ESTABLISHED LONG-TERM PARTNERSHIP, THE ENERGY BOND BETWEEN THE TWO, CREATES AN IMPORTANT ANCHOR IN YOUR ENERGY FIELD, WHICH ADJUSTS TO EACH OTHER'S NEEDS AND FUNCTIONING PATTERNS.

No relationship bond is without a challenge, since the main purpose of all our relationships is to learn and grow. There may be old patterns that continue through generations. If a person was deprived of love as a child, it may be very difficult for them to express love towards their own children. An established pattern is challenging, but not impossible to overcome. In fact, we need to master it for our evolutionary growth.

Regardless of who the loved one you are caring for is - your partner or your parent - it is possible that the relationship may not have always been entirely positive. Maybe it was somewhat challenging, restricting, codependent, perhaps even manipulative, at times abusive, draining and generally difficult.

Now you find yourself in a different set up. They are vulnerable, helpless and you are their caregiver. You may have overcome any negative dynamics that previously occurred with your loved one, however, when they become ill, their core character traits magnify and unfortunately some old negative qualities may reemerge. That can specifically occur with the parent-child relationship, and prove quite challenging.

IT IS MOST IMPORTANT THAT YOU DO NOT SLIP INTO YOUR OLD NEGATIVE PATTERNS WHILE TAKING CARE OF LOVED ONE.

You need to establish new boundaries that will help you maintain a healthy relationship in this new coexistent space. If they were excessively attached to you in the past, now they will be even more. They may persistently demand your energy and push the right trigger button in you, to make you react and appease them. If you don't resist this energy pull, you will become rapidly exhausted, constantly feel their energy tug and need of attention.

This interaction dynamic can occur with any other previous old tendency, such as being overly critical or scolding you, while you are taking care of them. You must distinguish if your loved one really needs your help, or is exceedingly demanding as part of their old pattern. Objectively assess their needs and follow your healthy boundaries, remaining calm, kind and loving. This will help diffuse old patterns. If you do not react in a negative way, you will remedy the situation and it shall pass.

KEEP IN MIND, SOMEONE CAN ONLY DRAIN YOUR ENERGY IF YOU ALLOW AND FACILITATE FOR THEM TO DO SO.

When your loved one enters the final phase, they often lose the ability to communicate or display any kind of emotion at all. Their energy field is seriously depleted and they cannot properly function without other people's vital energy. They will get that missing energy from an outside source - you.

AS A CAREGIVER, YOU ARE SUPPLYING YOUR LOVED ONE WITH YOUR OWN VITAL ENERGY, SIMPLY BY BEING NEAR THEM.

There is no coincidence that when caregiving, your energy is drained amazingly fast and you feel wiped out. Professional caregivers always suffer from burn out - exhaustion which is caused less by strenuous physical activity, and more by subtle energy drain. A hired caregiver may spend hours sitting nearby, slowly feeding or watching over loved one, as they nap. Therefore private caregivers spend a large amount in a passive state, yet still get exhausted.

When sitting next to someone who is terminally ill and lacking their own life energy, you can become inexplicably sleepy and drained. You wonder why and try to justify it with other contributing factors, when in fact you are being energetically wiped out by your loved one, who may be peacefully sleeping.

It is also no coincidence that caregivers often face a battle with weight gain. You will most likely also suffer from weight gain while strapped down with the caregiving duties. There are numerous stress consequences on your health that can contribute to weight gain as well. However, another cause for weight gain can be your body's natural attempt to protect your energy field from being drained by another person. The physical area where someone can unknowingly "hook" into your energy field is the solar plexus. It is the third energy center on a chakra scale connected to the emotions of fear, anger and ego. When one feels afraid or angry they often experience stomach problems.

OBSERVE YOUR BODY'S REACTION IN THE STOMACH AREA WHEN YOU ARE IN AN EXTRA CHALLENGING CAREGIVING SITUATION. IF YOUR STOMACH EXPANDS AND YOU FEEL BLOATED, YOUR ENERGY BODY IS TRYING TO PROTECT ITSELF.

This may suddenly occur for no apparent reason. You will feel bloated and your stomach will stick out. That is partially because your body is trying to defend itself from the outside energy drain that is attached to that area. You need to be aware of this energy drain dynamic and properly protect yourself from getting depleted without even knowing about it. What can you do?

Healthy children and animals have an excess of vibrant life force, so they can easily "feed" a weaker person. If you have children, encourage them to pay short visits to your loved one. Even a few minutes a day will make a difference. Your loved one will notice and enjoy their company and you will quickly observe a pick-up in their overall energy level. The children will not experience an energy drain.

THE IDEAL ASSISTANT THAT CAN HELP YOU IN THIS CIRCUMSTANCE IS A PET. ANIMALS HAVE AN EXTRAORDINARY ABILITY TO REPLENISH PEOPLE WITH THE VITAL LIFE FORCE.

Animal therapy is precisely that form of subtle energy exchange. If you have a well behaved pet, it would be very beneficial to have them regularly visit your loved one. You will notice a positive shift in their energy level, they will relax, feel more peaceful and content. In addition, I discourage you from sleeping in the same room with your loved one, not even a taking nap during the daytime.

WHILE YOU ARE SLEEPING, YOUR NATURAL PROTECTIVE SHIELD IS VULNERABLE AND YOUR ENERGY SOURCE IS MORE EASILY ACCESSIBLE.

It is also not advisable for you to aimlessly sit next to your loved one for hours at a time, reading or watching TV and the likes. When you are engaging in an activity where your attention is low, it is that much easier to tap into your energy field and deplete your power. Chances are, if you are sitting in your loved one's room for extended periods of time, you will doze off within minutes. Why? Because they are hooked onto your energy field and you are so depleted, you literally can't manage to stay awake.

So my suggestion is that you remain active and alert when you are near your loved one. If they are securely resting and napping in their recliner or bed after a meal, you can leave them for a bit, always checking on them and listening to your room monitor. When you are awake, aware and in charge, you are energetically stronger.

IT IS ALSO A GOOD IDEA TO WASH YOUR HANDS WITH SALT WHEN DONE WITH CAREGIVING DUTIES AT THE END OF THE DAY.

Place some regular salt into your hands, spread the fingers and gently massage your hands while washing them under running water. Salt has an especially cleansing effect and helps remove other people's subtle energy residues. This way you are properly protecting your energy field, so that you can be stronger and energetically more resilient. An evening shower will also help you cleanse your energy field, so try to keep a regular schedule and conscious tend to your delicate subtle field.

We assume that if something cannot be seen, it does not exist. But energy exchange very much does exist and needs to be properly understood. With these simple steps you can help protect as well as replenish your subtle energy field - aura.

CHAPTER SEVENTEEN

Final Weeks and Days

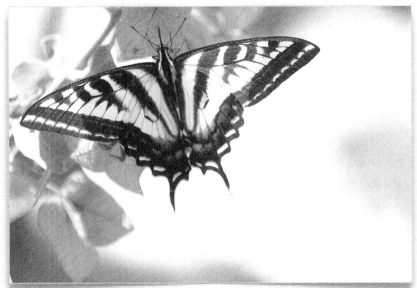

OUR LIFE JOURNEY IS A TRANSFORMATION

I will cherish my last days with my Mother forever. Even though my heart cried every second of those long never ending hours, in my spirit I prayed for her release. I felt and knew her soul would be free once she would transition.

I spoke to her words of encouragement and love whenever I had the strength. Her demeanor became very distant and removed and she was visibly slipping into a world I had no access to. But she was very peaceful and calm about it. It seemed that she was in deep thought and rather studious. That may seem strange, but it was how I perceived it.

I gently stroked her hair as she closed her eyes and was deeply relaxed. She never got any medication for pain or sedatives. Thankfully she did not need it and was transitioning with awareness, naturally. She was never alone and in the final moments of her life, Dad and I were with her, as always. I held her in my arms and spoke to her. I told her I loved her and will see her soon. She heard me.

I know when my moment of transition arrives, she will be there, in the next world, waiting for me, smiling and happy that we can speak again. I look forward to the rest of my life with joy and optimism. But equally so, I look forward to our reunion. Someday.

END OF LIFE CARE

It is beyond difficult to watch your loved one dwindle away to nothing as their final day of life approaches. There are many physical changes that will occur and you will often feel quite helpless and overwhelmed. The long journey is coming to an end and the relentless illness that you were so bravely battling is finally taking over.

You will have to prepare yourself to remain strong during this time and keep a steady spiritual perspective that will hold you thru. No matter what your belief system is, here is your loved one, disappearing right in front of your eyes. What can you do?

CONTINUE TO OFFER YOUR LOVED ONE OPTIMAL CARE, ATTENTION AND REMAIN A LOVING AND CALM PRESENCE.

It is very important to realize that even though their days might be numbered, you cannot be less attentive or dedicated with care. Quite to the contrary, you need to be even more diligent to help assure a gentle and peaceful final transition.

Changes will occur every day, some smaller and some drastic. Suddenly one day, their appetite will decline by half. Or they will become too weak to be given a proper shower. You need to be prepared to immediately adjust your care regimen and still offer the best care for their optimal comfort.

Some new declining health challenges will occur, but can often be quickly resolved, if you know how. Your main perspective remains to assure your loved one is pain free and not suffering.

KEEP THEM MAXIMALLY COMFORTABLE UNTIL THEIR CHOSEN MOMENT IN TIME, WHEN THEY FINALLY MAKE THEIR TRANSITION.

YOUR COMPLETE SURRENDER

No matter how hard you fought to save your loved one, how much you sacrificed and endured, there is a time when you need to surrender and stop tormenting yourself. All was done, and now make peace with the fact that they will be leaving, once and for all.

They say that Alzheimer's is the slowest, most challenging way of leaving this life. But suffering should never to be compared. I believe death and its final struggle is always difficult, no matter what the circumstances. It is absurd to decide what is worse. Everything is worse.

A gentle slipping away while falling asleep seems like a blessing of a departure, but there is so much we don't know about life and death. Our human life requires us to surrender to the irrevocable fact, that one day every and each one of us shall perish. This is a firm and nonnegotiable rule that governs here, in this world.

PRACTICE ONGOING MEDITATION OR PRAYER THROUGHOUT YOUR DAYS. IT WILL HELP KEEP YOU GROUNDED AND CENTERED.

So when you face the time of ultimate surrender, release the outcome of your loved one's battle. Keep a clear focus on being what your loved one needs at this time: an ever reliable, loving and capable caregiver filled with serene peace. Connect to God and ask for strength to help you get thru this assignment.

COMMUNICATION

In the final stage of dementia, your loved one will most likely have very little or no speaking or communication capacity. You will have to rely on your keen observation skills to know how they are doing, feeling and all their possible needs. This is going to be quite a challenge. The key is to not become frustrated, but remain calm, patient and reassuring. Even if you are uncertain about what is bothering them, your lovingly soothing voice and confidence will help calm them. They will relax and trust, that you are watching over them.

You will understand when they are comfortable, or when they need your attention. Just like you have been doing before, while you took care of them, your intuition will help you establish a general comfort zone.

PRESENT, BUT NON INTRUSIVE

Your approach to communication with your loved one will shift to complete peace at all times. They must see you when they are awake and hear your soft, soothing voice so that they never feel abandoned. Let them have the opportunity to be at peace. Time is almost standing still for them. They are entering a phase of readjusting to their new way of existence.

IN CERTAIN INVISIBLE WAY, YOUR LOVED ONE MAY ALREADY BE ENTERING THE SPIRIT WORLD THAT IS IMPERCEPTIBLE TO US.

When they look far into the distance, they should not be distracted. When they do not recognize you anymore, do not force them to do so. Put your personal feelings aside and allow them to simply be. Remain a pleasant loving presence and get out of the way. This is their time and space for the sacred transition that awaits.

If they look at you, gently assure them that you are here, with them, they are never alone and all is well. They have nothing to fear. Tell them you love them so very much. No matter how absent they may seem, these words will calm them down and help them find peace. They still hear you.

HOSPICE CARE

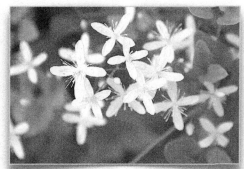

YOU ARE NOT ABANDONED, YOU ARE SUPPORTED

When it was time to engage the Hospice services, my soul felt absolutely crushed. In some distant corner of my heart, I felt as if I had given up. Through the years, I fought so hard to pull my Mother back from the abyss of this merciless illness and now, she was slipping away beyond any hope of return. I felt utterly helpless, overpowered and brutally conquered.

But Hospice nurses helped save me from crashing. They held my hand and in the final week of my Mother's life, they stood by her bedside through the night, so I could get a few desperately needed hours of sleep. They supported me and gently talked me through every step of this journey. Hospice service was a true blessing.

There will be a time when you will have to engage the Hospice services. I highly recommend you do so, as the Hospice nurses will be able to professionally assist you through the final steps of this demanding mission. They will provide you with physical, emotional and spiritual caregiver support, offer respite care and help with any paperwork or financial issues.

When engaging Hospice services you may feel like you've failed and given up, but in fact Hospice only represents the final stretch of the long journey. Do not misunderstand this as giving up, it is more about continuing to offer maximum comfort to your loved one, while making sure you don't get overwhelmed on your own.

It is important to understand that the purpose of Hospice is comfort care without curative intention, as a result, hospitalization or certain diagnostic medical tests are discouraged, and experimentation or tests trials are not allowed.

Engaging Hospice services requires specific paperwork as well as an in-person interview with you, in the presence of your loved one. This is necessary and a required step in Hospice approval process for eligibility. If your loved one's doctor usually pays home visits, it is very likely they will be present as well. Your loved one's personal physician or Hospice doctor has to assess that the life expectancy of your loved one is six months or less.

In the introductory interview, Hospice will inform you of their purpose and services they provide. This conversation will prove emotionally demanding. You will come face to face with the harsh reality, that your loved one is nearing the end of their life. During the course of the interview, you will verbally acknowledge that your loved one will pass away, since as a primary caregiver, you have to agree and accept the Hospice services. Uttering those actual words is heart wrenching.

Speaking of pending death can be most difficult. You have of course known in your mind for many years, that your loved one will eventually pass away, as we all shall. But it feels very differently when you are actually facing the final end and acknowledging that your loved one is on the threshold of a permanent departure. You are exhausted, vulnerable and overwhelmed.

ONCE THE HOSPICE PURPOSE AND SERVICES ARE ESTABLISHED, AND YOU HAVE ACKNOWLEDGED THE UNDENIABLE FACTS, YOU WILL FEEL A STRANGE SENSE OF RELIEF.

A big shift will occur and you will feel that you've entered a new phase of this journey. This is the most dreaded part, however once you face it, Hospice will help you feel supported and less alone. This can be a lifesaver. Yes, you were defeated, but you are not abandoned or alone.

Once the initial interview is concluded, Hospice will set up a schedule, according to the level of care your loved one requires. If they are in the early end-of-life stage, the Hospice nurse will come a few times a week for an hour, to check on your loved one, help with any caregiving issues and assess their overall a state. Once the actual dying process begins, Hospice nurses will be with you more frequently and at the very end, someone will stay with your loved one 24 hours a day.

The process will continue through various phases and Hospice will be extremely helpful in assuring your loved one's optimal comfort, while offering you their professional and knowledgeable support. You will be able to manage this journey considerably easier with their help at your side.

I suggest you remain very involved, present and well informed. Any information you can share with Hospice nurses regarding your loved one, will be extremely helpful. You can decide together how to proceed when certain choices have to be made. If your loved one is in any kind of pain or anxiety, Hospice nurse will provide, administer and help manage all necessary medication.

In the final days, a Hospice nurse will help watch over your loved one through the night, which will help you get a few hours of desperately needed sleep. With their help you will manage and survive through the most extreme ordeal of the dying process and the actual moment of death. They will also support you through the logistics of the period immediately after death, so you will not feel lost and alone. That is incredibly important and tremendously valuable.

HOSPICE SERVICES WILL OFFER YOU EMOTIONAL GUIDANCE, UNWAVERING SUPPORT AND KIND CARE THROUGH THIS CRUCIAL MOMENT OF YOUR LIFE.

PALLIATIVE CARE VERSUS HOSPICE CARE

Palliative care can begin at diagnosis, in coordination with any treatment. Palliative care addresses patient's overall comfort and wellbeing in all stages of illness. It uses life-prolonging medications and focuses on relief from physical suffering as well as curative measures.

Hospice care priority is patient comfort and end of life support for patient and family members. Hospice care begins only after it is clear the patient is not going to survive the illness and has less than six months to live.

BODY CARE IN LAST STAGE OF LIFE

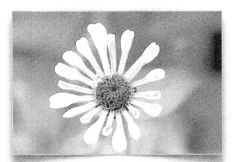

THIS TIME REQUIRES EXCEPTIONAL TENDERNESS

SPONGE BATH

When your loved one is too ill, weak and can't even hold up their head, it is obvious that you cannot give them a shower. It is time for a sponge bath. You may think that one can't properly clean someone with only a sponge. Well, you can. The key is being well prepared and having the right supplies.

You will need:
* At least two natural sea-sponges. You can get them in any health food store. When wet, they are incredibly soft and pleasant to the touch.
* A small bucket for rinsing the sponges as you go along
* A gentle hypoallergenic special rinse-free soap
* Three or four large towels
* Two small washcloths, designated for the groin area
* Plastic gloves
* Laundry basket for soiled towels, nightgown and bedding

I recommend that you give your loved one a sponge bath at least every other day. If they are perspiring a lot, wash them every day. Keep in mind the sponge bath will refresh them, but going thru it will definitely also wear them out a bit. That is why you need to be fast, organized and well prepared. You can't be running around the room looking for an essential item, while the loved one is exposed and waiting amidst the process.

HOW TO GIVE A SPONGE BATH

Sponge bath is given when the patient is bed bound and cannot be given a shower.

FOLLOW THESE STEPS FOR PREPARATION:

* Make sure the room is nice and warm, with no draft
* Put on your plastic gloves
* Place a laundry basket next to the bed
* Position a rolling over-bed table stand by the side of the bed for all your supplies
* Fill the bucket with very warm water and place it on the table stand beside the bed
* Immerse the washcloth and two natural sponges in the bucket
* Prepare all supplies for incontinence:
    * Fresh incontinence pad
    * At least two bed protection disposable pads
    * New mesh undergarment
    * Trash bag
    * Baby wipes
    * Protective cream for bed sore prevention
* Prepare the no-rinse soap next to the bucket
* Prepare hypoallergenic mild body lotion and place it on the stand

BEGIN THE PROCESS OF SPONGE BATH:

* Uncover the loved one
* Gently remove open-back nightgown
* Place towels under their head and around body on both sides, to help catch any excess water
* Cover the lower body with a towel, while working on upper body
* Take the wet sponge, apply some rinse free soap and gently wash upper body area
* Immediately lightly pat the moisture off and cover the washed upper body area
* Continue to use sponge on the entire body, except buttocks and groin area
* Wash the stomach and lower frontal area. Now go on and wash the front and back side of both legs. Avoid the frontal groin area at this time.
* Pat dry and cover lower body with a clean dry towel.
* Gently roll the loved one to the side - onto their hip and prop them with a pillow in front of their body, so they are comfortable and they don't roll over.

- ❀ Wash the back.
- ❀ Continue and wash down to their backside.
- ❀ Pat dry their back.
- ❀ Remove the old incontinence pad and dispose it into the trash bag
- ❀ Do not use sponge for any incontinence soiled areas, but instead first use the baby wipes if needed.
- ❀ Wash the backside - lower buttocks, with the specially designated washcloth.
- ❀ Lightly pat dry and return loved one to the original position on their back.
- ❀ Finally gently wash the frontal groin area with the second designated wash cloth. Always wash front to back.
- ❀ Pat dry and cover them with a clean dry towel.
- ❀ Gently turn them back onto the side
- ❀ Now apply the bedsore prevention cream to the buttocks
- ❀ Immediately place a new, clean incontinence pad in place.
- ❀ Take the mesh undergarment and gently place both feet into openings. Slowly and carefully pull it up to hold the incontinence pad in place.
- ❀ Apply hypoallergenic lotion to the entire body, starting with the upper body and going down.
- ❀ To apply lotion to their back, gently turn the loved one to the side
- ❀ Finally, dress your loved one in fresh open-back cotton nightgown.
- ❀ The sponge bath is completed.

WASHING HAIR WHEN BED - BOUND

You can wash your loved one's hair before or after sponge bath. If you do not want to tire them out, wash their hair on a separate occasion. You will need special No-rinse shampoo. The preparation process is similar as with the sponge bath. Simply begin by placing a dry towel under your loved one's head. Every movement you do, needs to be extremely gentle since your loved one's skin is very sensitive and can immediately get a scratch or a wound.

Apply the No-rinse shampoo, gently massage the head while you lather and then pat dry with a fresh towel. Repeat if necessary. When you finish, replace the towel under their head with a fresh, dry one. Check in a little while if the hair has dried and if needed, replace the towel gain to assure everything remains nice and dry.

INCONTINENCE DURING SPONGE BATH

You can prevent this from happening by eliminating time without an incontinence pad to a bare minimum. While you wash the rest of their body, keep the old incontinence pad in place until you get to that area. Then remove it, right away wash their buttocks and groin area, and then immediately place the new pad in place.

If however, your loved one has an incontinence mishap during the sponge bath, before a new incontinence pad is in place, simply clean everything as quickly as possible, clean the area with baby wipes, wash them again with a washcloth and immediately place the new incontinence pad and mesh undergarment in proper position. Make sure you also change the replaceable paper pad that is protecting the bed.

HOW TO CHANGE THE BEDDING
WITH LOVED ONE IN BED

Now you can begin to refresh the bedding:
- Remove all used towels and place them in the laundry basket.
- Move all but one pillow off the bed and change them into fresh covers
- While leaving the loved one on the bed with one pillow under their head, undo the fitted bed sheet on all corners of the bed. Gather the old fitted sheet next to the loved one in the center of the bed.
- Replace the fitted sheet with a fresh one, attaching it at upper and lower right corners and pull it towards the center of the bed.
- Gently and with one slow move, reposition the loved one over onto the clean side of the bed with the fresh fitted sheet, and fresh pillow case.
- Now that the loved one is off the old fitted sheet, pull it off the bed completely and place it the laundry basket
- Now stretch and tuck the new fitted sheet onto the upper and lower left-side bed corners. Your fitted-sheet change is now done.
- Place two new bed protective pads in the center of bed.
- Place the smaller paper disposable bed pad on top of them.
- Place a new sheepskin pad on top of protective pad.
- Gently reposition your loved one onto the sheepskin pad in the middle of the bed. Make sure their whole upper body, including hips are on sheepskin. This will greatly help prevent bedsores and assure maximum comfort.
- Cover your loved one so they are warm and comfortable.

This is a very demanding change, but when done well, you will have accomplished two things: a sponge bath and a bed change, while the loved one is lying on the bed. Always make sure that your loved one is nice and dry. Cover them well, turn the extra heating off or adjust the room temperature. In a little while, air out the room for a few moments. The loved one will fell much better after this procedure as they will be clean and refreshed. Most likely they will immediately fall into a comfortable sleep.

CONTINUOUS REPOSITIONING FOR BED SORE PREVENTION

Your loved one is more vulnerable than ever to getting bed sores. Keep in mind, a bedsore can occur also on the back of their head, at wherever point that is continuously pressed against pillows. It can occur on any body part that is left unattended and in the same position for an extended period of time.

> **IN THIS PARTICULAR PHASE AT THE END OF LIFE, THE BEDSORES CAN OCCUR QUICKLY, WITHIN HOURS. THEREFORE YOU NEED TO REPOSITION YOUR LOVED ONE EVERY TWO TO THREE HOURS.**

Sometimes, your loved one may be increasingly sweating in the dying process. This means you need to be more diligent than ever in helping prevent a bed sore. Keep them nice and dry and constantly check to make sure no place on the body is receiving pressure of the weight, for any extended period of time.

You need to continue to reposition them, ever so slightly, so they do not lie in one pose. This is the time to use all your supplies to help prop and situate their body into a most comfortable placement. Take a look at Chapter *Supplies and Safety* for a complete list of support pillows. You may want to add a very special foot pillow to help protect the heels.

As mentioned in same chapter, sheepskin is excellent in preventing bedsores and drawing away the moisture. In this final bed-bound phase, I strongly recommend having at least one medical sheepskin for your loved one.

PHYSICAL CHANGES IN FINAL PHASE

As your loved one goes through this end-of-life process, there will be daily physical changes. Here are a few suggestions to help ease any discomforts.

DECLINE IN APPETITE

During the final weeks and days of your loved one's life, there will be significant decline in their appetite. Feed your loved one with blended very easily digestible food, until they so desire and show interest. If they do not wish to eat, do not ever force feed them. Respect their body's natural process. When you feed them in bed, always prop them into a comfortable elevated half - sitting position. Feed them very slowly and cautiously.

DIFFICULTY SWALLOWING

Your loved one may have increasing trouble properly swallowing food. Always prop them up and never feed them or give them drink when they are lying down horizontally. Offer them very small amount of blended food and feed them with a teaspoon. Always wait to see that they have completely swallowed before proceeding. Be very patient and never rush them. Keep in mind, that even a small teaspoonful of blended food in their mouth, will help them absorb some liquid. Food should be cool and less liquid for easier swallowing

DRY MOUTH AND TONGUE REMEDY

In this final stage, your loved one may often breathe with their mouth open, which will create a very dry mouth and tongue and a gargling, rattling sound of heavy breathing. The best natural remedies are organic thick kefir drink, organic yogurt, or organic buttermilk. Kefir and buttermilk are fermented dairy products that contain gut healing probiotics. They help soothe and moisturize the mouth and prevent mouth sores. If your loved one can't swallow, you can take a large q-tip, dip it into the kefir, and gently moisten their lips and nearest areas in mouth cavity. The mouth will feel considerably more comfortable.

PAIN MANAGEMENT

Your loved one's doctor and Hospice services nurse will help administer any needed pain medication. To determine whether your loved one is in pain, use the same observation techniques as mentioned in Chapter *The Mind Communication*. Remember, as a long time primary caregiver to your loved one, your ability to interpret how they feel is at an advantage, because you have known them for a long time. Observe their facial expression, sounds and any gestures they make. Your observation and familiarity of what your loved ones expression conveys, can be very helpful to the Hospice nurse. Work with them.

CLEARING SUBTLE ENERGY SPACE
FOR A PEACEFUL TRANSITION

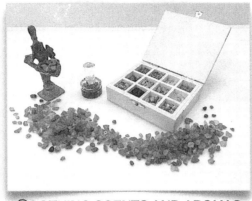

SOOTHING SCENTS AND AROMAS

If you are open to esoteric principles, I share with you some additional valuable insights. In Chapter *Self-care for Caregivers,* I spoke about you energy field - aura which is a very delicate and sensitive, invisible vibrational body.

We learned about how you as a caregiver, can best protect your energy field from feeling drained. You are very susceptible to becoming an energy recharging presence for your loved one, since they require constant subtle energy support in their considerably feeble state.

**NOW, AS THEY NEAR TRANSITIONING,
THEIR DEPLETED AURA IS MORE VULNERABLE THAN EVER.**

**TO HELP PROTECT THEM FROM ANY UNPLEASANT ENERGIES,
YOU CAN USE ADDITIONAL TOOLS TO KEEP THEIR ROOM
ENERGETICALLY CLEAN.**

Your loved one's room may feel saturated with heavy energy of sadness, grief and sorrow. In order to shift and improve the delicate energy state, you can energetically cleanse it. There are a few ways t accomplish this.

AROMATHERAPY

This is a most effective way to improve the vibrations in your loved one's immediate space. You have a wide selection of aromas that can be very pleasant, soothing and will immediately shift the general mood in the room. Take a look at the list of Essential Oils and their benefits, in Chapter *Holistic Caregiving Remedies,* and select according to your preference. Especially powerful aromas for this purpose and occasion are Frankincense, Thyme, Lavender, Cedar and Rose oil.

CRYSTALS

One technique is using quartz crystals and positioning them in the room. First, wash the crystals under running water, then position them by the windows, on the nightstand or anywhere where they may catch some light. You can use any crystal, but especially Amethyst and clear Quartz crystals are powerful and effective for the purpose of cleansing, healing and protecting the energy field.

INCENSE FOR CLEARING ENERGY

If your loved one's space feels extremely heavy and is difficult to tolerate, you may use another option for clearing subtle energy. Burning of sage for cleansing and healing purposes has been used by various cultures for thousands of years and is not tied to any specific culture or belief system.

You can open all doors and windows to your loved one's room, take a small sage smudge stick, and burn it for only a couple of minutes, while walking around the room. Then air out the room thoroughly and notice how the general sense of heaviness or sadness has shifted.

Use this technique only if your loved ones room is easily aired out. Optional herbs for burning incense are Frankincense, Sandarac resin, Styrax resin, Cinnamon, Myrrh and Sandalwood. Many of these extraordinary pleasant smelling herbs were used in Ancient Egypt and continue to be used in various religious ceremonies around the world.

**YOU MAY BE SURPRISED
HOW A VERY SMALL AMOUNT OF THIS SCENT
INTRODUCED INTO YOUR LOVED ONE'S SPACE
WILL HELP CREATE AN INSTANT FEELING OF SERENITY,
PEACE, LIGHTNESS AND COMPLETE CALM.**

FINAL ARRANGEMENTS

No matter how difficult this may seem, you need to get organized regarding the conclusion of life and funeral arrangements. If your loved one left specific instructions or last wishes, you will follow them. If you need to decide that part with your family or on your own, it is advisable to get it done in advance. At least that way, you won't have to deal with that aspect when you are in the midst of grieving. I strongly recommend that you organize all the arraignments ahead of time and engage Hospice service to help you with this final duty.

HOW LONG?

How long will the dying process take? This is the question that will be present every second of your final days. No one can tell you, and no one will ever want to tell you. They could be making a good guess, but that is all. This process can take weeks or days.

People that are inexperienced with this situation, assume a person can die easily and quickly. This is not usually the case with Alzheimer's dementia. This can vary, if you loved one suffers also from other illnesses.

The dying process is long and difficult. You need to know that. I do not believe it would benefit you to expect a quick ending. It is better to be informed and know that it could take a while. This way you can properly pace your energy and endurance, so you can last through his challenge. The best approach for you and the rest of the family members is to absolutely surrender.

YOUR LOVED ONE'S TIME OF DEPARTURE IS NOT UP TO YOU, IT IS UP TO THE UNIVERSE.

Your duty is to do the very best to prevent any suffering. That does not mean drugging your loved one when not necessary. It means taking care of them physically and emotionally while making sure they receive the highest level of care, until the very last minute of their life. You may hear many different opinions from people that may mean well, but are entirely uneducated in this area, and it will be challenging to tolerate them. But know in your heart and mind, that you need to be highly attentive to your loved one until the very end.

In this phase, their needs will escalate even more and become as unpredictable as ever. Your daily schedule will consist of accommodating your loved one's final journey and adjusting to their needs. Assure that your loved one does not suffer from any physical discomfort, implement great body care and mild food, if they so desire. As always, your care will play a crucial role in the way your loved one feels.

Surrender any anticipation and constant waiting, because it could take its tool on you. They could pass at any moment, or it could be weeks or perhaps a month. Even when things look very final, a sudden improvement can occur. Therefore your best mindset to navigate through this is complete and peaceful acceptance.

Remain a steady, constant, reliable and caring presence at your loved one's side and assure them most loving care. But know in your heart and mind, that they will most likely be gone within a few months. This will help you maintain the energy level needed, so you can manage. The Hospice nurse will be very helpful in assessing how your loved one is doing from week to week and day to day.

FOR NOW, LIVE IN THE MOMENT.

CHAPTER EIGHTEEN

Farewell and Departure

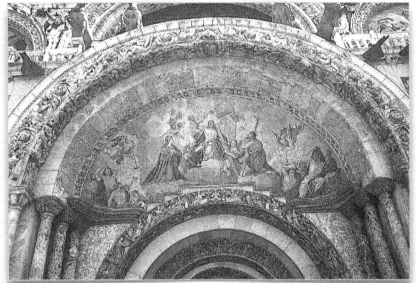

THE MYSTERIOUS GATEWAY OPENS ONLY TWICE IN OUR LIFETIME:
UPON OUR ARRIVAL AND INEVITABLE DEPARTURE.

FACING YOUR FEARS

One of the overwhelming fears that a caregiver will face towards the end of this journey is the fear of finding their loved one gone. Since you are on guard and know that the transition could happen at any time, this fear will naturally be present. Every time you enter their room, they could be gone. Every morning when you first lay your eyes on them, that could be the case.

That fear can be quite overwhelming and create a great sense of dread and anxiety. You will be sneaking into your loved one's room late in the evening to change them and fearfully listen, if they are still breathing. During the night, your ears will strain to hear the breathing on the room monitor. This kind of persistent ongoing fear can seriously increase your levels of anxiety and stress.

What can you do? Face this final fear head on. Yes, there is a possibility you will find them gone. The moment they leave this physical body will happen when it is meant to happen. So make peace with it. Obviously at one predestined moment, they will depart. Talk about it with the Hospice nurse, your friends or family members, and try to release this fear. Accept this as a possibility.

How can you release this dread? Accept that yes, if it is supposed to be that way, you will find them gone and you have absolutely no control over it. Remember that by enduring this long illness and care, you have already faced the worst. Be prepared for the final departure with all the technicalities that will be required to deal with, and then accept and surrender to it. You will notice a great weight and sense of pressure leaving you. A different kind of strength will carry you thru.

NOTHING HAS BROKEN YOU AND NEITHER WILL THIS MOMENT. YOU CAN FACE IT WHILE REMAINING CALM.

Hospice service will prove most helpful at this time of transitioning. If they are helping you around the clock, someone will hold vigil through the night. And if your loved one were to depart then, they will call you. Lean on them and their expertise and know you are not alone. During the day, you will be at your loved one's side almost constantly. If it is meant to be, you will hold their hand while they depart. And if they slip away quietly in a rare moment of solitude, know that the Universe wanted it just so.

LAST CONVERSATIONS

Every time you speak to your loved one, could be the last time. But then again, one could say that goes for everybody, any day. Certainly people die everyday, so every time you see someone, it could be the last time. However, with your loved one transitioning in your home, you are faced with that fact every single second. The positive side is, that you certainly have enough time to tell them anything you wish, and that can be very consoling.

> **YOU CAN TELL YOUR LOVED ONE THAT YOU LOVE THEM
> AT ANY MOMENT OF THE DAY OR NIGHT.
> AND THAT ALONE IS A GIFT.**

It is important that any kind of conversation is in no way upsetting. Your loved one cannot speak or respond to you, and you are having a one-way monologue. But there is a very good chance that they hear everything you say and also understand it, to a certain level. If you speak to them slowly, simply and clearly, they will understand you.

The sense of the sound is the last one to go. This is why your words matter a great deal. Your loved one is trapped in their body, robbed of their ability to speak, move about, or take care of themselves. It is an extremely challenging condition. However, at no time can you assume that they cannot hear you. Therefore your words must be soothing, loving, calming and reassuring. Your loved one is preoccupied with their own transition and that is their main concern. This must be a time of harmony, peace and total unconditional love.

If you feel weak and overwhelmed with sadness and emotions, do not expose your loved one to a big crying and sobbing outburst. It won't make them feel better in any way, but will most likely upset them and they will feel even more helpless. They do not want to see sorrow or worry about what is going to happen when they leave. They need to be at peace. Be the pillar of strength, harmony, love and comfort for them. Help them alleviate any worries they may feel about what they are leaving behind.

Assure them that all is well, they can completely relax, let go, not worry about anything and just feel tranquil. Anytime you speak to them, always be guided by those principles.

REMEMBER, EVEN IF YOUR LOVED ONE CANNOT SMILE AT YOU, YOU CAN STILL SMILE AT THEM.

No matter how sad it is see your loved one disappearing into the infinity, remain steady, loving and focused on easing their way through this decisive moment. If they feel worried, concerned or anxious about any family situations, it will make their transition more difficult. Use the last conversations to continuously establish an ease of mind and lightness of their heart.

ALLOW THEM TO DEPART AND RELEASE THEM TO THE UNIVERSE.

LAST VISITATIONS FROM OTHERS

Since you are the primary caregiver, you have a positive relationship with your loved one and feel at peace with the final transition. You have been able to speak with them about anything you wanted in a loving and kind way.

But this may be a difficult moment for others, who may have been partially or entirely absent from your loved one's life. They may not have that acceptance and peace. Perhaps there are unresolved issues or feelings of guilt. When seeing the loved one in their final weakened condition, they may feel overwhelmed. Everyone experiences grief and loss differently. A final visit will trigger an emotional reaction, for which they may not be sufficiently equipped to deal with.

Keep in mind, this is not the time to vent a decade old grudge, clear up an old conflict, make up for lost time, seek approval, forgiveness, praise or reach closure. Things may stay unresolved, words may remain unspoken. Some family members with unresolved issues, past conflicts and anger, may be very conflicted. They may stay away, holding on to their grievances and remaining entirely absent. If they did not manage to show any concern before, it won't be surprising if they'll stay in hiding, nowhere to be found.

More rare is the case when they reappear in an attempt to make peace, or get rid of their guilt. There may be remorse for completely abandoning the loved one during later years in time of illness. They will come to bid the final farewell in an effort to lay any past conflicts to rest.

EVEN A SIMPLE "I FORGIVE YOU " OR "PLEASE FORGIVE ME" "I AM SO SORRY" AND "I LOVE YOU," WILL HAVE THE POWER TO BRING SOME RESOLVE.

Hopefully the experience will be equally consoling for the loved one. Even if they don't say a word, or are sleeping and don't seem to register anyone, on some level they will sense that the person came and made an effort. However, there will be no lengthy conversations and goodbyes at this point. Your loved one's speaking capacity is so hindered, they are so weak and often lost in their own world, that they are unable to respond.

There may be circumstances where due to heavy family conflict, there will be no possibility for an in-person last visit and resolve. Time for that has come and gone. Any kind of confrontation is absolutely out of the question. If you have a difficult conflicts lingering within the family, I urge you to do everything possible to spare your loved one of any disruptive self-serving last moment visitations, that could potentially cause irreparable aggravation to your loved one.

YOUR FIRST PRIORITY REMAINS TO MAINTAIN AN OPTIMAL SAFE AND PEACEFUL ENVIRONMENT FOR YOUR LOVED ONE AND ELIMINATE ANY AND ALL SOURCES OF DISCOMFORT AND STRESS.

At this point, an agitation would be really dangerous and could trigger severe distress, which could result in definite need for medication. Your loved one's state is beyond delicate and they need to be protected from anyone who does not comprehend their vulnerability. If the conflicts could not be resolved when your loved one was still able to communicate, then this is no time to let an aggressive or conflicting person near them.

By seeing a person they have a conflicted relationship with, your loved one may feel frightened or start screaming in frustration of being unable to speak and properly express their feelings. There will be absolutely no positive accomplishment or outcome. One can only hope that all visits are harmonious and the relatives or family members come with loving and caring energy and can communicate in kind and amiable words. Instruct any visitors beforehand of what they can and cannot expect and what your loved one's needs are, so they don't come with a naive illusion or an unrealistic, self-serving expectation.

When your loved one is in their final stage of life, they are extremely weak and mostly sleeping. They cannot tolerate noise, any kind of loud conversations or constant presence of too many people in their room. What they need is total privacy in their own space and complete and utter tranquility. It is your duty to make sure the visits are cut to a minimum.

Allow the visitors a short time to say their farewell, and then lead them out of the room as soon as possible. Remember, your loved one is preparing for their final transition, any frantic energy around them may upset the sensitive nature of that delicate state.

Assure and protect their serene, peaceful environment and their own state of being, until their final moment arrives. If there is no friction with other family members, it will be fine to have them visit for a very short time and convey in kind, soft spoken words whatever they wish.

INSTRUCT THE VISITORS TO AVOID CRYING OR SAYING ANYTHING SAD OR UNSETTLING. THEY HAVE TO SAVE THEIR TEARS FOR LATER.

SUDDEN IMPROVEMENTS

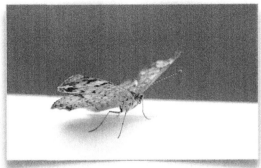

Oh, but I still want to fly...

Just when it seems that the final day of transition has approached, your loved one's condition may suddenly improve. It is very important that you are aware of this possibility. They could make an unexpected comeback, wake up in a more alert state, have increased appetite and show general signs of recovery. Before, their appetite may have been declining for a long while, finally reaching a really low level. And then one day, without any real explanation or drastic change in care, they could experience a sudden return of appetite.

Your loved one could suddenly appear much improved, filled with an amazing burst of energy, as if awakened from a deep sleep.

How can this happen? This is actually quite common. The dying process is about "reaching various plateaus." A steady decline may be interrupted with an unexpected turn-around, followed by a slow, short-lived improvement. This is why it is impossible to predict when your loved one will transition. No-one can foresee this sudden phase of improvement.

To clarify, your loved one will not suddenly get completely well. They are at a point of no return. But any improvements at all, may seem rather significant to you. When someone practically doesn't eat and then suddenly they have great appetite and eat two cups-full of food, the difference will seem enormous. And if you are not ready for this possibility, this new development may confuse you. In a way, you have emotionally prepared yourself that departure is near and now, it almost seems like the loved one has changed their mind and decided to stay and rally on.

Your sheer anticipation of an upcoming transition sets your entire being into a different mental and emotional place. Obviously, towards the end of this long journey you will feel considerably depleted. There will be little else to cram into a day except tending to loved one, staying at their side 24/7 and continuously assuring their comfort. Your life now really takes a back seat, as you are expecting the ending. But when circumstances change into an unforeseen opposite direction, it may emotionally overwhelm you. It is a true test of your endurance and capacity to surrender, once again.

Just remember, however long this final phase takes, it will eventually end. You know that your loved on is nearing the completion of their journey. They could be released any time, in five minutes or five days, or even five weeks. All that is possible. By being aware of this possibility, you do not expect a certain outcome on a certain day. And it is better that way. It will teach you to truly live in the moment. Trying to figure out why this is happening will not provide you with an easy answer. Let's just put it that way: everything has a reason.

> **SHIFT YOUR MIND INTO A CALM, NON-ANTICIPATORY STATE WHERE YOU ARE READY FOR ANYTHING, YET NOT WAITING FOR IT. IT REQUIRES MASTERY OF THE MIND TO ACCOMPLISH THAT.**

As far as this short-lived phase of improvement, it will eventually reverse and your loved one will rapidly decline. It is almost as if their body pulled out all the stops and gave it one more try, a genuine effort to conquer the battle. If your loved one is relatively younger, that may certainly be the case. If they are much older, their phase of improvement may last a day or two at the most, if at all.

At this time, I kept a 24/7 watch over my Mom, practiced surrender and took a nap whenever the circumstance allowed. Since I was waking up every three hours through the night, in order to turn her in bed to prevent bed sores, I was seriously sleep deprived.

But what helped me considerably was taking notes for this book. Every day as my Mother's condition revealed a new lesson, a new aspect or dynamic to me, I quickly wrote it down to make sure it won't be forgotten. I wanted to capture every possible piece of useful advice, so I could pass it on to someone special, like yourself. This is what saved me through those endless moments, days and weeks of dreadful waiting. It gave me the only glimmer of hope that something positive could emerge from all that pain and sorrow.

YOUR LOVED ONE'S FEARS

When one is nearing the end of their life, emotions resurface that may have been long ignored. The person may have old regrets, unfulfilled dreams and a reoccurrence of deep set fears. In the last moments of earthly life, we face the ultimate fear of death. It comes as no surprise, when even the most persistent atheist will call out to God, while facing the inevitable.

DEATH CHANGES EVERYTHING, INCLUDING SOMEONE'S BELIEFS.

Your loved one is in a different situation, since their illness has robbed them of the ability to express themselves, or their emotions. But this does not mean that they don't have feelings. In fact, quite the opposite is true. They may seem very much detached and not able to recognize those around them, but one overpowering, deep-set emotion that has always been a part of their basic character, may resurface and overrule all others.

IF YOUR LOVED ONE HAD A LIFETIME CONCERN OR AN OLD, UNRESOLVED FEAR THAT EXISTED DEEP IN THEIR PSYCHE AND PREOCCUPIED THEM THROUGH THEIR LIFE, IT MAY NOW REEMERGE AND RECLAIM A PRESENCE IN THEIR FINAL WOUNDED MINDSET.

A person suffering from dementia may fear death, just like someone who is mentally aware. But they can cannot express this fear, which makes it more challenging to deal with. You will be able to sense it in their look of concern, restlessness and a fearful facial expression. Perhaps they will moan or yelp in desperate attempt to communicate. Stay with them, console them as if you understood what they wanted to say. Establish a sense of peace while speaking to them in a loving and soothing manner. This will help them calm down.

It is also important to remember how they viewed death, mortality and spirituality when they were healthy. Your loved one's core belief stayed with them. If they had a specific religious belief that helped them through life, this may be the time to revisit it. It could be of great help.

In the final days of your loved one's life, you may find it appropriate to bring in a priest or their faith leader. This may help reduce fear or accept closure of their ultimate transition. I know it may appear as if they are not aware, but I believe that on some level they are. Hospice can be very helpful in this situation and upon your request, they can help secure the services of a priest, rabbi, minister or other faith leader.

This may seem trivial for some, but I believe that whatever faith your loved one belongs to, it could prove very reassuring for them to have a visit from such a pastoral representative. Even if they sleep through the visit and it seems they do not register the priest's presence, rest assured, on some level they will know. It may help them gain a sense of comfort and reduce distress and fear.

And finally, if they always feared death in the past, it is important you comfort them and help them ease and reduce such fears. The best remedy is a calm, gentle and soothing voice of guidance and reassurance.

> **KEEP REAFFIRMING TO YOUR LOVED ONE**
> **THAT THEY ARE NOT ALONE, THERE IS NOTHING TO FEAR,**
> **THEY ARE CHERISHED, CARED FOR AND LOVED.**

YOUR MENTAL STRENGTH

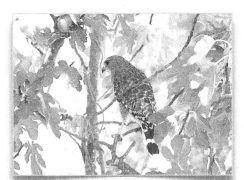

*B*eing the sole caregiver with no other help, except daily one-hour Hospice-nurse visitations, I had to work very hard not to break down. I changed my Mother around the clock every three hours, attempted to feed her, gave her sponge baths and witnessed her physical diminishment.

I spoke to her all the time, but lost all contact with her eyes, as they seemed to stare into nowhere. Every hour, I witnessed her disappearing and slipping further away. That can be too much even for the strongest person. Nobody wants to watch this sadness day and night. It become so overwhelming that I desperately needed to find a way to survive and cope with it.

As I reached a state of utter physical and emotional exhaustion, I struggled each day when the alarm clock woke me up for yet another change and preparation for the inevitable. I searched for answers on how to deal with this. I got well-meaning suggestions to have a good cry, but that didn't seem a sufficient answer to me. Sure, crying is cleansing, but it won't make it any easier.

An optimist by nature, I desperately searched for a tiny positive aspect of this experience. I wondered what kind of advice I could give to anyone going thru this. And I found the key to my answer, by realizing that at this point, it has to be all about the mind.

Now that you are witnessing and experiencing the brutal final chapter of this illness, you may feel completely defeated. You feel like all the love, care and effort seem to be dwindling away into the faraway past and all you are left with is a small, weak, emaciated body and a lost stare. These long final days will test your spirit and its strength to its core.

THE ONLY WAY TO SURVIVE THIS PERIOD IS TO ENGAGE THE POWER OF YOUR MIND TO ITS MAXIMUM CAPACITY.

What does that mean? It is important to understand that the dying process of a dementia patient is very different, than other terminal illnesses. Dementia patient's decline is generally so slow, that it is sometimes difficult to discern if they are in the active dying process. They seem to linger in the final days considerably longer. Just like the gradual process of the illness has taken years, so can the last phase.

No one can predict what is going to happen. One day may look like the end is near and then the next day things will turn around, and you could face another month of this agony. Obviously there is no place to hide as you live with this reality. Every time you enter your loved one's room could be the much dreaded moment when you find them gone, or they may be just peacefully sleeping, or staring into space and sleeping with their eyes open. And then there are moments when they stop breathing for what seems a very long time… and then they start again. To get thru this period as intact as possible, you need to prepare your mindset. If you don't, the situation will overpower you. So summon up your courage, steel yourself up and consciously ready your mind for this final effort. How can you accomplish this?

BECOME A VERY FOCUSED, CALM AND CAPABLE INSTRUMENT, A KIND OF A CAREGIVING GUARDIAN.

If I strengthened myself in my mind, before tending to my Mom, I transformed into an instrument for her care. I pushed my emotions aside and focused on the long list of tasks. I knew that this was the final stretch of the long caregiving process, so I became determined to see this through. My mission had been clear all these years, and I was not about to give up now.

I taped into the last reservoir of adrenaline and engaged my mind in high gear. I kept everything impeccably organized in her room, maintained a steady routine, remained precise and tenacious and methodically observed her, to detect any possible discomfort or a way to ease her situation.

I did everything as an instrument for her care, and not as a daughter watching her dying Mother. I left my emotions at the door of her room. Upon entering her space, I transformed myself into her caregiving guardian. Loving, caring, gentle and relentless, but just her nursing guardian. The part of me-the daughter who is witnessing her Mother's slow decay, was left outside. And that helped me immensely. Actually, it saved my heart.

THE TIBETAN TEACHINGS SAY HOW IMPORTANT IT IS TO KEEP THE DYING PERSON'S ROOM VERY PEACEFUL, CALM AND SERENE.

This is not a place for tears, sobbing, or any other kind of upsetting emotions. If you are falling apart at your loved one's bedside, drowning in tears and hanging on to them, how do you expect them to feel peaceful about moving on? The shedding of tears from your heart has to be done away from your loved one.

PEOPLE IN TRANSITION ARE ENTERING A DIFFERENT DIMENSION, WHICH MAKES THEM EXTREMELY SENSITIVE TO SUBTLE VIBRATIONS AND ENERGIES.

Upsetting energy could prevent them from experiencing peace on all levels. A departing soul must not worry about who is upset when they leave them behind. All the love you have for them should be shown throughout their life and not just now, in the final hours. It is too late for missed conversation or curing guilty feelings.

You should love your loved one when you can, every day, and not just at the end. Are your tears expressing love, or fear of abandonment? Are you are crying because you feel sorry for yourself or out of pure emotional agony? Your tears are well justified, but the place to express them is in private. No one near you will feel good when seeing you cry.

If someone decided to be absent from your loved one's life, that was their choice. Now is not the time to try and undo the past. You, as the primary caregiver are a strong pillar of peace, comfort and unconditional love. You will care for them till the very end. Make peace with it and engage in it fully and completely.

YOUR LOVED ONE'S DEPARTURE WILL FORCE YOU TO FACE SOME SERIOUS FEARS WITHIN YOURSELF. IT WILL MAKE YOU A CONSIDERABLY STRONGER PERSON.

Concentrate on your destined assignment to complete it as well as you can. Having a resolved and focused mind when caring for your loved one in these final days, will get you thru it.

Your job is clear, so don't you dare crack now. Pace yourself appropriately. It is not necessary to sit with your loved one for hours, if they don't specifically need you. They require peace, calmness and stillness. Give them space, check on them quietly without waking them up and regularly change them, reposition them, feed them if they wish, do everything that is necessary, but leave the room when they are comfortably in bed, napping and you are done with tending to them. Have a room monitor with you when you move about your home, so you can hear every sound and immediately tend to them. Check on them every few minutes and if they are sleeping, let them be.

Keep your mind the pillar of strength and remain stoic, tender, caring, acutely aware and ever present for them, while respecting their space and peace. You will get thru it all.

THE HARDEST MOMENTS ARE JUST THAT - MOMENTS.

Better times lay ahead for you somewhere in the future, even thou it may seem like an impossible dream. You will get thru it and when it is all done, you will have a treasured, peaceful and resolved feeling in your heart, by knowing that you have done absolutely everything in your power, to make their journey and transition easier.

YOUR LOVED ONE FEELS LOVED AND THAT IS A TREASURE YOU CAN'T BUY ANYWHERE IN THIS WORLD.

CRYING AND TEARS

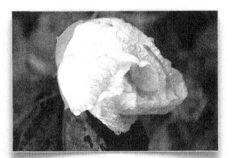

Crying is a powerful and healing emotional release. You have to get it out and let go of all the sadness and pain. This is why I would never suggest that you shouldn't cry. I just don't think it is a good idea to do it at the bedside, in the presence of your loved one. Other than that, you can cry all you want. Of course you can't always control when you're going to cry. Tears come when you least expect them or at a most inconvenient moment. Just stay brave and breathe. If you let yourself cry in peace when no one is around, you will regain some harmony and reestablish your inner calm.

CRYING IS A HEALTHY RELEASE OF TENSION AND PENT UP FEELINGS, THAT CAN BE TOXIC WHEN SUPPRESSED.

If you feel you must remain strong for the other parent or family members, then maybe you can cry at night. Then you have as many hours as needed. Many people cry at night. And they come to regain a peaceful and comfortable state that way.

It is better to cry freely and alone without someone consoling you. That way you don't have to keep yourself from crying, or justify or explain why you are crying. In this particular situation even a stone would understand your tears. This is possibly the saddest time in your life. You have been traveling this journey with your loved one and have sacrificed an enormous amount of your life to help them.

In a way, you feel robbed, destroyed, devastated, crushed, lonely, forgotten, irreparably exhausted and basically like your life is over, entirely and completely. You feel like you want to die and just forget everything. It seems that life punished you, somehow. You feel like you look terrible, have anciently aged and life just passed you by. And that my dear friend, is perfectly normal under these circumstances. But all is not lost.

SPIRITUAL ASPECTS OF DEATH

From a subtle energy perspective, our emotional connections with people and material attachments keep us bound to this world. Everything in this life that we are attached to, creates a bond. Throughout our lifetimes we meet, love, separate or reconnect with various people. These subtle energy bonds are like invisible cords of a mighty powerful force. A bond of love between parent and child can be extremely strong, likewise the love between two souls in a romantic connection. There are also strong bonds of friendship, but obviously love is the strongest bond that exists.

**THE MOST POWERFUL ENERGY THAT KEEPS US CONNECTED
TO THIS PLANE OF EXISTENCE,
IS THE BOND OF LOVE FOR ANOTHER SOUL.**

When your loved one senses that they will die, this long established emotional cord keeps them here and makes it more difficult to leave. However, if their bond is with someone who is no longer alive, this will make it easier for them to leave. On a subconscious level, they anticipate a pending reunion, once they transition to another plane of existence.

It can be very helpful to talk about this directly with your loved one, instead of pretending it does not exist. For example, when your loved one is in the final months or weeks of their life, you could openly remind them of a dear one that has already passed ahead of them, like their parent, partner, sibling or a dear friend.

You can mention that this person is waiting for them in Spirit world and will meet them as soon as they cross over. You are reminding them, that they will not be alone in their transition into a new world and there is nothing to fear. They may be stepping into the unknown, but their departed family and friends and familiar faces will be waiting for them on the other side.

These are the topics many people do not want to talk about, however I believe it can be very helpful. Openly speaking about their upcoming transition makes it less frightening, more real and acceptable.

Dying is a natural process that awaits us all, and eventually we shall die as a result of an illness, ailment or simply old age. Why avoid the subject or pretend it will never happen? Speaking openly about your loved one's next natural step can be healing. It may be hard for you to utter those words, or you may feel like crying, but that will not help your loved one. Talking about it openly is a positive and beneficial choice that can greatly diminish your loved one's fear and anxiety.

REMOVING PENDING OBSTACLES

Once your conversation with loved one addresses the spiritual aspects of crossing over into another world, you may want to make sure that any unresolved issues do not present an ongoing obstruction. For instance, if your loved one is worried about you or someone else that is dear to them, it will be more difficult for them to leave. They may not be able to speak and express themselves, but seeing their spouse or child suffering in grief, may evoke deep worry and concern.

In case of accidents when a person is in sudden danger of dying, they usually express concern about a loved one. When they survive, they often explain how they felt an urgent desire to consciously return avoid death, because they were so concerned about a dear one left behind.

This kind of a natural response is common and does not disappear, even if the person is memory impaired and suffering from dementia. Somewhere in the deepest corner of their mind, they carry this primary worry. And this deep-set concern becomes an obstacle that may keep them fighting for life and hanging on longer.

**IN ORDER TO HELP RESOLVE ANY KIND OF HESITANCY
ON YOUR LOVED ONE'S PART,
ASSURE THEM THAT EVERYONE WILL BE FINE,
EVERYONE IS TAKEN CARE OF AND
THERE IS ABSOLUTELY NO REASON TO WORRY.**

BECOME THE GUIDING LIGHT

More than ever, your loved one is leaning on your strength, support and guidance during this final days. You can take this opportunity and truly become their guiding light. The words you share with your loved one on these final days will have a profound effect on their ability to move on.

What should you say? You can tell them a simple set of sentences when you feel they may be receptive or even when they are peacefully sleeping. Speak clearly, slowly and softly close to their ear. Reassure them that all is taken care of and continuously encourage them to move towards the beautiful, bright light. Remind them who could be waiting for them on the other side. This could be anyone dear to them who has already departed.

> **SUGGEST THEY FEEL NO FEAR, STEP TOWARDS THE BRIGHT LIGHT AND REUNITE WITH THEIR DEPARTED LOVED ONES THAT AWAIT.**

Emphasize that you will be eventually joining them and expect they will wait for you on the other side, when your time comes. Mention that you will see them again, in a little while. Describe the next world as beautiful, filled with brilliant light. Tell them they will feel lightness and effortless ease. Here is a suggestion of your guiding words:

> **"I LOVE YOU.**
> **EVERYONE WILL BE FINE, YOU CAN RELAX,**
> **LET GO AND MOVE ON INTO THE LIGHT.**
> **DON'T WORRY ABOUT ANYONE, EVERYTHING IS TAKEN CARE OF.**
> **WE LOVE YOU AND ARE WITH YOU, UNTIL YOU ARE READY TO GO.**
> **YOU ARE NOT ALONE.**
> **YOUR DEAR ONE IS WAITING FOR YOU ON THE OTHER SIDE.**
> **THEY WILL BE SO HAPPY TO SEE YOU.**
> **THERE IS NOTHING TO FEAR.**
> **I WILL SEE YOU SOON AGAIN, WHEN IT IS MY TIME.**
> **WHEN YOU SEE A BRIGHT LIGHT, GO TOWARDS IT.**
> **I LOVE YOU SO MUCH AND WILL SEE YOU SOON AGAIN."**

THE LONG DYING PROCESS

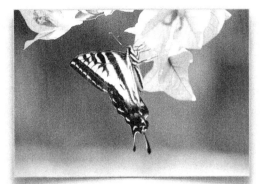

WE ARE ALL ON A JOURNEY TO ETERNITY

One of the biggest misconceptions is the belief, that as soon as someone stops eating, they will die. This is not the case. A healthy person cannot survive without water between eight or maximum twenty-one days, depending on the individual. But the dying process of a dementia patient can be very slow. People on their death bed who use minimal energy, may go on for a few days, or last a few weeks without food and water.

Just when you think that you have endured and overcome the worst and most exhausting experience of your life, you get to face the final superior challenging situation of the slow dying process of your loved one. What is worse in this life than watching a loved one dye slowly? Your inner strength, physical stamina and psychological endurance will be challenged in ways you have never imagined.

Why is the dying process so long? One could guess that if your loved one is in a relatively healthy physical shape, their body will endure and refuse to give up. Or we could take into account that the patient's character has to do something about it. If they have a vigilant warrior-like nature and have persistently endured battles, that may play a role. It is possible. But in the end, there may be invisible aspects we know so little about.

THERE ARE LEVELS OF CONSCIOUSNESS THAT ARE COMPLETELY UNKNOWN TO US.

There are also various ways of transitioning, that we have not even begun to study or research. Why do some people hang on and linger, while others simply close their eyes and are released?

> **FROM A SPIRITUAL PERSPECTIVE, PERHAPS THE DEMENTIA PATIENT'S SPIRIT NEEDS A BIT LONGER TO ADJUST TO THE NEW REALITIES OF THE NEXT REALM.**

By allowing a spirit to transition gradually, perhaps confusion is eliminated. I would assume that may be a positive circumstance.

But when your loved one is hanging-on in a semi comatose state, I can't seem to find anything positive there. While the loved one can be completely calm and seem peaceful in deep sleep, the caregiver will suffer while witnessing this act of nature.

> **LIFE IS CREATED AND GIVEN AND THEN LIFE IS TAKEN AWAY. THERE ARE NO MORE NEGOTIATIONS NOW.**

More than ever, you are made aware, that you are definitely not in control. There is a power so commanding and superior to our comprehension of it all, that we are truly blessed just by realizing it exists.

If you never paid much attention to spiritual aspects of life, at this moment in time, you will inevitably reassess your stand on the divine, God or Universal power. It is letting you know, that you are a small, tiny speck and life is precious. All you can do is serve your loved one as selflessly as possible, and continue to assure their optimal comfort. If you can alleviate any kind of suffering you are doing them a great favor.

If the dying process is long, you absolutely need to have assistance of Hospice nurses, especially thru the nights. This is not the time to lie awake with a room monitor and listen to the relentless loud breathing, rattling sound of irregular breath and gaps in between. You won't be able to rest. Thankfully, the Hospice services will offer assistance from the nighttime nurse, so you can catch the much needed sleep.

Your mental stamina is going to be your asset, but if you get too emotional, you will break. So I suggest that you honestly asses yourself and determine whether you can handle this part. Maybe you did good until now, but at this particular moment in the process, you just need to take a step back and preserve your energy.

Your loved one may be showing all the sighs of the oncoming death, but still won't depart. The dying can drag on for days that seem an eternity. This is not the time to make unnecessary appointments or try to explain the situation to friend on the phone. Very often a well-meant commentary could send you spinning into a complete state of devastation, or just simple plain break-down.

Why? Because you are in adrenal burnout and are emotionally highly sensitive. No one can understand what you are going thru, unless they have experienced it themselves. They may say a well-meant comment that you should "let go of your loved one and not hang on to them," but when you have said your final goodbyes a hundred times and made sure all was said that you could possibly think of to help release them, than you know very well, that such a comment is irrelevant. Again, nobody can truly put themselves into your shoes. They can guess, sympathize, but not advise. Take it in stride and not personally.

Instead, rely on the professional help and advice of the Hospice nurses. They will guide you and stand by your side. You have played a tremendous role in preventing suffering for your loved one, but don't allow yourself to be crushed and depleted at the end.

> ## CONSERVE YOUR ENERGY AND REMAIN DETERMINED
> ## IN UNWAVERING COMMITMENT TO ASSURE COMFORT
> ## FOR YOUR LOVED ONE, UNTIL THEIR LAST BREATH.
> ## WHEN YOU ACCOMPLISH THAT,
> ## YOU WILL BECOME A TRUE WARRIOR
> ## OF UNCONDITIONAL LOVE AND KINDNESS.

ENTERING THE LAST PHASE

After years of caregiving and all the resulting hardships and challenges, there is no doubt that this last phase is most difficult, exhausting, draining and sad. You may try to look at it from a different philosophical perspective or console yourself with the thought, that your loved one will finally be at peace and freed from the cage of their incapacitated, diseased body. But the fact remains, that you are coming face to face with death. Unless you have been through the experience of witnessing another person's transition or have lost a loved one before, this is entirely different from anything you've ever known.

If you are taking good care of your loved one, they are not suffering, but sleeping most of the day and night. The one that is really suffering now is you, while forced to watch closely the daily decline of the physical body thru this journey to its inevitable end. This can be emotionally overwhelming. What you will learn is that despite the fact that the person may be more than ready to leave, the physical body is an entirely different matter.

THE PHYSICAL BODY IS PROGRAMMED TO SURVIVE AND GO ON, NO MATTER HOW DIRE THE CIRCUMSTANCES.

In case of dementia, the imbalance of transitioning is startling, because we see a person who has lost the mental faculties, but the physical faculties continue to go on and on. This is why the illness is especially draining. The transitioning process is not natural, but out of synch. One part is incapacitated, while the others may continue to function quite well.

The opposite example would be when someone who is mentally very much aware and present, but their physical body is succumbing to an illness. There is no comparing of suffering or imagining what is worse. Either case is difficult.

The most natural process of transitioning would be death of old age, when all faculties would remain coordinated and eventually slow down and stop. Such death can occur naturally in sleep, which would be the gentlest of departures. This does not mean drug induced sleep, but natural, nightly sleep where the souls gently slips away before the sunrise.

PHYSICAL CARE IN THE LAST DAYS OF LIFE

Everything is magnified now a hundred fold. The danger for bed sores is tremendous, the demanding process of sponge bath becomes a true battle of endurance. The time when loved one does not eat or even drink is most difficult to endure. But you must respect that and never force them to eat. If their mouth is closed, respect it. There is a possibility that they will still take a few sips of some thickened liquid, like a kefir drink. That is about the only thing you can feed them, to help maintain the mouth and digestive flora in some kind of comfortable state. You may also try half a teaspoon of coconut milk or a freshly squeezed natural juice, just to moisten their mouth cavity and ease discomfort. Observe how they accept it. Avoid any juice or food that is acidic.

RELY ON PROFESSIONAL HOSPICE NURSE THROUGH THIS PERIOD.

When the food and liquid intake diminishes, you may start to witness the dramatic process that is so difficult. There could still be a lot of urine, even though there has been no drinking for a few days. The human body is quite amazing and incredibly programmed. The breathing could change, as could the pulse and oxygen levels. There is a possibility that it will seem like you are witnessing a steady decline and yet there could be a sudden holding pattern, that could endure a few days. The breathing and the relentless heart will go on, even with while there seems to be no life left in the body. The person seems to be completely gone, but the body will still function on. Remain calm and not too emotional. Stay focused, observe all body signs and continuously concentrate on optimal comfort.

CHALLENGES WILL MAGNIFY. DON'T LET YOUR GUARD DOWN. SOLDIER ON UNTIL THE END.

PERSPIRATION - There could be profuse perspiring, which means you need to be changing the nightgowns all the time. I suggest that you cut the back of regular nightgown and make it look like a hospital gown. It will make changes much easier for everyone involved. There could be a quick and sudden appearance of bedsores due to massive weight and muscle mass loss and perspiration. You need to change the person even more.

MOUTH - Hygiene must be maintained, as the body will go thru such dramatic changes that it is extremely important to keep it clean and free of toxic excretions. If they are breathing through their moth, it is vital to keep it moist. Dip a Q-tip into coconut butter and apply it all around the front of the mouth cavity, never reaching too far back. Apply it on the lips and keep them nicely moisturized at all times.

HEAD - Gently wipe the sweat off their face and keep them dry. Make sure they are not wet behind the neck and the back of the head. They can easily get a bedsore. Place a small fresh towel on the pillow under their head and change it every hour or two, as needed.

BODY TEMPERATURE - It could be completely erratic. That means that the face could be cold, nose freezing, while they sweat. Or the chest and upper body could be hot, while the feet and hands and knees are completely cold. One side of the face may be blushed and sweaty, while the other is yellow, pale-gray and cold.

SKIN TONE - The skin tone can change by the minute. The coloring could be anything from pale white to green, with overtones of gray and again blushed.

BREATHING - It could stop for what seems like an eternity, then accelerate to faster and again stop. Completely irregular breath can change into a continuous fast-paced breathing, as if they were jogging. Fast and short shallow breaths could go on for days. Imagine a marathon runner' a breathing and facial exhaustion. Your loved one could look just like that, while lying in bed motionless for days.

BLOOD PRESSURE - There could be complete unpredictability as of what is going on by blood pressure jumping up and down, oxygen level below 90 and a rapid heartbeat.

> ## COMPLETELY LET GO OF THE TIME FACTOR.
> ## KNOW THE TRANSITION IS VERY NEAR
> ## AND IT WILL COME WHEN IT IS MEANT TO COME.

By knowing these facts and various possibilities, you are hopefully better prepared to deal with this phase, instead of feeling surprised by the length of it. The journey will be completed when it is time. And that, my friend, you have nothing to do with. Respect the Universe, the loved one and their destiny and try to go with the flow. Have faith. Pray.

THE MOMENT OF DEPARTURE

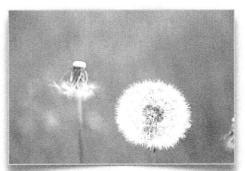

EVERY ENDING CARRIES HOPES OF A NEW BEGINNING

*T*his is the most unpredictable and difficult moment that awaits. If you are going to be present or not it is not for you to decide. It is a predestined moment and no one can tell you when it is going to happen. That means you may not be standing at your loved one's side, and no amount of planning can prevent that.

You could hold a vigil at their bedside for three days straight and when you run out for five minutes, this will be the destined time when they depart. That could happen.

In my Mother's case, she picked a moment when both my Father and I were present. That moment will stay with me forever. It was the most difficult and devastating moment of my life, but there was also an otherworldly beauty of such magnitude to it, that it cannot be explained.

I got to hold her in my arms while consoling and speaking to her till the end. She did not die alone, she knew she was loved and completely taken care of. She looked beautiful as always.

It is hard to see the life fade out of your loved one. The sadness in my heart was indescribable and overwhelming beyond words. I am grateful her suffering ended and her spirit is finally free to soar the way it did when she was healthy and alive. But her journey and final transition were beyond difficult.

Why does this have to happen? I can't give you the answer. I can only tell you that life is a balancing act of light and darkness. Do all you can to recognize and enjoy the light, and when you come upon dark moments, fly thru them as fast as possible. Always concentrate on the good.

They say the last sensory apparatus that endures till the end, even when someone is unresponsive, is the sense of hearing. At the moment of death, tell your loved one how much you love them and how they have nothing to fear. Hopefully they will be able to hear you. Stay strong and calm while your loved one is transitioning.

At this point your loved one's spirit is lingering between two worlds and there is just a smalls string of energy left here. Respect the timing that has been chosen for each and every one of us, and faithfully stand guard.

After your loved one crosses over and transitions into their next existence, their spirit will invisibly leave their body. The moment this occurs, you will feel a powerful shift of energy and their physical body will change dramatically.

If you are sensitive to subtle energies, you will feel that the body lost a mighty force that resided in it. Your loved one's spirit energy will feel completely different, but not extinguished. It will feel expanded and less constricted, as if liberated from the restraints of the physical body. Slowly it will feel increasingly more distant.

The body will appear very peaceful and a porcelain like glow will descend upon their face. You will clearly sense they are no longer with you. The body will seem like a shell that carried a glorious spirit. Stay with your loved one and care for them one last time. If necessary wash them, change their clothes, and make them ready for their final departure.

Hospice nurses will be of great help at this difficult time and will guide your through every step. Your loved one is gone and you are left with an overwhelming aftermath and indescribable void in your life and heart. You are relieved they are finally released and free of suffering, and you knew for many years that this moment was coming. You prayed it would be swift and painless. Yet when it finally happens, when the moment has arrived and they are forever departed, your heart will buckle under the weight of sadness.

If you bear witness to the process of dying and the final departure, it will forever alter your life and the perception of it. Life is incredibly precious. Every moment granted, should be spent mindfully and with an open heart.

LIFE'S JOURNEY IS BUT A BRILLIANT FLASH OF LIGHT IN THE MAZE OF STARS IN THE ENDLESS SKY.

CHAPTER NINETEEN

Free at Last

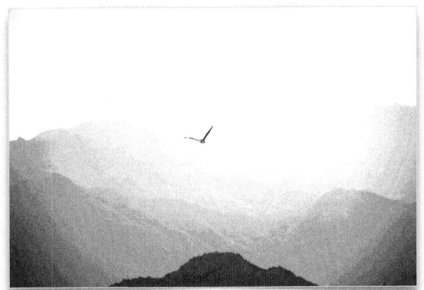

REBIRTH IS GRANTED UPON COMPLETION OF AN ASSIGNMENT

When my Mother died, I felt as if my heart broke into a million tiny pieces. Like a precious antique glass that cracks and is irreparable. I was truly relieved that her agony and suffering were over and she was free in spirit, which was surely a better place to be than being trapped in a useless body. But there was the other part of me, the part that could not really express the sadness and sorrow about all these years of my care for her. I had to be so very strong in order to get thru it all. Stoic resilience, that was my way of surviving thru this ordeal. But on the inside, I felt completely numb and exhausted. While she died physically, I died in my heart.

I still feel sad beyond words that my Mother is gone. But if I think more closely, she was really gone a long time before her actual physical departure. Nevertheless, her presence gave me strength. Having her in my home gave me the feeling that my wise, unbeatable and protective Mother was still with me. Even though she was completely helpless and depended on me for everything, I felt her spirit strength, that was always such a powerful part of her.

Now that she is gone, I miss the part of her that I lost years ago. It is strange how human psyche works. I miss that wonderful time in our lives, when we could still talk, laugh and have an absolutely fantastic time together. That is the part I miss the most. And I feel sad that we were both robbed of many happy years together.

I have given her so much of myself, that everything else in my life fell away. Afterwards, I saw myself standing at a new doorstep of my life and had to find the will to go on, move forward and explore a new chapter of my life. She would want me to get rested, recover, pursue my dreams and be happy. That's what she would want.

The day that she passed away, my engrained picture image of her changed. I suddenly felt her presence, but in a very different way. I felt her years younger, full of energy, passion and otherworldly wisdom. Now, she is my constant companion, somewhere in the invisible distance. I can feel her watching over me from afar. I talk to her, ask her for advice and when I am really still and focused, I hear her answers.

I imagine she has happily reunited with all her loved ones that departed before her. I pray she has peace about her long and difficult life journey and that she is content about how she valiantly fought her final battle. I am proud of her and sense that she is all right, very busy and engaged on many levels.

Sometimes I hear her words of caution, other times, her sparkling laughter. I trust her protection and ever present advice. She might be right next to me as I write these words, I just can't see her. She lives on, in a world unknown to me. But I certainly do feel her. She is filled with so much love and still very much a part of my life. She is with me, always and forever.

DEATH

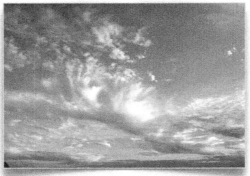

YOUR SPIRIT IS IMMORTAL

The final passage affects everyone differently. It helps if you do not look at death as the end, but as an act of transition, meaning, it is not the end of your soul's journey. It seems like this is the ending of a big chapter, but there are other chapters to unfold. I believe that when each one of us embarks on that lonely path of final passing, we rejoice with the loved ones that departed earlier. Maybe there is an incredibly beautiful, all-forgiving happy reunion and a brand new chapter begins. That sounds highly possible, don't you think?

DEATH IS BIG.

IT IS AS BIG AS BIRTH, WHEN WE ENTERED THIS UNKNOWN WORLD AND BRAVELY EMBARKED ON A DANGEROUS JOURNEY.

BIRTH IS THE SECRET ENTRY AND DEATH IS THE SACRED EXIT.

No one knows for sure what lies beyond this limited world of ours. We don't know the before or the after. We only know what happens here, in between these two mysterious gateways, while we travel through our limited time capsule. It makes us realize how helpless and small we are, and how we can't control much.

But what we can do is live life to the fullest, every and each day. We can make our very best effort to seize every opportunity, follow our dreams and strive to leave a positive trace of our existence. And even if we suffer while here, we can turn it into something positive. Every lesson we learn can help alleviate the suffering of those behind us. So while we travel towards the final threshold, we can make a difference.

Don't dismiss your presence in this crowded world as seemingly unimportant. Your journey, however small it seems, can ease the way for others behind you. The wisdom you gained through your experiences, can help prevent others from suffering like you did. To me this is the only way to reconcile what my darling Mother has endured.

I INSIST ON FINDING A RAY OF LIGHT.
I KNOW MY MOTHER FEELS THE SAME.

AFTER TRANSITION

This can be a time of utter confusion, emptiness and a sense of feeling lost. Especially if you were the primary caregiver for your loved one and you worked 24/7 non-stop. Your every day began and ended with caregiving. Your shopping for supplies and food was about caregiving. Your non-existent social calendar was about caregiving. Your evenings were about caregiving and your private and professional life were about caregiving. Your world revolved around the person you cared for.

Why? Because there is no other way to care for someone. You have to be truly totally involved and committed to it. Now your schedule, your duties and your every day world have fallen apart. Suddenly you are relieved of those obligations and responsibilities and you might find yourself at a loss.

It will take you a while to get your bearings. Your new life will linger in limbo, until you figure it out. You will talk to your friends, they may all offer loving suggestions and advice, but you alone must decide what is best for you and what you want. Unless someone has gone through a primary caregiving experience themselves, they really cannot begin to understand what you have been through. Their well intended input may not be very helpful. I highly recommend you remain connected with your Hospice services. They offer grief counseling after your loss and can be your great source of support. If you need to, rely on them and ask for help.

GIVE YOURSELF TIME.
BEFORE YOU CAN RECOVER, YOU NEED TO MOURN.
AND THERE IS NO TIMETABLE FOR THAT.

GRIEF

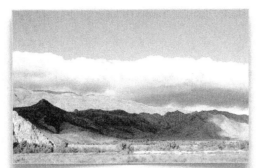

EVERY CLOUD EVENTUALLY DISAPPEARS

Grief has no schedule, no rules and no warning. Grief comes and goes as it pleases.

**GRIEF MAY STAY WITH YOU FOREVER,
BUT HOW YOU MANAGE TO COEXIST,
WILL DETERMINE THE QUALITY OF THE REST OF YOUR LIFE.**

If you thought that caregiving and the dying process were the most difficult times in this entire process, you are in for a surprise. After it is all concluded and your loved one is gone, you will find yourself in completely unknown territory. The freedom you suddenly gained will be so new and foreign to you, that it could overwhelm you. Your entire life, every hour of your schedule had a purpose. And it all revolved around the loved one, because they required it. Even if you had caregiver help, you were still there for your loved one, supervising and participating all along.

Now your every hour will only remind you of that loss. Every morning you will be reminded that this is the time you checked on your loved one how they slept and if they were still breathing. During the day at particular time, you will be reminded of the changing time, meal time and so on. It will be a constant battle of memories, of duties that had enveloped and taken over your life.

Do not think that this would have been preventable, had you spent much less time with your loved one. It is impossible to be an absent primary caregiver. Being present is part of the assignment. So now you will endure the consequences of your selfless serving. It will be a period of adjustments and the best advice I can give you is to let your tears flow.

You will be sad, angry and devastated all over again for all the years you have lost to this disease. All the moments you were robbed off, all the times you could have been happy and were instead dealing with the torment of incontinence or aggravation and agitation that the illness caused.

> ## TO HELP COUNTERACT PERSISTENT AND UNPLEASANT EMOTIONS, TRY TO REMEMBER THE GOOD AND HEALTHY TIMES YOU HAD WITH YOUR LOVED ONE, BEFORE THE ILLNESS SET IT.

This may require some deep effort, since that was years ago. But it is necessary to revive those good, old, happy memories. If you were present at their final transition, this will stay with you forever and you need to work thru it all. Let yourself grieve, do not hold it all pent up. Those days where you had to be strong are now finally over. You have another job to do, paying attention to you.

> ## IT IS YOUR DUTY TO GIVE YOURSELF PROPER TIME TO RECOVER.

I encourage you to cry as much as you feel the need to. Talk about everything that makes your heart heavy with your friends and family. Seek professional counseling, if you feel you need additional help. Hospice services will guide you through this process. Grieve as much as you can bear, but do not wallow in it. Look ahead and consciously open the door to new possibilities to enter your life. That's what your loved one would want you to do. Be good, kind and gentle with yourself. Don't chase grief away and pretend it is not there. Grief wants attention, it requires it.

> ## RESPECT GRIEF, HONOR IT, AND IT WILL RETRIEVE INTO THE FAR AWAY CHAMBERS OF YOUR HEART.

It may reappear when you least expect it, but with your acknowledgement, it will not disrupt your life. Oddly enough, it will enrich it and help you understand the endless spectrum of love.

> ## GRIEF IS ON THE OTHER SIDE OF LOVE, BUT IT IS STILL A PART OF LOVE. AND LOVE IS EVERYTHING.

RELEASING GRIEF

The time has come when you have to face yourself, your life and all that's happened. This will not be easy. It is the price of caregiving. You cannot change the past, but you can change the present and the future. In order to feel some enthusiasm and cheer about your life, you need to make space in your heart for new happiness and joy.

The grief that you have been carrying in you heart, has accumulated. You maybe stayed cheerful on the surface, especially in your daily care and interaction with your loved one. But the deep sadness, sorrow and helplessness, have left an indisputable imprint on your entire being. Don't fight it. Release it.

The ongoing business and responsibilities may have helped you avoid facing the sadness of the situation and unfulfilled personal life. That is entirely understandable. There was no choice, but now you are faced with a clear decision to move forward. You still have a life ahead of you, but it may take a while for it to show up.

Remain open and patient. Dedicate some time to consciously clearing all that has been burdening you. Perhaps you can talk about it with a friend, a support group or a therapist. However, do not expect everyone to understand your heartache and grief. There is simply no rule how long your grief is going to last. It has an open-end run. Assuming you will bounce back in matter of weeks is unrealistic.

How long will it take? As long as necessary. If you carried this heavy burden all on your own, then longer. If you had a strong support group or a great family and helpful siblings, then considerably shorter. Since everyone's circumstances are different, each one of us processes sadness and grief differently.

Find and engage in all possible activities that help you unburden your heart. They should be healthy, revitalizing, regenerating, creative and inspiring. The most important step to begin cleansing your grief, is your willingness to do so. This may take some effort. Why?

BECAUSE GRIEF HAS BECOME YOUR STEADY COMPANION. IT IS TIME TO OPEN YOUR HEART AND FIND A NEW, HAPPIER ONE.

DEPRESSION AND RECOVERY TIME

After my Mother left, I felt like I wanted to die as well. I was exhausted, crushed, severely burned-out and felt that I was really done with life. It seemed that I was barely hanging on for such a long time, and now my purpose was lost. There was seemingly nothing left of me.

I was fighting with determination to see my Mother thru it all and assure her a comfortable end at home. I refused to let this cruel illness rob her of that comfort, and nothing was going to prevent it from happening. But in all honesty, I don't think I could have lasted much longer.

They say that life's biggest tests push us to the edge. Well, I felt I was way over the edge, hanging by one last straw. I was in danger of falling into the abyss.

Part of you dies with your loved one and that is understandable. You may not be able to recognize whatever is left of you. It doesn't resemble the old-you anymore. So, this is a challenging passage for you, dear caregiver. All I can say is to take your time, be still and just breathe.

THERE WILL BE WEEKS, MOSTLY LIKELY MONTHS, BEFORE YOU REGAIN ANY SENSE OF WHAT YOUR NEW LIFE IS ABOUT. IT DOESN'T MATTER HOW LONG IT TAKES, THIS IS YOUR RECOVERY TIME.

You need to have no pressure. You are experiencing a complete shock to your system that was exclusively geared around this intense situation. Your every hour and energy supply went into sustaining and maintaining proper care. Your endurance has been stretched to its limits. Living in this fight or flight state for such an extended period of time, will leave consequences. Most likely, you are suffering from adrenal burn out. It is also very possible that you have been depressed for the majority of time during your caregiving duties.

IF YOU CAN'T SEEM TO MANAGE YOUR DEPRESSION, SEEK PROFESSIONAL HELP.

If you feel you can manage on your own, embark on a mission to heal, recharge and reset your entire life. Use the suggestions in this book from Chapters: *Healthy Diet* and *Holistic Caregiving Remedies* and supplements.

HEALING YOUR HEART

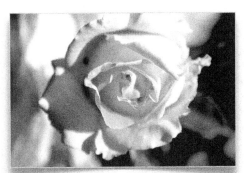

FLOWERS HOLD A HIGH HEALING FREQUENCY

A week after my Mom was gone, I went into complete shock. My system was so geared to work around her 24/7 and have no days or evenings off, that I barely maintained the schedule of care. Once she was gone, I was completely lost and broken.

My healing process took some serious time. I required complete peace and absolutely no pressure from anyone. The years of caregiving had been so draining, that I needed to stop my wheels to a total standstill. The sadness came in waves. The overwhelming moments where I felt I could not bear it, twisted me into a nerve bundle.

But I took a deep breath and got thru it. Slowly, I felt better. It took me quite a while to be able to sleep. As exhausted and sleep deprived as I was, I could not sleep during the night. So I allowed myself to take naps during the day.

One activity that truly helped me was gardening. For hours at a time, I embarked on long gardening escapades. Alone with nature I managed to calm down, bit by bit. Meditation and breathing exercises definitely helped as well, but I also needed a physical outlet. You can get into a very meditative state in nature surrounded by flowers. For me that was heaven-sent.

My garden had been somewhat neglected, since I had no time to tent to it. So I embarked on rose clipping, clearing ways and old pathways and trimming trees to help them breathe easier. I could feel their thankful and loving energy towards me. I cleansed the garden and healed my heart. Trees have always been my best friends. I would hug a tree and feel a big surge of energy flow thru my entire body. Such power and so generous with their love. That is what I needed. Care and loving energy. After all the years of caregiving to others, I needed to give care to myself.

We are all different and we all suffer in different ways. You may deal with the pain by crying or may completely withdraw and go into hiding. There is no wrong or right way to be. Just be yourself. This may take some time to remember and rediscover. You may be suddenly overcome by profound feelings of sadness and despair. They may overpower you like an ice storm that freezes everything in sight. Your recovery may feel at a standstill. But in fact, this is a part of the process. Just remain still and eventually, the frozen icicles will melt and give way to a new spring.

There may be much well intended advice coming your way, but you need to listen to your own heart and inner voice. Find out what calms you down. If you feel like sleeping until you feel rested, do that. If you cannot sleep at night, try to make up for it during the day. Your body clock will go through a massive withdrawal and the most important fact is to remember to be patient with yourself. If you feel anxious and frustrated with the slowness of your healing process, learn to be still, breathe and go within.

> **TALK TO YOURSELF WITH A GENTLE AND LOVING VOICE.**
> **ASK YOURSELF QUESTIONS AND LISTEN TO YOUR ANSWERS.**
> **THE RESTLESS AND STORMY OCEAN INSIDE YOU WILL SUBSIDE**
> **AND EVENTUALLY BRING YOU ASHORE.**

Dealing with paperwork, phone calls and such matters is beyond exhausting at this point. Try to cut it to a minimum. You will call people when you are ready to go thru the conversations. Everything and everyone else can wait, but your healing time cannot. Sleep as much as you can.

Let the nature help you. And then just be quiet and peaceful for as long as possible. Slowly but surely you will regain your inner tranquility and higher awareness.

WHAT ABOUT YOUR HEALTH?

That is the question that will become a big part of your life now. No matter how strong and resilient you are, the consequences of caregiving years have made an impact. You need to seriously concentrate on your physical recovery. First of all, get an assessment of your current state. Are you overweight, sleep deprived, depressed, burned out, nervous and restless?

The complete physical exhaustion may hit you weeks after. Your whole physical body will go thru a massive change. You are in true danger of getting sick and need complete and absolute rest.

IN ALL HONESTY, IT WILL TAKE AT LEAST SIX MONTHS TO A YEAR, TO GET TO A BETTER PLACE AND RECOVER.

You will have to engage in self-study, go on a healing journey, explore acupuncture, homeopathy, chiropractic adjustments or massage treatments. A very healthy diet will be essential and a good selection of supplements and herbal remedies will help you relax and de-stress. You will require unlimited patience with what will seem like the slowest recovery process on earth. But you owe it to yourself. It is very likely you are suffering from adrenal burn out. This will demand complete peace and no exertion.

VIGOROUS EXERCISE IS NOT RECOMMENDED, IN FACT, QUITE THE OPPOSITE. ALLOW YOURSELF ABSOLUTE REST.

It may take you a month or so, before you feel ready to do a little bit of stretching and gentle exercise. Perhaps a short walk, a swim or a gentle yoga class. Do not pressure yourself, just take it slow and be very self-loving. The patience you learned while tirelessly taking care of your loved one, needs to be used for dealing with yourself. Be generous with time, attention, loving care and tend to all your needs.

And finally, make it a rule to go to bed early and allow for a very generous amount of regular uninterrupted sleep. You will recover and you will heal. But remember the length of time you were a caregiver. That is the time you were burning the candle on both ends. In all fairness, you cannot expect to recover and undo all that overnight. You deserve an abundance of healing time. You simply must give yourself that luxury.

WILL THIS HAPPEN TO ME?

It is a question any child of Alzheimer's or dementia patient lives with. It is also an ongoing concern and worry of every partner that cared for their loved one.

HERE IS MY SHORT AND HONEST ANSWER.
NO.
HOW AM I SO SURE ABOUT THIS?
BECAUSE YOU HAVE THE GREATEST ADVANTAGE OF INFORMATION.

You know what is healthy for you and what is not. You are aware of natural remedies you can take to fortify your brain's natural elasticity. You know the foods you should stay away, the lifestyle you should lead in order to avoid an onset of this illness.

You may hear stories how someone was incredibly health conscious and still got this illness. Fact is, the inflammation of the brain is preventable, if you tend to it properly. And Alzheimer's is very much connected to inflammation of the brain.

Read, research, follow a very conscious and healthy lifestyle. Get enough sleep, avoid stress at all cost and take good care of yourself. You will stay healthy. Even if you have a predisposition and feel the early onset of this illness, you can turn around the boat and come ashore, stopping it in its tracks.

INFORMATION IS POWER.
YOU ARE NOT POWERLESS.
YOU ARE WAY AHEAD OF THE GAME.
TAKE ADVANTAGE OF THIS BENEFIT.

REDEFINE YOUR IDENTITY

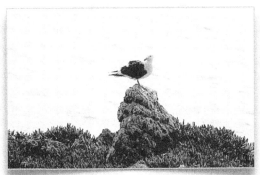

WHO ARE YOU TODAY?

*W*hen I went through this period, I was in quite a difficult place. There was so little of my own life left, that I did not know where to begin. There were periods where I was very upset and impatiently wanted to catch up for all the lost time, and do a million things at once. The I realized I was simply out of energy.

For a little while I entertained the idea of creating a senior-care wellness center. But that was only a temporary phase, since I had been in that word for so long, it seemed like a natural next step. I quickly realized that was not what I wanted at all. I needed to reinvent myself completely.

It took me two years of slow stop-and-go steps, before I re-launched myself into he world. It was my luck that I did everything in my life very early on and had accomplished so much at a very young age. So when I recovered and returned into the world, I was better, more mature and serious. I had gained some hard earned wisdom and could pick up the pieces of my previous accomplishments and rebuild my new reinvention on that.

I knew exactly what I wanted, what I was willing to tolerate, and what was absolutely out of question. This was a very good new rulebook. I finally stepped into my abundant power. It soon became clear that by taking care of my dear Mother for all those years, she had gifted me with one final parting gift - self empowerment.

I became the powerhouse she always told me I was. I became the resilient lioness of a woman that she exemplified. I carry her heart on my wings of desire, to be the best version of myself.
I make her proud.

Of course your life has changed forever. Going back to business as usual is a far and impossible thought. Most likely there is no usual business to get back to. If you were the primary caregiver, you have no business left. That is a fact. The difficult and confusing phase of trying to reassemble your life will begin. You might have to start from scratch.

Why? You are a very different person now and nothing is the same anymore. Things change, people change and undoubtedly the world has changed. You need to be very gentle and patient with yourself as you begin some deep soul searching.

What to do? Where to begin, and more importantly what is left of you? If you were a full time caregiver you need to allow yourself to go through a serious period of adjustment. I am afraid to say, this shall not be easy. I am saying this, so that you are prepared, fair and patient with yourself.

> **REVISIT YOUR OLD DREAMS AND WISHES.**
> **ANYTHING YOU WANTED TO DO IN THE PAST BUT DIDN'T, TRY IT NOW.**
> **EVENTUALLY YOU WILL FIND YOUR NEW CALLING.**

Just follow your heart and know that there is no better time than now. Use this opportunity as a launch-pad for a new chapter of your life.

FINANCIAL ABYSS

It is no secret that caregiving is an under-appreciated job. It is also no secret that the entire ordeal is known to financially wipe out not only one person, but entire family estates. It is incredibly expensive, financially crippling and can throw you into a perpetual financial hardship. You are trapped in a no-win situation.

> **UNDERSTANDING THAT CAREGIVING IS A LONG-TERM SITUATION**
> **IS CRUCIAL FOR YOUR FINANCIAL ENDURANCE.**

Know that once you are in it, your ability to earn money will significantly diminish, if not entirely disappear. It will force you to become very creative, smart and resilient with your finances. As soon as you find yourself in the caregiving situation, reach out to all possible government agencies, that offer resources and support. There is help out there, but you have to find it. Read more in Chapter *Your Loved one and Your Past - Financial Ability.*

Consider creating your own online business, or finding and maintaining an earning position in the vast world of online employment. You don't have to leave the house and can adjust your working schedule. It is an excellent solution. Stay active, be extremely well organized and prioritize well. You will learn a lot and find that you have an incredibly resilient spirit.

YOU WILL RECOVER, IF YOU STAY VERY ENGAGED.
GIVING UP IN NOT AN OPTION.
PERSISTENCE AND PERSEVERANCE IS.

Remain balanced in your core and the world around you will adjust. You will survive and in some time you shall flourish again. Have faith, my dear.

DOES TIME REALLY HEAL?

I do not have the answer to that. I guess in a way, time does heal old wounds. But I can also say that ignoring pain will not make it go away, no matter how much time goes by.

NOT DEALING WITH GRIEF WILL NOT MAKE IT DISAPPEAR.
SO IN THIS CASE, TIME DEMANDS TRUTHFULNESS.

It has taken me over ten years to find the strength to be able to complete this book.
Why so long?
I needed time to recover. When I am writing a book, I want to enjoy the process and until now, that was simply not possible. Now, I have distanced myself from the deepest valleys of my grief and have climbed back onto a mountaintop with a new view of the horizon. My life is a bit more peaceful and settled. I have managed to breathe through some of that grief and made enough room in my heart to be able to tackle this valuable material and prepare it for you, dear reader. But truthfully, I could have waited another ten years. The main reason why I pushed myself to complete it, is quite simple. The hardship that caregivers endure is enormous. You need all the help you can get right away.

I also made a promise to myself that one glimmer of good that must come out of my Mother's journey is to offer the valuable information I gained, and the specifics of the holistic caregiving I created. I have to share with you with my hard earned wisdom, so that hopefully you can navigate through your caregiving journey with wind in your sails.

Did time heal my wounds?

Not entirely, but it granted me space to reflect and decide on my own, that this information is too valuable to remain dormant. It reminded me that every passing day another caregiver could gain some precious information that would help them breathe easier, sleep sounder and feel more informed.

> **TIME IS AN ENIGMA.**
> **THE ONLY TRUTH ABOUT IT THAT WE KNOW,**
> **IS THAT IT IS PRECIOUS AND FLEETING.**

INNER PEACE

This is your reward, it is what you have gained as a result of your caregiving journey. It is priceless. You may think you can buy it, but you cannot. You may be able to buy physical solitude and enjoy a worry-free financial state. But that may all be fleeting, if inner turmoil occupies your mind.

> **BUT THEN THERE IS INNER PEACE.**
> **THAT, YOU CANNOT BUY WITH ALL THE FORTUNES OF THE WORLD.**
> **YOU MUST LEARN IT AND EARN IT.**

Once you do, you become untouchable to the pressures of ever present worldly disarray. After you've been the loving caregiver to your loved one, there will be one assurance you will have; inner peace that you offered everything you could to them.

There should be no regrets, for you have done your very best. You were there for them and cared for them with love and dedication. For that my dear, you will forever enjoy a sense of serenity that is invaluable.

> **RECOGNIZE YOUR HARD-EARNED INNER PEACE AND ENJOY IT.**

LOOKING AT YOUR PAST AND TOWARDS YOUR FUTURE

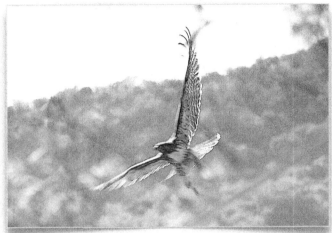

YOU SHALL SPREAD YOUR WINGS ONCE MORE
AND SOAR INTO THE SKY

For me personally, as agonizing and difficult that my Mother's journey was, I remember her smile, the way she touched my cheek and looked at me lovingly with her hazel eyes.

In the last days of her life I asked her, as countless times before, if she knew how much I loved her. Even though she seemed hardly present anymore, at that particular moment she looked me straight in the eye and answered with a resounding "Yes!" That was her last spoken word to me.

As I promised, I stayed with her till her last breath, until she died in my arms. It consoles me greatly that she was not alone when she passed away, and that I could offer her the very best of everything in my dedicated care for her. To me, she was the best Mother in the world and deserved the very best of everything.

And after this great loss, I still see my immense blessings. I am most fortunate to still have my dearest Father, who is healthy and vibrant in body, mind and Spirit. I am forever grateful to him, for he has given me the purpose to carry on, the encouragement to reinvent myself and the unconditional love of the best Father in the world. And aren't I the lucky one, after all?

My hope for you is that you will look back at this entire caregiving experience as a special gift bestowed upon you, where you were able to do an incredibly generous, loving and sacred service for someone you love. You may got thru a phase where it really hits you how many years went by and how you of lost a big part of your life. But that is really an illusion.

**WHAT IS THIS LIFE REALLY WORTH,
IF WE DON'T DO ANYTHING GOOD FOR ANYONE ELSE WHILE HERE?**

There is an interesting thing that happens after we've gone through a difficult and painful experience. With time the pain seems to fade away and we remember only the good. Selective memory like that, can help you enjoy life and not dwell and hang onto old pain and disappointments. Instead, remember the precious tiny moments where you could exchange a word, smile, touch or a caress with your loved one. These are the memories worth keeping alive.

I believe the true meaning of our life is to learn and experience unconditional love. Receiving it and selflessly offering it in return, makes you a meaningful and useful spark of life in the universal wheel of life. You are an intricate part of the everlasting Light force. You matter, your actions and words can change someone's life. You had the opportunity to make a gigantic positive difference in eliminating suffering, and you accomplished this task with excellence. I congratulate you, my dearest caregiver. May all the loving forces of this Universe protect, guide and enlighten every day of your beautiful life.

When you complete your caregiving journey, your perception of life will change forever. You will understand that it doesn't matter what others think, believe or expect of you. All that matters is that you can look in the mirror and know in your heart, that you did everything you possibly could for you loved one. Inner peace and closure will be granted to you. You satisfied an old contract, a commitment given before you reentered this world.

**YOU FULFILLED A PROMISE, COMPLETED YOUR ASSIGNMENT
AND SUCCEEDED IN YOUR MISSION.
YOU ANGEL WINGS AWAIT.**

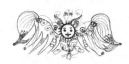

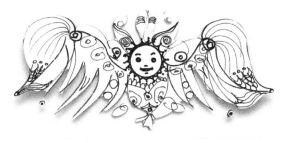

When your caregiving journey comes to an end,
you will understand that this is just a new beginning
in the circle of your Soul's grand travels.

You will know that our time here is very fleeting,
that every precious moment matters
and life is too short to dwell on darkness.

Each one of us shall leave someday,
and probably return again.
Our loved ones share this travels with us,
from life to life we meet again.

And if in this lifetime you care for someone,
perhaps in the past they cared for you.
Maybe they saved your life,
or loved you more than life itself.

Perhaps you are simply returning the favor,
fulfilling an ancient promise,
following your heart and teaching others about love.

And maybe this has been your final mission
to master selfless love and unconditional devotion,
give kindness, compassion and protection,
just like the Gods offer you all day and night.

Rest assured, you are never alone.
Know that you are loved more than you can imagine.
You are precious, special and adored.
You are a true Angel of the sky.
You are blessed.

ABOUT THE AUTHOR

SABRINA MESKO Ph.D.H. is a recognized Mudra authority and International and Los Angeles Times bestselling author of the timeless classic *Healing Mudras - Yoga for your Hands* translated into fourteen languages. She authored over twenty books on Mudras, Mudra Therapy, Mudras and Astrology, spirituality and meditation techniques.

Sabrina holds a Bachelors Degree in Sensory Approaches to Healing, a Masters in Holistic Science, and a Doctorate in Ancient and Modern Approaches to Healing from the American Institute of Holistic Theology. She is board certified from the American Alternative medical Association and American Holistic Health Association. Sabrina is also a Certified RCFE - Residential Care Facility for the Elderly - Administrator.

She has been featured in media outlets such as The Los Angeles Times, CNBC News, Cosmopolitan, the cover of London Times Lifestyle, The Discovery Channel documentary on Hands, W magazine, First for Women, Health, Web-MD, Daily News, Focus, Yoga Journal, Australian Women's weekly, Blend, Daily Breeze, New Age, the Roseanne Show and various international live television programs. Her articles have been published in world-wide publications. She hosted her own weekly TV show educating about health, well-being and complementary medicine. She is an executive member of the World Yoga Council and has led numerous international Yoga Therapy educational programs. She directed and produced her interactive double DVD titled *Chakra Mudras* - a Visionary awards finalist. Sabrina also created award winning international Spa and Wellness Centers and is a motivational keynote conference speaker addressing large audiences all over the world. Sabrina is the founder of Arnica Press, a boutique Book Publishing House. Her mission is to discover, mentor, nurture and publish unique authors with a meaningful message, that may otherwise not have an opportunity to be heard.

She is the founder of world's only online Mudra Teacher and Mudra Therapy Education, Certification, and Mentorship program, with her certified graduates and therapists spreading these ancient teachings in over 26 countries around the world.

Sabrina has created special programs for Holistic Caregiving and is very popular in the health care community. She has spoken at caregiver support organizations such as Lezza Gibbon's *Care Connection* in Los Angeles, and to large international audiences of nurses, hospice and healthcare workers who truly appreciate and need the holistic caregiving techniques to help prevent burnout and maintain highest level of caregiving while implementing effective self-care principles.

WWW.SABRINAMESKO.COM

Made in the USA
Monee, IL
10 April 2022

94386202R00240